The Stress Response of Critical Illness: Metabolic and Hormonal Aspects

Jean-Charles Preiser
Editor

The Stress Response of Critical Illness: Metabolic and Hormonal Aspects

Springer

Editor
Jean-Charles Preiser
Brussels
Belgium

ISBN 978-3-319-27685-4 ISBN 978-3-319-27687-8 (eBook)
DOI 10.1007/978-3-319-27687-8

Library of Congress Control Number: 2016935706

Springer Cham Heidelberg New York Dordrecht London

Printed on acid-free paper

Springer International Publishing AG Switzerland is part of Springer Science+Business Media
(www.springer.com)

Foreword

Life is like riding a bicycle. To keep your balance, you must keep moving.

Albert Einstein

All living organisms share common biological characteristics, developed over hundreds of millions of years, which have allowed them to adapt and survive since the beginning of life on earth. This is particularly true for human beings, so weak and frail before the occurrence of organized civilizations. The importance of effective adaptation abilities was recognized very long ago by the Chinese and Greek physicians, although it was not before the nineteenth and twentieth centuries that the real importance of the stress response with its complex multisystem mechanisms was discovered. Claude Bernard recognized the importance of a constant *milieu intérieur*, insuring the function of body cells in a changing environment via adaptive mechanisms in the vital organs. Later, Walther Cannon developed further the concept of *homeostasis*, leading in case of failure of the homeostatic mechanisms to disequilibrium and illness.

In 1936, Hans Selye published the historical Letter to the Editor of Nature, "A syndrome produced by diverse nocuous agents," describing stress as the consequence of an inadequate response to harmful physical and psychological agents. The stress response was originally believed to be mainly related to the neuroendocrine system activation, but Selye later realized that nearly all systems were involved and the concept of a multisystem general response was developed.

Although the clinical relevance of such adaptive mechanisms in trauma and acute conditions was long recognized, their long-term effects on the mood and behavior were not acknowledged before the second part of the twentieth century: the post-traumatic stress disorder was only included in 1980 in the third edition of the DSM of the American Psychiatric Association. This underlines the central role of the brain in the response to stress, as a regulation but also as a target organ, when its vulnerability to emotional and psychological challenges, exceeds its resilience capacity and induces undesirable emotional and behavioral symptoms.

In the field of stress response, the critical care environment is unique, since it gathers individuals with different kinds of stress: patients with life-threatening conditions, health-care professionals, mainly physicians and nurses, as well as family members. In the early phase of critical illness, the patients are submitted to acute challenges such as hemorrhage, ischemia, hypoxia, sepsis and pain, as well as psychological or emotional threats. The initial adaptation to the critical illness is mainly related to the multiple autonomic, endocrine, tissue, and immune mediators; it promotes survival and recovery. However, when the critical illness is prolonged, inadequate regulation of this response may occur, inducing damaging effects, such as depressed immunity, metabolic dysfunctions, and malnutrition. At longer term, patients with prolonged or complicated stay are at risk to develop post-traumatic stress disorder, mainly characterized by psychological, emotional, and behavioral symptoms.

The family is submitted to intense psycho-emotional stress, leading to adverse psychological responses, the so-called post-intensive care syndrome-family. The latter is mainly characterized by insomnia, anxiety, depressive symptoms, inability to perform the grief, and difficulty or inability to work. Surprisingly, the clinical importance of post-intensive care syndrome-family was only discovered about 20 year ago, despite quite a high prevalence: about a third of family members are affected by PTSD symptoms in both pediatric and adult ICUs. The process of decision making involving families and proxies plays a critical role, particularly the methods of communication and inclusion. Various strategies of communication with family members have shown to be associated with decreased anxiety, improved resilience, and coping.

In addition to emotional, psychological stress, the health-care givers are submitted to work-related stress, promoting burnout symptoms, as emotional and physical exhaustion, inability to work, depersonalization, and depression. The prevalence of PTSD in ICU nurses is particularly high, due to the daily contact with suffering, uncertainty of therapy, and death. This is also the case of health-care professionals working in emergency and mental health care, which in addition are often submitted to violence and physical assaults. The occurrence and severity of work-related stress is affected by several factors, the type, nature, and severity of the stressor, the presence of a team support, and the quality of professional training, as well as by individual factors, such as the individual personality, mental health, and social-family support.

The publication of *The Stress Response of Critical Illness: Metabolic and Hormonal Aspects* by Jean-Charles Preiser and more than 20 top-level scientists must be highlighted, since it constitutes a remarkable high level and original contribution. This book comes at a right stage, as a large body of recent information has brought new insights on the metabolic and endocrine aspects of the stress response during the last decade, such as the corticoadrenal response in sepsis, the regulation of blood glucose, and substrate metabolism in the settings of critical care.

Lausanne, Switzerland René Chioléro

Contents

Part II Hormonal Regulation

Part III Particular Clinical Situations

Chapter 1
Introduction

Jean-Charles Preiser

The important thing in science is not so much to obtain new facts as to discover new ways of thinking about them. William Henry Bragg

One of the most challenging tasks on earth is to bring people together and to build bridges to promote the cross-fertilization of knowledge!

In the field of care of the critically ill, this statement can be translated into the integration of new discoveries or major advances in the understanding of physiology into unbiased evaluations of new therapeutic strategies adapted from novel experimental findings. Conversely, basic science should be open to clinical data and able to understand and to integrate clinical concerns into research questions. This book aims to bridge the new knowledge gathered in experimental research with new clinical results.

Historically, the *"stress response"* was quoted by the Canadian physiologist Hans Selye, who discovered the mechanisms of the "fly or fight response" designed to restore the homeostasis needed for an independent life, as described by Claude Bernard. Some of the basic and adaptive mechanisms were preserved over the evolution, in keeping with the Darwinian theory of evolution.

Now, the changes and improvements in the practice of medicine allow patients to survive critical illness, allow surgeons to perform risky interventions, allow anesthesiologists to sedate very weak patients, etc. The support of the vital functions prolongs the lifespan of a critically ill thanks to improvements in pharmacological agents, in the technology of ventilators, renal replacement therapies, and extracorporeal membrane oxygenators. However, the metabolic and functional consequences of the critical illness can last weeks or months, representing a major burden for the society and cannot be supported by any dedicated device. Only a few drugs

J.-C. Preiser, MD, PhD
Department of Intensive Care, Erasme University Hospital, Université Libre de Bruxelles, 808 route de Lennik, Brussels 1070, Belgium
e-mail: Jean-Charles.Preiser@erasme.ulb.ac.be

J.-C. Preiser (ed.), *The Stress Response of Critical Illness: Metabolic and Hormonal Aspects*, DOI 10.1007/978-3-319-27687-8_1

and nutritional formulas can slightly influence metabolism. Therefore, a detailed knowledge of the intimate mechanisms of the stress response is warranted to help clinicians to support the adaptive and desirable metabolic responses while trying to minimize the maladaptive ones.

In this book, several world-leading experts accepted to share their knowledge and to summarize the current understanding of the metabolic response to stress, including the cellular and subcellular mechanisms, the use of macro- and micronutrient as energy substrates during catabolism or anabolic resistance typically associated with critical illness. The roles and patterns of endocrine mediators will be discussed in detail. The final section will address difficult clinical situations, as examples of how the new findings can be translated into daily practice.

Specifically, in the first section, the bioenergetics of the stress response has been revisited in detail by C Faisy, using the concept of stress as a challenge to the equilibrium at each level of the body. The successive phases of the metabolic response to stress were being reviewed in a temporal and clinically relevant sequence. Novel insights as hibernation and mitochondrial mechanisms of adaptation have been updated by J Grip, N Tardif, and O Rooyackers, while the development of anabolic resistance has been reviewed by JP Thissen. The ensuing alterations in the use of lipids, carbohydrates, and protein metabolism were updated by Ph Calder, P Singer, L Tappy, A Norberg, F Liebau, and J Wernerman, whereas the current roles of micronutrients have been reviewed by MM Berger. A Thooft, R Machado, and myself summarized the related issue of stress hyperglycemia.

In Part 2, the current understanding of the functional changes of hormonal systems has been described by L Langouche and G Van den Berghe for the thyroid axis and P Marik for the adrenal system. The roles and relevance of new important endocrine mediators, the enterohormones released from the gastrointestinal tract, and the adipokines released from fat tissue have been reviewed by M Plummer, A Reintam, A Deane, K Robinson, J Prins, and B Venkatesh.

In Part 3, the clinical views and attitudes in situations accompanied by challenging metabolic alterations have been addressed. The issue of severe undernutrition was revisited by P Singer and J Cohen; the specificities of traumatic brain injury by H Quintard, C Ichai, and JF Payen; the particular aspects of sepsis and organ failures by V Fraipont and myself; morbid obesity by M Coeffier and F Tamion; and the issues related to burn injury by A Abdullahi, D Patsouris, SR. Costford, and MG Jeschke.

I would like to thank wholeheartedly each one of the authors who brought his own contribution and his personal stone to the huge enterprise of understanding the metabolic response to stress, an indispensable step to improve the quality of care and the quality of the lives of the survivors of critical illness.

Part I
Metabolic Changes

Chapter 2
Successive Phases of the Metabolic Response to Stress

Jean-Charles Preiser, Carole Ichai, and A.B. Johan Groeneveld

Abstract The metabolic response to stress have been selected as an adaptive response to survive critical illness. Several mechanisms well preserved over the evolution, including the stimulation of the sympathetic nervous system, the release of pituitary hormones, a peripheral resistance to the effects of these and other anabolic factors are triggered to increase the provision of energy substrates to the vital tissues. After an acute insult, alternative substrates are used as a result of the loss of control of energy substrate utilization. The clinical consequences of the metabolic response to stress include sequential changes in energy expenditure, stress hyperglycemia, changes in body composition, psychological and behavioral problems. The loss of muscle proteins and function is a major long-term consequence of stress metabolism. Specific therapeutic interventions, including hormone supplementation, enhanced protein intake and early mobilization are investigated.

2.1 Introduction

The understanding and knowledge of metabolic response to critical illness has dramatically changed during the last decade, following several important discoveries in line with the findings of pioneering scientists of the nineteenth and twentieth

J.-C. Preiser, MD, PhD (✉)
Department of Intensive Care, Erasme University Hospital, Free University of Brussels, 808 route de Lennik, Brussels 1070, Belgium
e-mail: Jean-Charles.Preiser@erasme.ulb.ac.be

C. Ichai, MD, PhD
Department of Anesthesiology and Intensive Care, Hôpital Saint-Roch, University of Nice, Nice, France

A.B.J. Groeneveld, MD, PhD
Department of Intensive Care, Erasmus Medical Center, Rotterdam, The Netherlands

J.-C. Preiser (ed.), *The Stress Response of Critical Illness: Metabolic and Hormonal Aspects*, DOI 10.1007/978-3-319-27687-8_2

century. In his theory of the evolution, Charles Darwin reported that "It is not the strongest or the most intelligent that survives. It is the most adaptable to change." This statement is particularly relevant after any life-threatening injury triggering a "critical illness," when survival in a hostile environment strongly relies on the ability to mount an appropriate adaptive response. In terms of the metabolic response to stress, the principle of homeostasis of Claude Bernard ("The constancy of the internal environment is the condition for a free and independent life") is highly relevant to the critically ill whose homeostasis must be restored as rapidly as possible to survive the injury. The mechanisms allowing the maintenance of homeostasis, vital functions, and ultimately survival in a hostile environment have been unraveled by Hans Selye, who described the "fight or flight" response, "a nonspecific response to a wide variety of stimuli." Sir David Cuthbertson described several phases of the metabolic response over time, including the ebb phase and the flow phase. A third sequence, the chronic phase, preceding recovery, was more recently suggested and is probably relevant to the post-injury phase frequently encountered in modern intensive care [1, 2]. The mechanisms of these successive adaptive changes mounted to survive a stress are increasingly understood and are now gathered into a general theory.

2.2 Pathophysiological Mechanisms

The metabolic response to stress involves a neuroendocrine and an inflammatory/immune component. Recent data suggest that hormones released from the adipose tissue and from the gastrointestinal tract can play an important role as well (Fig. 2.1).

The neuroendocrine component is triggered in a region located near the hypothalamus, paraventricular nucleus/locus coeruleus. When a stressor is detected and signaled to the central nervous system, a prototypical response will be triggered, resulting in the activation of the sympathetic nervous system (SNS), the hypothalamic-pituitary axis, and later by behavioral changes. Many different stressors can be sensed and transmitted; for instance, a peripheral tissular injury induced by a trauma will activate afferent nerves, hypoxemia or hypercapnia will trigger chemoreceptors, hypovolemia will activate baroreceptors, and inflammatory mediators will change the phenotype of microglial cells.

The SNS is involved in the fast control of most of the body's internal organs, via the activation of adrenergic receptors. After any stress, an immediate release of norepinephrine occurs from the postganglionic neuron in response to the stimulation of its nicotinic receptors by acetylcholine released from the preganglionic neurons [3]. The adrenal medulla is a functional sympathetic ganglion, where chromaffin cells release norepinephrine and epinephrine into the bloodstream upon stimulation by the preganglionic neuron.

The activation of the hypothalamus-pituitary axis results in the release of adrenocorticotropic hormone, thyroid-stimulating hormone, growth hormone, and follicle-stimulating and follicle-luteinizing hormones by the anterior pituitary gland. The circulating levels of hormones released from peripheral glands in response to these

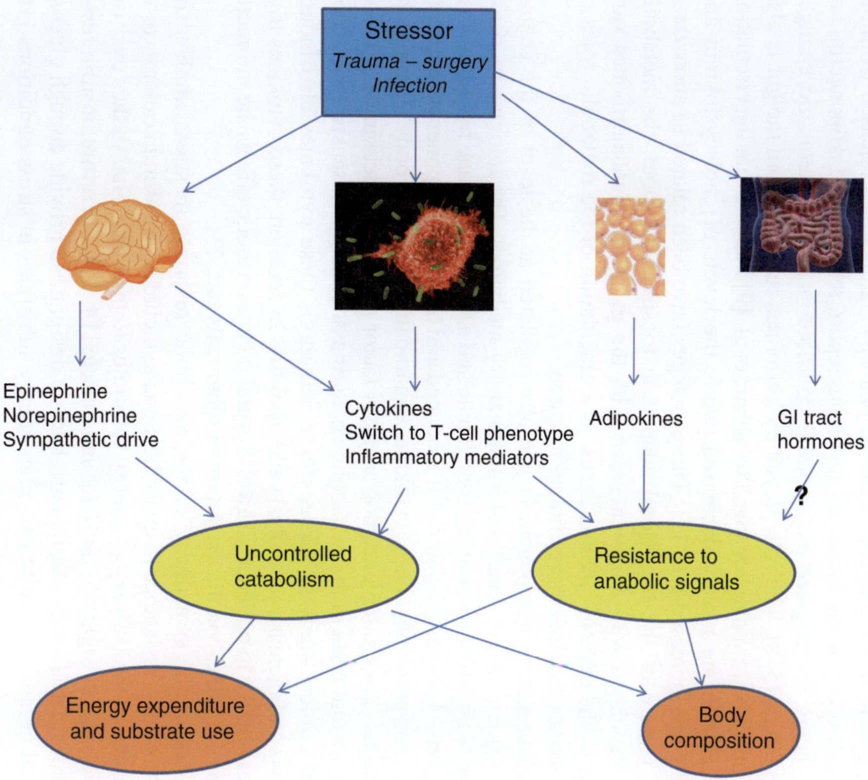

Fig. 2.1 Different levels of the metabolic response to stress. Once a stressor has been sensed, systems/organs are activated (first level). Mediators are released upon activation (second level). Physiological and phenotypical changes are triggered (third level)

pituitary factors are decreased, with the notable exception of cortisol. Peripheral inactivation of the active hormones is the likely mechanism [2], while recently reported alterations in the cortisol breakdown [4] could account for its increased concentration. During the chronic phase, the plasma levels of both pituitary factors and peripheral hormones are lowered, while a peripheral resistance to the effects of growth hormone, insulin, thyroid hormone, and cortisol persists. These hormonal alterations profoundly and sequentially affect the energy, protein, and fat metabolism. The metabolic response to stress thus depends on the time lag after the initial insult.

In addition to these well-characterized pathways, adipokines released from the different cell types of the fat tissue, including leptin, resistin, and adiponectin, are currently being investigated as potential contributors to the metabolic changes related to sepsis [5–8]. The role played by hormones released from the gut is also under scrutiny. Recent data reviewed by Deane et al. [9] indicate that the circulating levels of ghrelin are mostly decreased, while the levels of cholecystokinin and peptide YY are increased [10, 11]. These changes have been related to anorexia, a common feature of the behavioral adaptation to stress. Of note, the metabolic changes associated with adipokines and with the gastrointestinal hormones vary according to the clinical circumstances. The elucidation of the metabolic roles of these hormones requires more clinical research.

The inflammatory component is partially regulated at the level of the central nervous system, via cytokines and inflammatory mediators. The immune response of the host to an infection comprises an innate and a specific immune response. This latter response is subdivided into cell-mediated and humoral components, including antibodies and cytokines. These cytokines can impair some of the body's physiological functions. For example, tumor necrosis factor (TNF), interleukin (IL)-1, and IL-6 play pivotal roles in the metabolic changes associated with sepsis. In addition to typical clinical signs of sepsis (fever, lethargy), these cytokines also induce weight loss and increase proteolysis and lipolysis. In addition, these cytokines trigger anorexia at the hypothalamic level. Several other metabolic effects are indirectly exerted by cytokines via the activation of other cells [12, 13].

The final common pathway of the metabolic response to stress implies the development of a resistance to anabolic signals, including insulin, in order to reset the hierarchy of the delivery of energy substrates to prioritize vital tissues over the insulin-dependent organs, mainly fat and muscle [14, 15]. Therefore, insulin resistance is considered as an adaptive mechanism designed to provide enough glucose to the vital organs, unable to use other energy substrates in stress conditions [16, 17], which results in the inability to suppress central hepatic glucose production [14, 18] and to a decrease of insulin-mediated glucose uptake in the periphery. Insulin resistance is mediated through the reduction of post-receptor insulin signaling defects and downregulation of glucose transporter (GLUT)-4, especially in skeletal muscle. Moreover, impaired nonoxidative glucose disposal results from a reduction in skeletal muscle glycogen synthesis. Despite decreased insulin-mediated glucose uptake, there is an early increase in whole-body glucose uptake, primarily a result of cytokine-mediated upregulation of GLUT-1 [18].

The complexity of the metabolic response is further enhanced by the currently increasing prevalence of obesity and the (type of) metabolic and nutritional support that is given and may either attenuate or aggravate some of the metabolic responses to stress. The latter depends, among others, on the level of feeding – under- and overnutrition – as well as, indirectly, the level of inflammation that is either evoked or attenuated by nutrition. Also preoperative fasting is a metabolic stress, and losses of energy and proteins following bleeding, hemofiltration, gastrointestinal dysfunction, and others may further compound the metabolic response to stress [19]. Some of the hormones released early from endocrine glands such as (nor)epinephrine, cortisol, thyroid hormone, and glucagon are clearly associated with hypermetabolism aimed at survival, whereas the later changes, with impaired production and/or increased resistance, are more likely adaptive and aimed at a long-term protection of the organism. The latter may, theoretically, be associated with mitochondrial changes, some type of hibernation, and a shutdown of excessive organ function and may thereby, together with an inflammatory response, herald development of multiple organ dysfunction syndrome [19]. Some of these chronic hormonal changes may, however, be regarded as maladaptive when contributing to ultimate mortality by increasing organ dysfunction, immunodepression, and wasting [20–25].

2.3 Clinical Consequences

The clinical consequences of the metabolic response to stress include several different aspects, from changes in resting energy expenditure, use of macronutrients as sources of energy, stress hyperglycemia, and changes in body composition to behavioral changes (Table 2.1 and Fig. 2.2).

2.3.1 Energy Expenditure (EE)

Traditionally, the EE is thought to be lower during the first ebb phase described by Cuthbertson. During the later flow phase, EE is considered to be higher than the EE predicted for a matched healthy subject [26–28]. During the third chronic phase of critical illness, EE decreases slightly. Kreymann et al. serially measured EE in patients with sepsis and septic shock and found lower values during severe sepsis

Table 2.1 Typical patterns of metabolic changes

	Usual patterns of change
Energy expenditure	Decrease (ebb phase or early phase) followed by increase (flow phase or late and recovery phases)
Use of energy substrates	Increased oxidation of carbohydrates, more than lipids/proteins Use of alternative substrates (lactate)
Stress hyperglycemia	Systematic
Changes in body composition	Decreased active cell mass Decreased fat-free mass, increased or unchanged fat mass
Behavior	Lethargy, anorexia

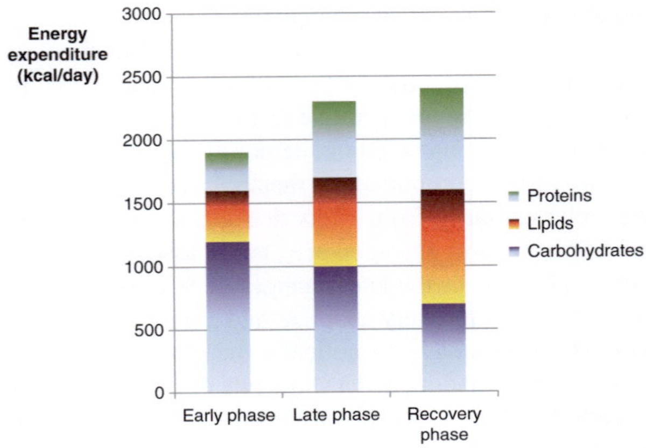

Fig. 2.2 Schematic representation of the three successive phases of the metabolic response to stress, depicting the changes in energy expenditure, and use of energy substrates occurring during the early, late, and recovery phases

[29]. Due to these temporal changes, the actual EE is extremely difficult to predict during critical illness [30]. Indeed, EE is influenced of several physiological derangements, such as fever of hypothermia, changes in heart rate, shivering, agitation, as well as by therapeutic interventions such as sedative agents, nonselective beta-blockers, and active cooling. The use of indirect calorimetry is the best way to assess EE, even though its use to guide the caloric prescription is debatable [31–34].

2.3.2 Use of Energy Substrates

The metabolism of macronutrients is altered at several levels, including the digestive absorption, the intracellular intermediate metabolism, and the oxidation of substrates.

Facing the increased requirements, the oxidation of macronutrients is largely increased during critical illness, and the relative contribution and metabolism of each type of macronutrient is regulated by the circulating hormones (Table 2.2). Overall, the oxidation of carbohydrates is globally more increased than the oxidation of lipids and proteins [35]. Later on, decreased glucose utilization, increased fat turnover, and loss of muscle and visceral (organ) protein mass with wasting occur. A negative nitrogen balance – pointing to increased protein breakdown over protein synthesis – is the ultimate result, even when reprioritization leads to an increased overall hepatic protein synthesis. Indeed, muscle may lose amino acids at the benefit of the liver. These changes are hardly amenable to any fruitful intervention to improve protein synthesis, attenuate lipogenesis, and thereby conserve lean body mass needed for rehabilitation.

Carbohydrates Glucose is the preferential energy substrate during critical illness and will be able to yield 2 ATP after anaerobic glycolysis and 36 additional molecules of ATP by the Krebs cycle when the mitochondrion is functional. At the whole-body level, changes in the metabolism of carbohydrates include the rapid

Table 2.2 Use of substrates during the successive phases

Macronutrient	Anabolic	Catabolic
Carbohydrates	Insulin	Cortisol Glucagon Growth hormone Catecholamines
Lipids	Insulin	Catecholamines
Proteins	Insulin Growth hormone – IGF-1 Testosterone Catecholamines	Cortisol Glucagon Catecholamines

utilization of the glycogen stores, followed by a high level of endogenous glucose production from lactate, glycerol, and alanine in the liver, the kidney, and the intestine [36, 37]. As the turnover of glucose is increased, plasma concentrations of glucose will rise, resulting in the typical stress hyperglycemia [18]. While nonoxidative metabolism (e.g., glycogen synthesis) is impaired, oxidative glucose metabolism is upregulated early [38]. Alterations in the digestion of dietary carbohydrates occur as well: once ingested, the long molecules of polysaccharides are cleaved into oligosaccharides (3–10 sugars) by the amylase enzymes. The resulting oligosaccharides will be cleaved by enzymes of the intestinal brush border. The activity of one of these enzymes, lactase, can be inhibited in the critically ill, thereby reducing the absorption of enteral carbohydrates [39].

Use of lactate as an alternative substrate Alteration of lactate metabolism is one of the prominent component of the metabolic stress response. Lactate is a physiological substrate (carbohydrate) issued from pyruvate reduction during glycolysis. In stable conditions, lactate production and elimination are equivalent, i.e., 1200–1500 mmol per day, leading to a stable blood lactate concentration of 0.8–1.2 mmol/L [40]. Most organs, except those without mitochondria, simultaneously release and take up lactate. As a result, the net flux of lactate depends on the difference between release and uptake and varies upon organs and their energetic condition [41]. In stable conditions, the brain, muscles, and digestive tract are producing lactate organs, whereas the liver is responsible for more than 70 % of lactate clearance. Lactatemia and lactate metabolism (turnover) are often confused. Lactatemia indicates an instantaneous equilibrium between total body lactate production and clearance. Accordingly, lactatemia can be in a normal value, while lactate turnover can be normal, high, or low, just indicating that there is an equilibrium between production and elimination.

Lactate, is a physiological intermediate energetic substrate. The Cori cycle (conversion of lactate into glucose) confirms the ability of lactate to serve as a very efficient interorgan shuttle, allowing to provide fuel useable by organs in various stress conditions [42]. For instance, red blood cells not equipped with mitochondria produce ATP only *via* an anaerobic glycolysis leading to lactate production, the latter being further metabolized in glucose in the liver in the presence of oxygen. Growing data support that these exchanges are favored during stress condition and that lactate "per se" is at least a useful if not an obligatory substrate used by organs and tissues during energetic crisis conditions and has been particularly demonstrated to fuel the heart and brain.

At rest, the heart consumes energy issued for 60–90 % from fatty acids ß-oxidation. But in case of hypoxia such as during myocardial ischemia, increased O_2 consumption, or decreased O_2 delivery, metabolic pathways shift toward a preferential use of carbohydrate oxidation for ATP production [43]. The role of lactate as a myocardial fuel has been confirmed experimentally during septic and hemorrhagic shocks [44, 45].

Stress hyperglycemia The etiology of hyperglycemia in type 2 diabetes is a combination of insulin resistance and beta cell secretory defects [14, 18]. The development of stress hyperglycemia involves a much more dramatic, complex interplay of counterregulatory hormones such as catecholamines, growth hormone, and cortisol, and cytokine resulting in excessive hepatic glucose production (from gluconeogenesis and glycogenolysis) and insulin resistance. Increased hepatic output of glucose, particularly through gluconeogenesis, appears to be the most important contributor to stress hyperglycemia (see Chap. 8 for further discussion).

Numerous association studies [46, 47] confirm the presence of a U-shaped relationship between admission BG value and outcome, i.e., low and high BG are associated with poor outcome. An admission BG value of 5.5–6.1 mmol/L is associated with the lowest mortality rate. Similarly, high GV and low BG complexity are also associated with a worsened outcome.

Lipids The use of lipids as energy substrate is relatively less increased than carbohydrates, during critical illness [35]. Indeed, the conversion of lipids into ATP requires large amounts oxygen and functional mitochondria. During critical illness, endogenous triglycerides stored in the adipose tissue and exogenous triglycerides released from chylomicrons and other lipoproteins are avidly hydrolysed to release FFAs and glycerol into the bloodstream. In contrast to physiological conditions, this increased lipolysis cannot be efficiently inhibited by infusion of carbohydrates. The oxidation of FFAs is increased in peripheral tissues, while in the liver they are converted to ketone bodies or re-esterified to triglycerides and released into the bloodstream as very-low-density lipoprotein (VLDL), which is subject to impaired clearance. However, the production of FFAs from exogenous and endogenous triglycerides still exceeds the utilization of FFAs, and plasma FFA levels are typically increased in critically ill patients. Overall, the metabolism of lipids is increased, although complete oxidation can only be achieved in tissues where mitochondria are functional.

Proteins Under normal conditions, proteins are constantly broken down and replaced in a highly selective and closely balanced process. The majority of intracellular proteins are degraded via activation of the ubiquitin-proteasome pathway. In a series of enzymatic reactions, ubiquitin forms a chain on a protein to be degraded. Once tagged, the protein is recognized by a proteasome. The protein unravels and is injected into the central core of the proteasome where it is broken down into peptides.

Stress metabolism is characterized by over-activation of the ubiquitin-proteasome pathway that causes excessive protein degradation and muscle wasting.

Overall, the large increases in protein breakdown are partially balanced by increased protein synthesis (of inflammatory mediators). The amino acids released during the degradation of proteins will be either reused (cf. alanine, glutamine) or oxidized and will provide waste products: urea and ammonium. The nitrogen balance will be negative, with a rate of breakdown largely exceeding the rate of synthesis. Consequently, the stores of proteins, i.e., the skeletal muscles, will be rapidly depleted. These losses are related to the large wastage of muscles, which is involved in ICU-acquired weakness [48–52]. This is one of the most devastating consequences of the metabolic response to stress. A major complaint of patients who had a prolonged stay in an ICU is weakness, even a considerable time after discharge. In a study by Herridge et al., survivors of an acute respiratory distress syndrome had persistent muscle wasting and weakness 5 years after discharge from the ICU [48]. Thus, it is essential to take muscle function into consideration when assessing and monitoring the nutritional status of ICU patients.

2.3.3 Changes in Body Composition

The changes in body composition systematically found during critical illness include a loss of lean body mass and a relative preservation of the fat tissue [6]. As a result, body cell mass is typically decreased, while extracellular fluid is increased. Recently, functional and morphological changes of the fat tissue have been identified. These changes can be summarized as a preservation of the fat mass, with increased number of small adipocytes and increased infiltration of the fat tissue by macrophages [53]. Functionally, these changes result in increased lipid storage.

2.3.4 Psychosocial and Behavioral Problems

Long-term psychosocial and behavioral issues have been consistently reported in different cohorts of critically ill patients [54]. Some of these changes, such as prolonged catabolism, are clearly related to the metabolic response to critical illness. Behavioral changes, including anorexia, might be related to changes in the release of gastrointestinal hormones [10].

2.4 Therapeutic Implications

Generally speaking, hormone repletion in the chronic phase by exogenous administration, even though attempted in the past on numerous occasions, has not been successful in attenuation morbidity and mortality of the critically ill, even though successful from a metabolic point of view [55]. For instance, growth or thyroid hormone suppletion may have anabolic effects by increasing protein synthesis and ameliorating protein breakdown in the critically ill but may even increase morbidity and mortality because of other unwanted effects [56–59]. Although insulin may have some albeit controversial anabolic effects and may help, by overcoming resistance and glucose control, the patient-centered outcome effects are highly controversial. Recently, expert guidelines recommend to avoid severe hyperglycemia, although an universally acceptable high limit to titrate insulin therapy cannot be defined [60–62]. Sex steroid hormones are still explored to increase anabolism [63]. Intervening with intermediary metabolism by administering (pharmacologic quantities of) substrates, often together with other nutritional supplements seemed promising in the last decades, but recent evidence suggests that this may be less helpful. For instance, glutamine supplementation of nutrition improved immunologic, gut function and protein metabolism, and even patient-centered outcomes in prior studies, but recent, large studies demonstrate that this may be associated with worse rather than better vital outcomes [64]. This is not to say that adequate nutrition lacks sufficient evidence in improving patient outcomes. Whatever route, quantities, or composition is chosen – these issues remain highly controversial – there is no doubt that prolonged starvation and resultant malnutrition in the critically ill substantially contribute to morbidity and mortality. The question, however, remains whether altered composition – branched chain amino acids, immunonutrition with L-arginine and glutamine, antioxidants, and others – is meaningfully contributing to altered utilization and metabolic processes, particularly in sepsis and trauma patients where metabolism is driven by underlying inflammatory and host defense mechanisms rather than by exogenous supply. Then, metabolic or nutritional support may have some cosmetic effects, including normalization of altered plasma and tissue amino acid and protein levels, but without large effects on gluconeogenesis from protein breakdown, protein synthesis and lean body mass, and even in the presence of hyperinsulinemia. Early mobilization and the avoidance of prolonged sedation are other daily therapeutic measures that are likely to attenuate catabolism.

Hence, other interventions include raising ambient temperature (to decrease energy-consuming heat production) and administering beta-blockers to attenuate sympathetic overstimulation, inflammation, and protein breakdown and to improve organ and muscle function, particularly in burns and sepsis [65, 66]. The latter is still under investigation and certainly not uniformly and routinely accepted. Animal studies suggest that gut-derived ghrelin has anabolic properties, and studying its administration in critically ill patients has been proposed, since circulating levels have been found to be increased or lowered depending on the phase of disease.

2.5 Conclusion

The metabolic response to stress is a complex combination of neurological, endocrine, immune, and inflammatory mechanisms which lead to multiple functional changes in each tissue of the body. A better understanding of the physiology of this response is needed when the progresses of intensive care medicine allow the survival of patients whose adaptive metabolic mechanisms are developing. Therapeutic interventions need to account for the complexity and sequential pattern of the metabolic response to critical illness.

References

1. Preiser JC, Ichai C, Orban JC, Groeneveld ABJ (2014) Metabolic response to the stress of critical illness. Br J Anaesth 113:945–954
2. Van den Berghe G, de Zegher F, Bouillon R (1998) Clinical review 95: acute and prolonged critical illness as different neuroendocrine paradigms. J Clin Endocrinol Metab 83:1827–1834
3. Hamill RW, Woolf PD, McDonald JV, Lee LA, Kelly M (1987) Catecholamines predict outcome in traumatic brain injury. Ann Neurol 21:438–443
4. Boonen E, Vervenne H, Meersseman P, Andrew R, Mortier L, Declercq PE, Vanwijngaerden YM, Spriet I, Wouters PJ, Vander Perre S, Langouche L, Vanhorebeek I, Walker BR, Van den Berghe G (2013) Reduced cortisol metabolism during critical illness. N Engl J Med 368:1477–1488
5. Koch A, Gressner OA, Sanson E, Tacke F, Trautwein C (2009) Serum resistin levels in critically ill patients are associated with inflammation, organ dysfunction and metabolism and may predict survival of non-septic patients. Crit Care 13:R95
6. Marques MB, Langouche L (2013) Endocrine, metabolic, and morphologic alterations of adipose tissue during critical illness. Crit Care Med 41:317–325
7. Hillenbrand A, Weiss M, Knippschild U, Wolf AM, Huber-Lang M (2012) Sepsis-induced adipokine change with regard to insulin resistance. Int J Inflam 2012:972368
8. Fantuzzi G (2009) Adiponectin and inflammation. Am J Physiol Endocrinol Metab 296(2), E397
9. Deane A, Chapman MJ, Fraser RJL, Horowitz M (2010) Bench-to-bedside review: the gut as an endocrine organ in the critically ill. Crit Care 14:228
10. Nematy M, O'Flynn JE, Wandrag L, Brynes AE, Brett SJ, Patterson M, Ghatei MA, Bloom SR, Frost GS (2006) Changes in appetite related gut hormones in intensive care unit patients: a pilot cohort study. Crit Care 10:R10
11. Nematy M, Brynes AE, Hornick PI, Patterson M, Ghatei MA, Bloom SR, Brett SJ, Frost GS (2007) Postprandial ghrelin suppression is exaggerated following major surgery; implications for nutritional recovery. Nutr Metab (Lond) 4:20
12. Losser MR, Damoisel C, Payen D (2010) Bench-to-bedside review: glucose and stress conditions in the intensive care unit. Crit Care 14:231
13. Plank LD, Hill GL (2000) Sequential metabolic changes following induction of systemic inflammatory response in patients with severe sepsis or major blunt trauma. World J Surg 24:630–638
14. Lena D, Kalfon P, Preiser JC, Ichai C (2011) Glycemic control in the intensive care unit and during the postoperative period. Anesthesiology 114:438–444
15. Biolo G, Grimble G, Preiser JC, Leverve X, Jolliet P, Planas M, Roth E, Wernerman J, Pichard C, European Society of Intensive Care Medicine Working Group on Nutrition and Metabolism (2002) Position paper of the ESICM Working Group on Nutrition and Metabolism. Metabolic basis of nutrition in intensive care unit patients: ten critical questions. Intensive Care Med 28:1512–1520
16. Soeters MR, Soeters PB (2012) The evolutionary benefit of insulin resistance. Clin Nutr 31:1002–1007
17. Marik PE, Bellomo R (2013) Stress hyperglycemia: an essential survival response! Crit Care 17:305

18. Dungan KM, Braithwaite SS, Preiser JC (2009) Stress hyperglycaemia. Lancet 373:1798–1807
19. Singer M, De Santis V, Vitale D, Jeffcoate W (2004) Multiorgan failure is an adaptive, endocrine-mediated metabolic response to overwhelming systemic inflammation. Lancet 364:545–548
20. Desborough JP (2000) The stress response to trauma and surgery. Br J Anaesth 85: 109–117
21. Siegel JH, Cerra FB, Coleman B, Giovannini I, Shetye M, Border JR, McMenamy RH (1979) Physiological and metabolic correlations in human sepsis. Surgery 86:163–193
22. Wilmore DW (2000) Metabolic response to severe surgical stress: overview. World J Surg 24:705–711
23. Kyle UG, Jolliet P, Genton L, Meier CA, Mensi N, Graf JD, Chevrolet JC, Pichard C (2005) Clinical evaluation of hormonal stress state in medical ICU patients: a prospective blinded observational study. Intensive Care Med 31:1669–1675
24. Donatelli F, Corbella D, Di Nicola M, Carli F, Lorini L, Fumagalli R, Biolo G (2011) Preoperative insulin resistance and the impact of feeding on postoperative protein balance: a stable isotope study. J Clin Endocrinol Metab 896:E1789–E1797
25. Hoffer LJ, Bistrian BR (2013) Why critically ill patients are protein depleted. J Parenter Enteral Nutr 37(3):300–309
26. Magnuson B, Peppard A, Auer Flomenhoft D (2011) Hypocaloric considerations in patients with potentially hypometabolic disease States. Nutr Clin Pract 26:253–260
27. McClave SA, Martindale RG, Kiraly L (2013) The use of indirect calorimetry in the intensive care unit. Curr Opin Clin Nutr Metab Care 16:202–208
28. Siirala W, Olkkola KT, Noponen T, Vuori A, Aantaa R (2010) Predictive equations over-estimate the resting energy expenditure in amyotrophic lateral sclerosis patients who are dependent on invasive ventilation support. Nutr Metab (Lond) 7:70
29. Kreymann G, Grosser S, Buggisch P, Gottschall C, Matthaei S, Greten H (1993) Oxygen consumption and resting metabolic rate in sepsis, sepsis syndrome, and septic shock. Crit Care Med 21:1012–1019
30. Uehara M, Plank LD, Hill GL (1999) Components of energy expenditure in patients with severe sepsis and major trauma: a basis for clinical care. Crit Care Med 27:1295–1302
31. Vincent JL, Preiser JC (2013) When should we add parenteral to enteral nutrition? Lancet 381:354–355
32. Heidegger CP, Berger MM, Graf S, Zingg W, Darmon P, Costanza MC, Thibault R, Pichard C (2013) Optimisation of energy provision with supplemental parenteral nutrition in critically ill patients: a randomised controlled clinical trial. Lancet 381:385–393
33. Casaer MP, Mesotten D, Hermans G, Wouters PJ, Schetz M, Meyfroidt G, Van Cromphaut S, Ingels C, Meersseman P, Muller J, Vlasselaers D, Debaveye Y, Desmet L, Dubois J, Van Assche A, Vanderheyden S, Wilmer A, Van den Berghe G (2011) Early versus late parenteral nutrition in critically ill adults. N Engl J Med 365:506–517
34. Schetz M, Casaer MP, Van den Berghe G (2013) Does artificial nutrition improve outcome of critical illness? Crit Care 17:302
35. Tappy L, Schwarz JM, Schneiter P, Cayeux C, Revelly JP, Fagerquist CK, Jéquier E, Chioléro R (1998) Effects of isoenergetic glucose-based or lipid-based parenteral nutrition on glucose metabolism, de novo lipogenesis, and respiratory gas exchanges in critically ill patients. Crit Care Med 26:860–867
36. Watford M (2005) Is the small intestine a gluconeogenic organ. Nutr Rev 63:356–360
37. Battezzati A, Caumo A, Martino F et al (2004) Nonhepatic glucose production in humans. Am J Physiol Endocrinol Metab 286:E129–E135
38. Shangraw RE, Jahoor F, Wolfe RR, Lang CH (1996) Pyruvate dehydrogenase inactivity is not responsible for sepsis-induced insulin resistance. Crit Care Med 24:566–574
39. Burgstad CM, Besanko LK, Deane AM, Nguyen NQ, Saadat-Gilani K, Davidson G, Burt E, Thomas A, Holloway RH, Chapman MJ, Fraser RJ (2013) Sucrose malabsorption and impaired mucosal integrity in enterally fed critically ill patients: a prospective cohort observational study. Crit Care Med 41:1221–1228

40. Orban JC, Leverve X, Ichai C (2011) Lactate: métabolisme et physiopathologie. In: Ichai C, Quintard H, Orban JC (eds) Désordres métaboliques et réanimation : de la,physiopathologie au traitement. Springer, Paris, pp 181–198
41. Van Hall G, Stromstadt M, Rasmussen P et al (2004) Blood lactate is an important source of energy for the human brain. J Cereb Blood Flow Metab 29:1121–1129
42. Leverve XM (1999) Energy metabolism in critically ill patients: lactate is a major oxidizable substrate. Curr Opin Clin Nutr Metab Care 2:165–169
43. Ichai C, Armando G, Orban JC, Berthier F, Rami L, Samat-Long C, Grimaud D, Leverve X (2009) Sodium lactate versus mannitol in the treatment of intracranial hypertensive episodes in severe traumatic brain-injured patients. Intensive Care Med 35(3):471–479
44. Stanley WC, Recchia FA, Lopasschuk GD (2005) Myocardial substrate metabolism in the normal and failing heart. Physiol Rev 85:1093–1129
45. Levy B, Gibot S, Franck P, Cravoisy A, Bollaert PE (2005) Relation between muscle Na + K+ ATPase activity and raised lactate concentrations in septic shock: a prospective study. Lancet 365:871–875
46. Krinsley JS, Egi M, Kiss A, Devendra AN, Schuetz P, Maurer PM, Schultz MJ, van Hooijdonk RT, Kiyoshi M, Mackenzie IM, Annane D, Stow P, Nasraway SA, Holewinski S, Holzinger U, Preiser JC, Vincent JL, Bellomo R (2013) Diabetic status and the relation of the three domains of glycemic control to mortality in critically ill patients: an international multicenter cohort study. Crit Care 17:R37
47. Falciglia M, Freyberg RW, Almenoff PL, D'Alessio DA, Render ML (2009) Hyperglycemia-related mortality in critically ill patients varies with admission diagnosis. Crit Care Med 37:3001–3009
48. Herridge MS, Tansey CM, Matte A et al (2011) Functional disability 5 years after acute respiratory distress syndrome. N Engl J Med 364:1293–1304
49. Hill GL (1992) Jonathan E. Rhoads Lecture. Body composition research: implications for the practice of clinical nutrition. JPEN J Parenter Enteral Nutr 16:197–218
50. Lecker SH (2006) Protein degradation by the ubiquitin-proteasome pathway in normal and disease states. J Am Soc Nephrol 17:1807–1819
51. Mitch WE, Goldberg AL (1996) Mechanisms of muscle wasting. The role of the ubiquitin-proteasome pathway. N Engl J Med 335:1897–1905
52. Hill NE, Murphy KG, Singer M (2012) Ghrelin, appetite and critical illness. Curr Opin Crit Care 18:199–205
53. Langouche L, Perre SV, Thiessen S, Gunst J, Hermans G, D'Hoore A, Kola B, Korbonits M, Van den Berghe G (2010) Alterations in adipose tissue during critical illness: an adaptive and protective response? Am J Respir Crit Care Med 2010(182):507–516
54. Broomhead LR, Brett SJ (2002) Clinical review: intensive care follow-up – what has it told us? Crit Care 6:411–417
55. Ligtenberg JJ, Girbes AR, Beentjes JA, Tulleken JE, Van der Werf TS, Zijlstra JG (2001) Hormones in the critically ill patients: to intervene or not to intervene ? Intensive Care Med 27:1567–1577
56. Takala J, Ruokonen E, Webster NR et al (1999) Increased mortality associated with growth hormone treatment in critically ill adults. N Engl J Med 341:785–792
57. Ruokonen E, Takala J (2002) Dangers of growth hormone therapy in critically ill patients. Curr Opin Clin Nutr Metab Care 5:199–209
58. Voerman HJ, Strack van Schijndel RJM, Groeneveld ABJ, de Boer H, Nauta JJP, van der Veen EA, Thijs LG (1992) Effects of recombinant human growth hormone in patients with severe sepsis. Ann Surg 216:648–655
59. Schulman RC, Mechanick JI (2012) Metabolic and nutrition support in the chronic critical illness syndrome. Respir Care 57:958–978
60. Ichai C, Preiser JC, Société Française d'Anesthésie-Réanimation; Société de Réanimation de langue Française; Experts group (2010) International recommendations for glucose control in adult non diabetic critically ill patients. Crit Care 14:R166
61. Groeneveld ABJ, Beishuizen A, Visser FC (2002) Insulin: a wonder drug in the critically ill? Crit Care 6:102–105

62. Whyte MB, Jackson NC, Shojaee-Moradie F, Treacher DF, Beale RJ, Jones RH, Umpleby AM (2010) Metabolic effects of intensive insulin therapy in critically ill patients. Am J Physiol Endocrinol Metab 298:E697–E705
63. Maggio M, Nicolini F, Cattabiani C, Beghi C, Gherli T, Schwartz RS, Valenti G, Ceda GP (2012) Effects of testosterone supplementation on clinical and rehabilitative outcomes in older men undergoing on-pump CABG. Contemp Clin Trials 33:730–738
64. Heyland D, Muscedere J, Wischmeyer PE, Cook D, Jones G, Albert M, Elke G, Berger MM, Day AG, for the Canadian Critical Care Trials Group (2013) A randomized trial of glutamine and antioxidants in critically ill patients. N Engl J Med 368:489–497
65. Kelemen JJ, Cioffie WG, Mason AD, Mozingo DW, McManus WF, Pruitt BA (1996) Effects of ambient temperature on metabolic rate after thermal injury. Ann Surg 223:406–412
66. De Montmolin E, Aboab J, Mansart A, Annane D (2009) Bench-to-bedside review: ß-adrenergic modulation in sepsis. Crit Care 13:230

Chapter 3
Bioenergetics of the Stress Response

Christophe Faisy

Abstract Energy is a property of matter which obeys the two principles of thermodynamics: energy conservation within a given system and the general trend toward a higher degree of disorder, i.e., the concept of entropy (diminution of the amount of energy available within a given system). Chemical reactions in biological and biomolecular systems are based on a succession of energy transmission provided by redox reactions involving the exchange of electrons between the oxidized and the reduced organic substrates. The major energy source of all cells in aerobic organisms is adenosine triphosphate (ATP). Oxidation reactions in nutrients allow ATP synthesis by oxidative phosphorylation. The most common chemical reaction to produce energy in cells is the hydrolysis of ATP to ADP and inorganic phosphate. Before the formalization of the principles of thermodynamics, Antoine-Laurent de Lavoisier (1743–1794) has already anticipated the key principle of bioenergetics among living organisms: "Life is a slow combustion sustained by respiration. Animals are composed of fuel elements. The food replaces loss of substances arising from the combustion of matters present in the body." Indeed, living systems are open systems drawing their energy from substrates like nutrients. This is why living organisms are fundamentally different from inert material: biochemical reactions lead to an increase in energy availability, i.e., negative entropy. What has perhaps best characterizes a living system is the negative entropy to allow a dynamic and unstable balance between this open system and its environment. See from this thermodynamic perspective, homeostasis (degree of organization of the organism) is only the consequence of the accumulation of negative entropy. It should be therefore possible to consider the frontier between life and dying processes by estimating negative entropy. This opens up new prospects in fields like critical care medicine.

C. Faisy, MD, PhD
Service de Réanimation Médicale, Hôpital Européen Georges Pompidou, Assistance Publique – Hôpitaux de Paris, University Paris Descartes – Sorbonne Paris Cité, Paris, France
e-mail: christophe.faisy@wanadoo.fr

J.-C. Preiser (ed.), *The Stress Response of Critical Illness: Metabolic and Hormonal Aspects*, DOI 10.1007/978-3-319-27687-8_3

3.1 Introduction

Energy is a property of matter which obeys the two principles of thermodynamics: energy conservation within a given system and the general trend toward a higher degree of disorder, i.e., the concept of entropy (diminution of the amount of energy available within a given system). Chemical reactions in biological and biomolecular systems are based on a succession of energy transmission provided by redox reactions involving the exchange of electrons between the oxidized and the reduced organic substrates. The major energy source of all cells in aerobic organisms is adenosine triphosphate (ATP). Oxidation reactions in nutrients allow ATP synthesis by oxidative phosphorylation. The most common chemical reaction to produce energy in cells is the hydrolysis of ATP to ADP and inorganic phosphate. Before the formalization of the principles of thermodynamics, Antoine-Laurent de Lavoisier (1743–1794) has already anticipated the key principle of bioenergetics among living organisms: "Life is a slow combustion sustained by respiration. Animals are composed of fuel elements. The food replaces loss of substances arising from the combustion of matters present in the body." Indeed, living systems are open systems drawing their energy from substrates like nutrients. This is why living organisms are fundamentally different from inert material: biochemical reactions lead to an increase in energy availability, i.e., negative entropy [26]. What has perhaps best characterizes a living system is the negative entropy to allow a dynamic and unstable balance between this open system and its environment. See from this thermodynamic perspective, homeostasis (degree of organization of the organism) is only the consequence of the accumulation of negative entropy. It should be therefore possible to consider the frontier between life and dying processes by estimating negative entropy. This opens up new prospects in fields like critical care medicine.

3.2 Cellular and Molecular Aspects: Toward New Paradigms

The survival of living organisms depends on the interactions with their environment to which they must adapt. As an open system, living organisms must maintain three functions or functional complexes: Physical composition (homeostasis), form or size (heterostasis), and permanence or temporal evolution (teleostasis) [18, 19, 21]. Homeostasis refers to the maintenance of the physicochemical characteristics like ion concentration, temperature, or pH. It is therefore the functions of the metabolism. According to the duality of energy–matter, anabolism refers to the assimilation and transformation of nutrients in own structures, whereas catabolism is the degradation of such structures to produce the energy required for the physiological functioning. The most important elements of metabolism are carbon, hydrogen, and oxygen, which represent the physical aspect of metabolism (Fig. 3.1). Indeed, these elements constitute carbohydrates and fats which are the major energy reserves (close to 100,000 kcal in healthy human). At the cell level, the metabolism ensuring homeostasis took place in the cytoplasm and is carried

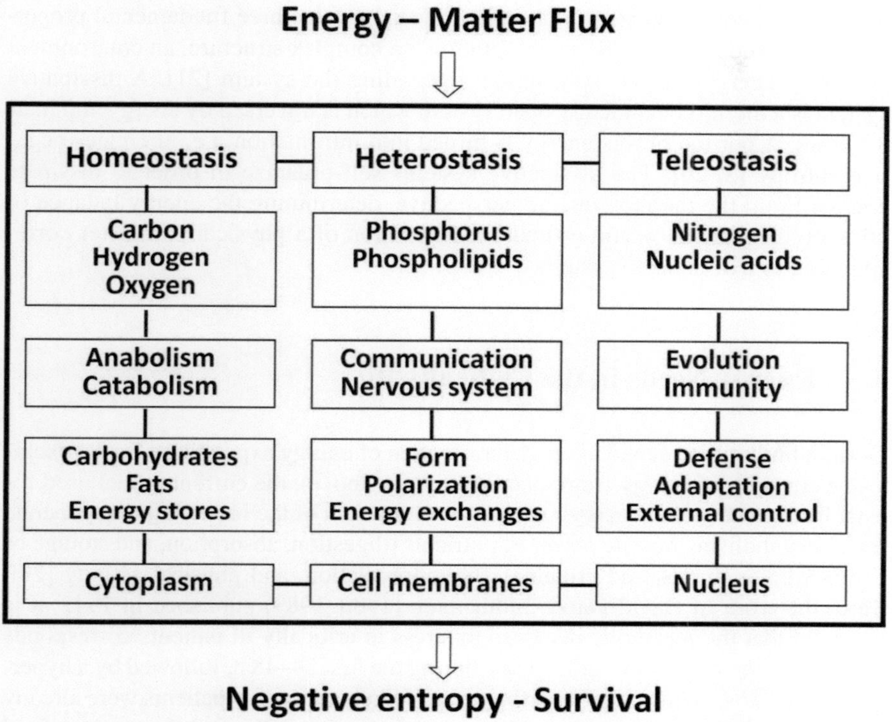

Fig. 3.1 Systemic model of functional integration: the three main biological functions. The black rectangle in bold represents a dissipative structure, i.e., a system open to its environment and traversed by a flux of energy or matter, increasing information and negative entropy into the system. Living organisms are dissipative structures

out by redox reactions (Fig. 3.1). Pertinently, indirect calorimetry, the "gold standard" for the assessment of resting energy expenditure in critically ill patients, merely measures energy produced by metabolism (first column in Fig. 3.1), but does not give direct information on the energy flows required to support the functions of heterostasis and teleostasis. This point may explain why the balance between energy expenditure and energy intakes is very difficult to estimate; thereby the aim of reducing energy deficit in critically ill patients cannot be achieved with the current methodology. All functions related to heterostasis (cross talk and environment delimitation) are provided at the cell level by the membrane, especially its polarization. The element phosphorus from membrane phospholipids plays a crucial role in the energy exchanges during polarization–depolarization processes. A typical example is the information transmission by nervous system. Teleostasis is the adaptation functions devoted to the evolution of living organisms, i.e., genetic and immunologic properties. At the cell level, this corresponds to the nuclear functions (nucleic acids). At the organ level, this corresponds to the reticuloendothelial system (Fig. 3.1). According to Ilya Prigogine (1917–2003), the conditions of evolution by self-organization of matter depend on the three fundamental properties of the model of "functional integration": a complex structure, an environment providing energy, and an information integrating the system [21]. A dissipative system is a thermodynamically open system which is traversed by energy and matter flows. A portion of this energy is turned into information, i.e., it creates negative entropy [2, 26]. The dissipative systems self-organize in order to dissipate energy. From the thermodynamic perspective, determining the energy balance of critically ill patients would estimate the variation of a physical parameter corresponding to a dissipative system.

3.3 Energy Needs in the Critically Ill

Despite limitations related to the determination of energy expenditure by the exclusive estimation of energy from metabolism (see above), the current model used for establishing the global energy expenditure is the sum of the following components: Basal metabolism, thermic power of nutrients (digestion, absorption, and storage of carbohydrates, lipids, and proteins), thermoregulation, and physical activity [29]. Since the work of David Paton Cuthbertson (1900–1989) published in 1942, it is accepted that the metabolic response to stress in critically ill patients corresponds firstly to a hypometabolic "ebb" phase during the first 24–48 h, followed by a hypermetabolic "flow" phase [5]. Nevertheless, it is likely that many patients were already in the "flow" phase by the time they were admitted to ICU, and the modern fluid resuscitation would shorten the period of hypotension resulting in a short "ebb" phase [9, 30]. The magnitude and the duration of energy expenditure fluctuations are highly variable and influenced by the underlying disease, body composition, medications, or therapeutic procedures (sedatives, analgesics, curare, catecholamines, cooling, physiotherapy, and nursing), dietary carbohydrate-to-lipid ratio, and genetic factors [1, 6, 15, 23, 28, 29, 32, 33]. Similarly, substantial adjustments occur during denutrition, leading to a reduction of energy expenditure. To that must be added the effect of mechanical ventilation on oxygen consumption [16]. All these factors make estimating resting energy expenditure very complex in the critically ill. Another critical point is the estimation of the energy cost of metabolic interconversion of substrates, such as gluconeogenesis, ketogenesis, lipogenesis, or lactate production (any situation where the respiratory quotient is outside the range 0.7–1) [27]. For example, indirect calorimetry can only measure the total (or apparent) but not the real oxidation rate of glucose (Q_{ox}): Q_{ox} (total) = Q_{ox} (real) + Q_{ox} (lipogenesis) − Q_{ox} (gluconeogenesis). Interestingly, body cell mass, a component of the fat-free mass, is associated with oxygen consumption and resting energy expenditure [12, 13]. Body cell mass is altered by changes of nutritional status and the catabolic effects of disease. Therefore, development of clinical tools for evaluating body composition, especially body cell mass/weight ratio, could help demonstrate the relevance of the concept of energy balance by patients hospitalized in intensive care units (ICU) [8, 14, 25].

3.4 Energy Balance in the Critically Ill

Perturbations of the normal metabolic response to starvation with hyperglycemia, high lactate level, hypertriglyceridemia, and high level of nonesterified fatty acids due to insulin resistance characterize the hypermetabolic state of the critically injured patients [20, 22]. Energy deficit results from a combination of hypermetabolism and reduced intake due to frequent interruptions in feedings because of gastrointestinal intolerance and diagnostic and therapeutic procedures. In intubated and mechanically ventilated patients, the great variability of resting energy expenditure and nutrient delivery compared to prescription, partly due to frequent use of sedatives, analgesics, or vasoconstrictors, increases the risk of mismatch between energy requirements and intakes [9]. According to the current model used, energy balance corresponds to energy (calorie) really delivered minus resting energy expenditure. Total energy delivered must also take account of glucose infusions and propofol used for continuous sedation [29]. However, stored energy (adipose tissue, intramuscular triglycerides, and blood fatty acids or triglycerides) is ignored for the calculation of energy balance by using this method. From a thermodynamic point of view, it would be more appropriate to have a measurement tool integrating the overall energy dissipated by an individual patient.

3.5 Energy Deficit in the Critically Ill

Protein–energy malnutrition is commonly associated with impaired immune responses and affects the clinical course of some infections, such as pneumonia or bacteremia [3, 4, 24]. ICU patients are prone to develop early protein–energy deficit. The latter is associated with a higher rate of nosocomial infections, longer ICU stays, and higher healthcare costs. Energy deficit in ICU patients is mainly caused by reduced intake due to underprescribed calories and frequent feeding interruptions because of gastrointestinal intolerance or diagnostic and/or therapeutic procedures. Energy deficit results in an early energy gap during the first week of ICU stay, which is never overcome thereafter [31]. Cumulated energy deficit buildup during the first days of ICU stay appears to be an independent factor contributing to nosocomial infections [7, 10]. In addition, a large negative energy balance was observed during prolonged acute mechanical ventilation in the most critically ill patients and might affect their ICU outcomes. However, randomized intervention studies limiting energy deficit by combining parenteral nutrition with insufficient enteral nutrition have yielded conflicting results among ICU-acquired nosocomial infections [17]. Indeed, limiting early energy deficit in ICU patients might be reserved for those that are in a situation of chronic critical illness, i.e., patients with prolonged acute mechanical ventilation and severe energy deficits are likely to benefit most from preventive measures [7, 10].

3.6 A Dissipative System: Body Cell Mass

A dissipative system is a physical (inert or living) structure open to its environment and traversed by a flux of energy or matter. During its passage through the system, a fraction of this energy is transformed into information, creating negative entropy. The most obvious example is food consumption by living organisms. The energy flux through a dissipative structure is an increasing function of its information content [2, 21]. Therefore, per unit of mass, the energy expanded by the human brain is 5000 higher than the sun (Fig. 3.2). Body cell mass is the metabolically active compartment of fat-free mass that reflects the body's cellular components involved in oxygen consumption, carbon dioxide production, and resting metabolism. Body cell mass also interacts with energy stores (Fig. 3.3) and is altered by denutrition [11]. To

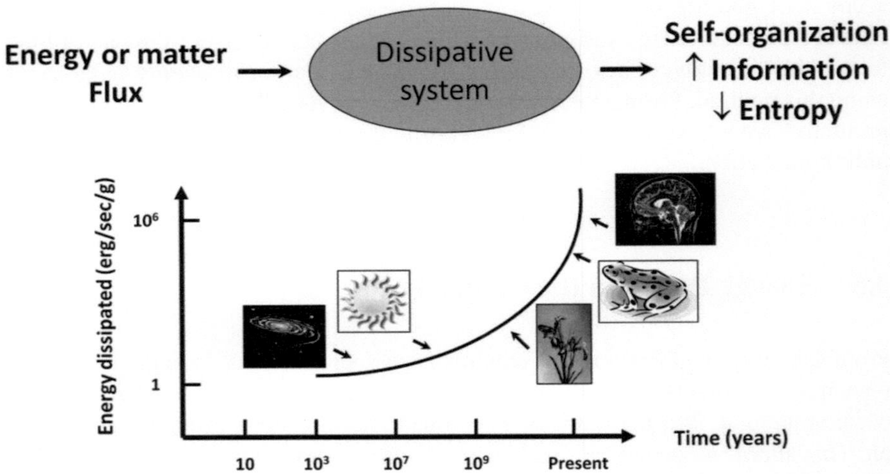

Fig. 3.2 Evolution of dissipative structures in the history from the universe (Adapted from [2, 21])

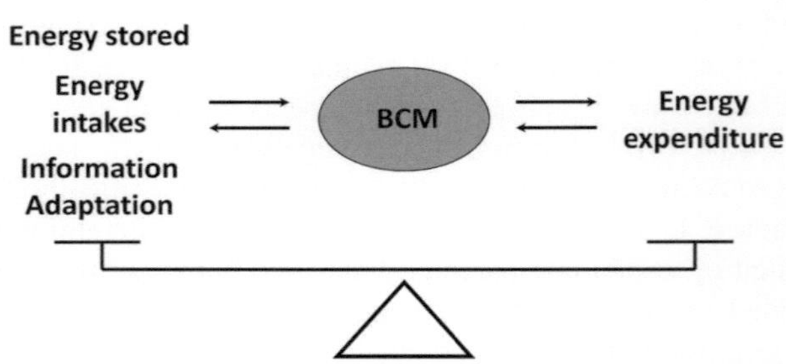

Fig. 3.3 Body cell mass (*BCM*) can be regarded as the reserve of negative entropy in living organisms. Estimating body cell mass would make it possible a thermodynamic approach of the nutritional assistance in critically ill patients

put in a simplified way, body cell mass corresponds to a dissipative system, i.e., a negative entropy reserve. Body cell mass could be a relevant tool for estimating nutritional status and prognosis in the critically ill patient, making it possible to override the uncertain estimate of energy balance by current models (Fig. 3.3).

Conflict of Interest The author has not disclosed any potential conflicts of interest.

References

1. Askanasi J, Rosenbaum SH, Hyman A, Silverberg PA, Milic-Emili J, Kinney JM (1980) Respiratory changes induced by the large glucose loads of total parenteral nutrition. JAMA 243:1444–1447
2. Chaisson EJ (2002) Cosmic evolution: the rise of complexity in nature. Harvard University Press, Cambridge
3. Chandra RK (1997) Nutrition and the immune system: an introduction. Am J Clin Nutr 66:S460–S466
4. Cunningham-Rundles S, McNeeley DF, Moon A (2005) Mechanisms of nutrient modulation of the immune response. J Allergy Clin Immunol 56:S73–S76
5. Cuthbertson D (1942) Post-shock metabolic response. Lancet 1:433–437
6. Drolz A, Wewalka M, Horvatits T, Fuhrmann V, Schneeweiss B, Trauner M, Zauner C (2014) Gender-specific differences in energy metabolism during the initial phase of critical illness. Eur J Clin Nutr 68:707–711
7. Ekpe K, Novara A, Mainardi JL, Fagon JY, Faisy C (2014) Methicillin-resistant Staphylococcus aureus bloodstream infections are associated with a higher energy deficit than other ICU-acquired bacteremia. Intensive Care Med 40:1878–1887
8. Faisy C, Rabbat A, Kouchakji B, Laaban JP (2000) Bioelectrical impedance analysis in estimating nutritional status and outcome of patients with chronic obstructive pulmonary disease and acute respiratory failure. Intensive Care Med 26:518–525
9. Faisy C, Lerolle N, Dachraoui F, Savard JF, Abboud I, Tadie JM, Fagon JY (2009) Impact of energy deficit calculated by a predictive method on outcome in medical patients requiring prolonged acute mechanical ventilation. Br J Nutr 101:1079–1087
10. Faisy C, Llerena C, Savalle M, Mainardi JL, Fagon JY (2011) Early ICU energy deficit is a risk factor of ventilator-associated pneumonia by Staphylococcus aureus. Chest 140: 1254–1260
11. Fiaccadori E, Morabito S, Cabassi A, Regolisti G (2014) Body cell mass evaluation in critically ill patients: killing two birds with one stone. Crit Care 18:139
12. Frankenfield DC, Cooney RN, Smith JS, Rowe WA (1999) Bioelectrical impedance plethysmographic analysis of body composition in critically injured and healthy subjects. Am J Clin Nutr 69:426–431
13. Gallagher D, Belmonte D, Deurenberg P, Wang Z, Krasnow N, Pi-Sunyer FX, Heymsfield SB (1998) Organ-tissue mass measurement allows modeling of REE and metabolically active tissue mass. Am J Physiol Endocrinol Metab 275:E249–E258
14. Ismael S, Savalle M, Trivin C, Gillaizeau F, Dauzac C, Faisy C (2014) The consequences of sudden fluid shifts on body composition in critically ill patients. Crit Care 18:R49
15. Long CL, Schaffel N, Geiger JW, Schiller WR, Blakemore WS (1979) Metabolic response to injury and illness: estimation of energy and protein needs from indirect calorimetry and nitrogen balance. JPEN J Parenter Enteral Nutr 3:452–456
16. Manthous CA, Hall JB, Kushner R, Schmidt GA, Russo G, Wood LD (1995) The effect of mechanical ventilation on oxygen consumption in critically ill patients. Am J Respir Crit Care Med 151:210–214

17. Pichard C, Oshima T, Berger MM (2015) Energy deficit is clinically relevant for critically ill patients: yes. Intensive Care Med 41:335–338
18. Pischinger A (2007) The extracellular matrix and ground regulation: basis for a holistic biological medicine hardcover. North Atlantic Book, Berkeley
19. Popp FA (1987) Neue Horizonte in der Medizin. Karl F. Haug Verlag, Heidelberg
20. Preiser JC, Ichai C, Orban JC, Groeneveld ABJ (2014) Metabolic response to the stress of critical illness. Br J Anaesth 113:945–954
21. Prigogine I, Stenger I (1988) Entre le temps et l'éternité. Fayard, Paris
22. Reid CL (2004) Nutritional requirements of surgical and critically-ill patients: do we really know what they need? Proc Nutr Soc 63:467–472
23. Roza AM, Schizgal HM (1984) The Harris Benedict equation reevaluated: resting energy requirements and the body cell mass. Am J Clin Nutr 40:168–182
24. Rubinson L, Diette GB, Song X, Brower RG, Krishnan JA (2004) Low caloric intake is associated with nosocomial bloodstream infections in patients in the medical intensive care unit. Crit Care Med 32:350–357
25. Savalle M, Gillaizeau F, Puymirat E, Maruani G, Bellenfant F, Houillier P, Fagon JY, Faisy C (2012) Modeling body cell mass for a relevant nutritional assessment in critically ill patients. Am J Physiol Endocrinol Metab 303:E389–E396
26. Schrödinger E (1944) What is life? The physical aspect of living cells. Cambridge University Press, Cambridge
27. Schutz Y (1995) The basis of direct and indirect calorimetry and their potentials. Diabetes Metab Rev 11:383–408
28. Swinamer DL, Phang PT, Jones RL, Grace M, King EG (1988) Effect of routine administration of analgesia on energy expenditure in critically ill patients. Chest 92:4–10
29. Taylor SJ (2007) Energy and nitrogen requirements in disease states. Smith-Gordon and Company Limited, London
30. Trager K, DeBacker D, Radermacher P (2003) Metabolic alterations in sepsis and vasoactive drug-related metabolic effects. Curr Opin Crit Care 9:271–278
31. Villet S, Chiolero RL, Bollmann MD, Revelly JP, Cayeux RNM, Delarue J, Berger M (2005) Negative impact of hypocaloric feeding and energy balance on clinical outcome in ICU patients. Clin Nutr 24:502–509
32. Weissman C, Kemper M, Damask MC, Askanasi J, Hyman A, Kinney JM (1984) Effect of routine intensive care interactions on metabolic rate. Chest 86:815–818
33. Weissman C, Kemper M, Askanazi J, Hyman A, Kinney JM (1986) Resting metabolic rate of the critically ill patients: measured versus predicted. Anesthesiology 64:673–679

Chapter 4
Mitochondrial Adaptation and Hibernation

Jonathan Grip, Nicolas Tardif, and Olav Rooyackers

Abstract Stress in the form of critical illness and organ failure is associated with damaged and dysfunctional mitochondria. However, actual function of mitochondria in sepsis and their role in the development of organ failure are not fully characterized, partly due to the heterogeneity of the disease, variation and difficulties in methods for studying mitochondrial function, and the problem that available animal model does not seem to represent the human situation very well. On the other hand, it seems that the mitochondrial dysfunction is accompanied by decreased metabolic demands or oxygen consumption, and it has therefore been hypothesized that a mitochondrial downregulation and hypometabolism are adaptive responses in order for the organ to survive the stressful event, similar to hibernation seen in some animals. Even though this theory is interesting and there is support for decreased metabolism in critical illness, the response does not mimic the regulatory mechanism seen in "true" hibernation that, e.g., is accompanied with a drop in body temperature. We look forward to further studies that may lead to a stronger rationale for, or disproves, the theories of metabolic downregulation in critical illness-related organ failure.

4.1 Introduction

Severe stress in the form of shock or sepsis often leads to critical illness that requires intensive care. Many patients with persisting stress will develop multiple organ failure. Without support of the failing vital organs in an ICU, patients will not survive. The development of multiple organ failure is the leading cause of death in these patients. The cellular mechanisms causing these organs to fail in not well known. Several theories including reduced oxygen delivery, impaired autophagy or decreased mitochondrial function have been proposed. About a decade ago, the

J. Grip • N. Tardif • O. Rooyackers (✉)
Department of Anesthesiology and Intensive Care,
Karolinska University Hospital and Karolinska Institute,
Huddinge, Sweden
e-mail: Olav.Rooyackers@ki.se

J.-C. Preiser (ed.), *The Stress Response of Critical Illness: Metabolic and Hormonal Aspects*, DOI 10.1007/978-3-319-27687-8_4

mitochondrial changes have been suggested as a state of hibernation in which the failing organs are reducing their mitochondrial function as a survival strategy [1]. In this chapter we will focus on the mitochondrial function in organs during severe stress and critical illness with organ failure and discuss the hypothesis that the reduced mitochondrial activity is a strategy for long-term survival, as with hibernation. We will describe normal mitochondrial function, how this can be assessed in studies, what goes wrong during stress and critical illness, and what the mitochondrial adaptations are during hibernation, and finally we will discuss the hibernation theory during organ failure.

4.2 Mitochondria

4.2.1 Mitochondrial Metabolism

Mitochondria are known as the power plant of the cell since they are involved in the majority of the energy conversion needed for cellular processes. Besides their role in energy production, mitochondria are also involved in calcium signaling, ROS balance, and apoptosis. Mitochondria are double-membrane organelles composed of the outer membrane and the inner membrane. The inner membrane is folded, creating the structure called cristae where the enzymes involved in oxidative respiration are located. These two membranes delimitate two compartments: (1) the intermembrane compartment where the H^+ gradient in the electron chain is created and (2) the matrix where the Krebs cycle enzymes and beta-oxidation take place and where the mitochondrial DNA (mtDNA) is located (Fig. 4.1).

The main function of mitochondria is to degrade energy-rich substrates, thereby creating energy-rich ATP. The majority of ATP is synthesized by oxidizing substrates via different pathways (glycolysis and beta-oxidation) and entering the Krebs cycle which will provide energy-rich intermediates for ATP production in the oxidative phosphorylation (Fig. 4.1). The different substrates for the energy production come from carbohydrates and fats, but also the carbon skeleton of the amino acids can be used for producing energy. The oxidative phosphorylation contains five complexes of the electron transfer chain, complex I (ubiquinone NADH dehydrogenase), complex II (succinate dehydrogenase), complex III (ubiquinol-cytochrome c reductase), complex IV (cytochrome-c oxidase), and complex V (F1F0ATPsynthase). This transfer of electron between the complexes is coupled with transport of hydrogen ions (H^+) out of the matrix, creating a gradient of protons (H^+) between the matrix and the intermembrane space (Fig. 4.1). The last electron acceptor is a molecule of oxygen, which is reduced to a molecule of water by complex IV. The proton gradient, also called mitochondrial membrane potential ($\Delta\psi_m$), is the driving force for ATP production by complex V. Some electrons escape during their transport between the complexes leading to the production of reactive oxygen species (ROS). Complex I and III are the main sites for ROS formation.

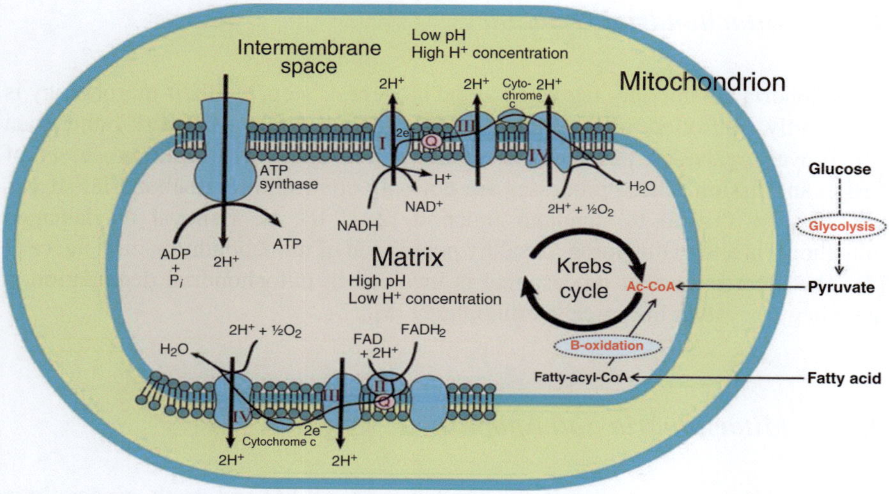

Fig. 4.1 Mitochondria oxidative respiration. Aerobic respiration corresponds to a transfer of energy from the substrates to the synthesis of ATP. The first reactions are the degradation of the energetic substrates, glucose, and fatty acids, respectively, by glycolysis (cytosolic) and beta-oxidation (mitochondrial matrix). These pathways lead to the synthesis of acetyl-CoA which feeds the Krebs cycle. The Krebs cycle is a series of reactions that notably provide reduced electron donors, i.e., NADH and $FADH_2$ which are essential for the oxidative phosphorylation. These molecules will provide electron for the complex I and II, who will transfer these electrons to the complexes III and IV. Unidirectional transport of the electrons between the complexes is achieved by the electron carrier's ubiquinone (Q) and cytochrome c. This flow of electrons is coupled with the pumping of protons (H+) creating a gradient of H+ between the matrix and the intermembrane space. Finally, the complex IV will reduce oxygens to form molecules of water. In the final step, the complex V (ATP synthase) uses the energy stored as the H+ gradient to synthetize ATP. *Ac-CoA* acetyl coenzyme A, *FAD* flavin adenine dinucleotide, *NAD* nicotinamide adenine dinucleotide

4.2.2 Mitochondria Biogenesis

Mitochondria cannot be synthetized de novo in the cell. Mitochondrial biogenesis is the growth and division of preexisting mitochondria. Regarding their importance in the cell, mitochondria biogenesis is tightly regulated. Mitochondria possess their own DNA (mtDNA) and their own replication machinery, coded for by the mtDNA. Information contained in the mtDNA is essential for mitochondrial respiration. Several copies are present in each single mitochondrion and encode for 14 proteins involved in the respiratory complexes and Krebs cycle enzymes. Still, the vast majority of the mitochondrial proteins are encoded in the nucleus and imported to the mitochondria via a specific import system. One of the main regulators of mitochondrial biogenesis and respiration is the peroxisome proliferator-activated receptor γ co-activator-1α (PGC-1α). PGC-1α governs the expression of nuclear-encoded mitochondrial proteins, like the nuclear respiratory factors (NRF1 and 2). These transcription factors NRF1 and NRF2 activate the mitochondrial transcription factor A (TFAM) that will initiate the transcription and the replication of the mtDNA.

4.2.3 Mitochondrial Dynamics

Mitochondria are not only regulated at the biogenesis step, but their morphology is also tightly controlled. Mitochondria in the cells constitute a network rather than single oval organelles, and their morphology is a result of dynamic processes of fusion and fission. These processes are not only controlling mitochondrial shapes but are also critical to maintain function [2–4] by the removal of damaged mitochondria and maintaining a healthy population of mitochondria within the cells [4]. The other important process that is involved in mitochondrial degradation is autophagy, or rather the so-called mitophagy [5].

4.2.4 Mitochondria and Apoptosis

Mitochondria are main actors in the regulation of cell life and death, especially in apoptosis (programmed cell death). Mitochondria's primary function in the maintenance of the energetic status of the cell is a critical factor in the regulation and activation of the apoptotic processes. But mitochondria are also an important direct intermediate in the apoptosis pathway regulation. Apoptosis is governed by a fine-tuning between pro- and anti-apoptotic molecules from the BCL-2 family [6]. When this balance is in favor of an apoptotic fate, pro-apoptotic factors, mainly Bcl-2-associated x protein (BAX) and Bcl-2 antagonist killer 1 (BAK 1) proteins, will accumulate on the outer membrane of the mitochondria and lead to the permeabilization of the membrane. This process, also called mitochondrial outer membrane permeabilization, results in the release of cytochrome c into the cytosol. Once in the cytosolic compartment, cytochrome c will activate the caspases which will trigger cell death via apoptosis [7–9]. Mitochondria also mediate apoptosis via caspase-independent pathways, by the release of apoptosis-inducing factor (AIF) and endonuclease G (EndoG) proteins, which lead to the apoptotic degradation of DNA [10].

4.3 Measuring Mitochondrial Function

Several methods exist to investigate mitochondrial function. The aim of this chapter is not to address all techniques for the investigation of mitochondrial function but rather to describe the methods that have been mainly used in the field of critical illness. In the first part, we will describe the markers used to assess mitochondria content and the in vitro measurement of the mitochondrial activity. In the second part, we will briefly describe the potential approach that could be used in vivo in humans.

4.3.1 Mitochondrial Content

In research involving mitochondria, the quantification of mitochondrial content has been widely used as an indicator for the oxidative capacity of a tissue. In addition, mitochondrial content is used as a normalization factor for many mitochondrial functional measurements (see Sect. 4.3.2).

The gold standard technique to assessed mitochondrial content is transmission electron microscopy (TEM) to measure mitochondrial volume or cristae area [11]. However, the costs and the requirement for highly specified skills for this method have led to the development of surrogate markers for mitochondria content. Also the volume measurements could be compromising in some situations with mitochondrial damage leading to mitochondrial swelling. The most often used marker for mitochondrial content is the measurement of citrate synthase (CS) activity, a mitochondrial enzyme present in the Krebs cycle. However, also maximal activities of other mitochondrial enzymes (e.g., complex IV) have been used. The maximal activity of CS is assumed to be stable is most situations. However, some acute changes have been described with exercise and an endotoxin challenge [12, 13].

Mitochondrial DNA (mtDNA) content, cardiolipin levels, or complex IV activity are commenly used markers. The reliability of these markers has recently been assessed in comparison with the TEM imaging [11]. Results showed that CS activity and cardiolipin are reliable markers for mitochondrial content. mtDNA content showed not to be a good marker. This latter observation could be explained by the fact that the number of mtDNA copy per mitochondria is variable.

4.3.2 Mitochondrial Function Measurements

4.3.2.1 In Vitro Approach

Mitochondrial Enzyme Activities or Expression

Spectrophotometric-based enzymes assays have been develop to measure the activity of each respiratory complex and other mitochondrial-located enzymes. The details for these measurements will be not described here, but one of the main advantages of these assessments is that they do not require large amounts of biological material, so they can be realized in tissue crude homogenates. A major disadvantage of this method is that maximal activities are measured, which represents more the total amount of the enzyme than actual in vivo activity. These enzymatic activities are often related to the mitochondrial content via the normalization by, for instance, CS activity. In addition Western blot analyses can be used to assess the total amount of the complexes and other mitochondrial enzymes.

Mitochondrial Respiration Rates

The reduction of the oxygen by complex IV is the last step before the synthesis of the ATP by the mitochondria. By measuring the consumption of oxygen in mitochondria ex vivo, the respiration rate can be assessed, which gives an idea of mitochondria function. Respiration is measured during the addition of specific substrates and inhibitors giving rates for the different complexes or the whole process. State 1 respiration is the basal O_2 consumption in absence of any substrates. State 2 respiration is measured in the presence of substrates and specific inhibitors but in the absence of ADP, reflecting the basal proton conductance. State 3 is obtained by the addition of ADP, giving the maximal respiration rate. State 4 is observed when all ADP has been completely consumed to form ATP. An increase in state 4 respiration is related to uncoupling of the respiration from ADP phosphorylation due to proton leak and most likely ROS formation. Detailed protocols for respiration measurements have been published [14–16].

Mitochondrial 0_2 consumption can be assessed by different systems; amperometric measurement based on a Clark electrode has initially been the method of choice. Amperometric measurements are assessing respiration at supramaximal ADP levels, thereby measuring maximal respiration rates which most likely are different from what happens in vivo. Initially measurements were done using isolated mitochondria. Isolated mitochondria are the simplest model to study mitochondrial respiration. However, mitochondria are integrated in a network and also work as an organized network with other organelles like the endoplasmic reticulum. This level of regulation is lost when studying isolated mitochondria. Furthermore, the isolating procedures are based on differential centrifugation, which will lead to the selection of a subpopulation of mitochondria and most likely over representing intact and healthier mitochondria [17]. To circumvent this problem, permeabilized cell models have been developed. The permeabilization process is used to allow the substrates to pass the plasma membrane. In this model, even if the cytoplasmic components are lost, the network of the mitochondria and the other organelles is maintained. Another advantage of this model is that all the mitochondria are studied and not a subpopulation like with the isolated mitochondria [18].

In the respiration measurements, temperature and agitation are critical factors. These should be kept constant to avoid any methodological bias, like a suboptimal enzyme activity or the presence of an oxygen gradient. The initially available equipment, like the Clark chamber, require a high amount of biological material and only allow short analyses time, due to the rapid decline in oxygen in the chamber. Therefore, high-resolution respirometry apparatus have been developed. With these new systems, a minimal amount of biological material is needed, and the time of analysis is longer, allowing for better assessment of mitochondrial respiration.

Recently fluorometric modules have been added to the high-resolution respirometers to monitor ROS production. Mitochondria produce ROS in the form of superoxide anions. These are unstable and are almost immediately converted into hydrogen peroxide (H_2O_2). H_2O_2 is stable and can be detected by fluorescent probes and measured in the respiration chamber of the high-resolution respirometers. The advantage of this method is possibility to measure mitochondrial respiration and ROS production at the same time in the same mitochondria or cells [19].

The development of specific oxygen-sensing fluorescent probes (XF flux analyzer or Luxcel MitoXpress) introduced the possibility to measure respiration in vivo in intact cells. However, this method is mainly dedicated to cultured cells and has not yet been used to study mitochondrial respiration in critical illness experiments.

ATP Measurement

The main function of mitochondria is the production of energy via the synthesis of ATP. ATP concentrations or production can be measured to see the energetic state of the cells/tissue.

ATP concentrations in tissues samples can be measured by enzymatic or chromatographic methods. However, except for skeletal muscle, the ATP pool is very unstable, and if no care is taken for immediate freezing, unreliable concentrations can be obtained [20]. In addition, measurement of ATP levels can disguise whether this is the result of a reduction in the total pool of energy-rich phosphates or an actual change in energy charge. To be able to distinguish between these, ATP levels should ideally be measured in relation to ADP and AMP levels [21].

ATP synthesis can be assessed by luminometry via a firefly luciferase enzymatic reaction. Photons released by the enzyme due to the degradation of ATP can be measured and calculated to assess ATP production rates [22]. This method allows the measurement of ATP production rate in fresh tissue ex vivo. As for the respirometry assessments, ATP production is measured by the addition of specific substrates and inhibitors in the presence of an excess of ADP. ATP produce via complex I (glutamate and malate) and complex II (succinate and rotenone) and from fatty acid via the beta-oxidation (palmitoylcarnitine and malate) can be measured at state 3.

4.3.2.2 In Vivo Approach

Near-infrared spectroscopy (NIRS) can measure the tissue oxygenation levels in vivo by measuring the optical absorption of the oxy-heme and deoxy-heme groups. This method allows for the continuous measurement of oxygenation of a tissue. Oxygenation level is the result of a balance between the use (oxygen consumption) and the supply (oxygen delivery) of oxygen. By applying local ischemia, which blocks the oxygen supply, oxygen consumption can be calculated, reflecting respiration [23].

Phosphorous magnetic resonance spectroscopy (31P-MRS) is a noninvasive technique to estimate tissue ATP and phosphocreatine (PCr) levels. The maximal ATP synthesis rate is calculated from the PCr recovery rate following depletion by an intense bout of exercise. But this method is only valid for the exploration of skeletal muscle. Coupling of the mitochondria can be measured by combining both the 31P-MRS and the NIRS to assess the P/O ratio representing the ATP produced per atom of oxygen reduced by the respiratory chain.

These methods are not easily applicable to a clinical setting especially for the measurement of ATP synthesis in critically ill patients and have therefore not been used in these situations.

4.4 Mitochondrial Adaptations During Critical Illness and Stress

Critical illness is one of the most severe forms of stress on the human body, with huge surges of stress hormones and inflammatory mediators being released into the circulation. Severe sepsis and septic shock remain the leading causes of morbidity, mortality, and costly ICU care, and as such a lot of resources have been put in to understanding its pathophysiology in the last decades. The septic condition is associated with metabolic disturbances, and mitochondrial dysfunction/depletion has been a subject for scientific interest as it has been hypothesized to play a major role in the organ dysfunction seen in severe forms of septic illness.

4.4.1 Animal Models

Despite large efforts, causality between organ failure and mitochondrial dysfunction has been difficult to show, and data from animal experiments shows great inconsistency. Most animal studies have been performed on rodents with insults ranging from 3 h to a few days, but also porcine models with insults up to 14 days have been used. Other than different time spans, various organs have been analyzed using different methods. These differences in term of methodologies, experimental model, and kinetics have resulted in great variation and discussion about the role of mitochondrial disturbance in sepsis. Animal studies are difficult to interpret because of the heterogeneity in the pathophysiology of the condition. Sepsis requires aggressive resuscitation, and whether or not the septic animals receive this will affect the outcome as well as the treatment given to the control animals. Two recent reviews conclude that the tendency points towards an acute initial increase followed by a decrease in function and content of mitochondria. However, altogether the data from the animal experiments are difficult to translate to what actually happens in various organs of the severely septic patient during an ICU stay [24, 25]. In addition, the main question whether mitochondrial dysfunction is related to or causing organ failure can only be studied in models with ongoing organ failure that are kept alive in a dedicated animal ICU, as is the situation for critically ill patients with multiple organ failure. Very few long-term animal studies including ICU treatment are available.

4.4.2 Clinical Studies

The studies performed on actual critically ill patients are fewer in numbers and are also stained by methodological difficulties, and the number of studies examining mitochondrial content and/or function from solid organs are even smaller. A summary of the human studies with the patients included, the methods used, and the main findings can be found in Table 4.1.

In 2002 Brealey et al. [26] demonstrated a decrease in ATP concentration and complex I activity (as a ratio of CS activity) in leg skeletal muscle for non-survivors of septic shock as compared to survivors and controls undergoing elective surgery. In contrast, we, in general, observe that mitochondrial content (CS activity) is lower in the skeletal muscle (both serratus anterior and vastus lateralis) of ICU patients with sepsis-induced organ failure, but that the activities of the complexes expressed per CS are not affected [27–29]. However, our samples were taken at different days of ICU treatment, whereas Brealey's patients were being studied during the first 24 h. When we combined the results from our studies, it becomes clear that mitochondrial content is lower in the skeletal muscle of critically ill patients with organ failure and that it decreases with prolonged ICU stay (Fig. 4.2). This decreased content is however not due to decreased synthesis rates of mitochondrial protein or an overall downregulation of signaling (mRNA expression of PGC-1α, NRF1, NRF2, and TFAM) for mitochondrial biogenesis [29]. On the other hand, it seems that an early activation of mitochondrial biogenesis signaling is associated with better outcome in critically ill patients [30]. In mixed ICU patients, markers for biogenesis in skeletal muscle showed no difference from surgical controls even though postmortem biopsies showed increased levels in liver tissue [31].

Since sepsis is an acute condition that presents itself clinically in a heterogeneous manner, it is difficult to say what phase of the condition a sample represents. In an attempt to standardize timing and examine the immediate response in a model of sepsis, Fredriksson et al. gave healthy volunteers a standardized injection of endotoxin. After 2 h CS and complex I activity had increased significantly, and a tendency toward an increase remained after 4 h, as compared to the muscle biopsies taken before the endotoxin challenge [12]. This would rather indicate an initial upregulation of mitochondrial activity in the very early phases of sepsis, which may be consistent with the observations on mitochondrial biogenesis in critically ill patients [30] and data from animal studies [32]. In a similar manner a 3-h continuous infusion of adrenaline increases mitochondrial ex vivo state 3 respiration by 30 % in the skeletal muscle [33]. The respiratory function is arguably a more complete measurement of mitochondrial function than enzyme activity, and even though not exactly a septic model, the stress response to adrenaline in some way mimics the hyperdynamic early phase of severe sepsis which is also characterized by a surge of catecholamines and pro-inflammatory mediators.

Due to the invasiveness of biopsies, difficulties of controlling time from onset, and individual treatment, several groups have incubated isolated mitochondria and various tissues with plasma or serum from septic patients as well as triggers of

Table 4.1 Summary of literature on mitochondrial changes due to sepsis and critical illness in humans

Author	Patients studied	Controls	Organ	Method/measurements	Main finding
Brealey et al. (2002)	Twenty-eight septic patients within 24 h of ICU admission	Nine patients undergoing elective hip surgery	Skeletal muscle (*vastus lateralis*)	Complex I–IV activity, intracellular ATP, glutathione, and nitrite/nitrate concentration	Non-surviving patients had lower ATP conc and complex I activity but higher complex IV activity than survivors and controls
Fredriksson et al. (2006)	Ten septic patients within 24 h of ICU admission	Ten age- and sex-matched controls undergoing elective surgery	Skeletal muscle (*vastus lateralis* and *serratus anterior*)	Complex I and IV and CS activity. ATP concentration. Morphological examination	VL: 30 % lower comp IV. Comp I and CS no difference. ATP lower SA: CS and Comp I lower but Comp IV and ATP similar
Fredriksson et al. (2008)	Seventeen severely septic ICU patients	Ten patients undergoing elective surgery	Skeletal muscle (*vastus lateralis*)	In vivo protein synthesis rate. Activity of CS and comp I and IV. mRNA	Comp I and IV decreased, but not when corrected for CS (which also decreased). Mitochondrial synthesis rate were the same
Carre et al. (2010)	Sixteen severely septic patients within 48 h of ICU admission	Ten patients undergoing elective hip surgery	Skeletal muscle (*vastus lateralis*)	Activity of CS comp I and IV. Real-time PCR for RNA. Morphology. Transcription factors. ATP conc	ATP higher in survivors to ns. Morphological differences. No complex activity differences when corrected for CS. Mitochondrial biogenesis factors correlated to survival
Sjövall et al. (2010)	Eighteen severely septic patients within 48 h of ICU admission	Eighteen healthy blood donors	Platelets and plasma at various time points throughout the first week	Respiration of intact cells. Mitochondrial DNA	Respiration increased throughout the first week of sepsis and was increased compared to controls. Content did not change
Sjövall et al. (2013)	Twenty severely septic patients within 48 h of ICU admission	Thirty-one healthy volunteers	Peripheral blood immune cells (PBIM) at various time points throughout the first week	Respiration of intact and permeabilized cells. Mitochondrial DNA and CS activity	Respiration of whole and permeabilized cells increased throughout the first week of sepsis and mitochondrial content and CS activity increased compared to controls

Belikova et al. (2007)	Eighteen severely septic patients within 48 h of ICU admission	Thirtytwo healthy volunteers	Peripheral blood mononuclear cells (PBMC) and plasma	Ex vivo respiration of PBMC with and without stimulation of ADP Ex vivo respiration after incubation in plasma	Septic PBMC had higher oxygen consumption but lower after stimulation with ADP. Healthy PBMC:s showed a similar pattern after incubation with septic or healthy serum
Japiassu et al. (2011)	Twenty severely septic patients within 48 h of ICU admission	Eighteen postoperative patients	Peripheral Blood Mononuclear Cells (PBMC)	*Ex vivo* respiration of permeabilized PBMC	State 3 respiration lower in septic cells, and reduction was correlated with severity of disease
Garrabou et al. (2012)	Nineteen septic ICU patients	Twenty healthy volunteers (blood) Five patients undergoing elective hip surgery (muscle)	Peripheral blood mononuclear celles (PBMC), plasma and muscle for incubation	Comp I, III, and IV and CS act and oxygen cons. of PBMC. Respiration of healthy muscle mitochondria after incubation with septic or control plasma	Oxygen consumption and complex activities were lower in septic PBMC. Septic plasma showed tendency to decrease respiration in incubated muscle mitochondria
Boulos et al. (2003)	Ten septic critically ill	Seven critically ill non-septic Ten normal control subjects	Umbilical endothelial cells incubated with serum from septic patients	Mitochondrial respiration after incubation with septic or control serum	Septic serum decreased mitochondrial respiration as compared to controls
Vanhorebeek et al. (2012)	Thirty-six postmortem surgical ICU patients Twenty-four medical ICU patients	Eighteen patients undergoing surgery (liver /rect abd) Five healthy controls (*vastus lateralis*)	Post mortem: Liver and skeletal muscle (*rectus abdominis* and *vastus lateralis*) ICU: *vastus lateralis*	Analysis for proteins biogenesis, fusion, and fission of mitochondria	Mitochondrial biogenesis and fusion/fision markers are upregulated in post mortem liver and *rectus abdominis*, but not *vastis lateralis*

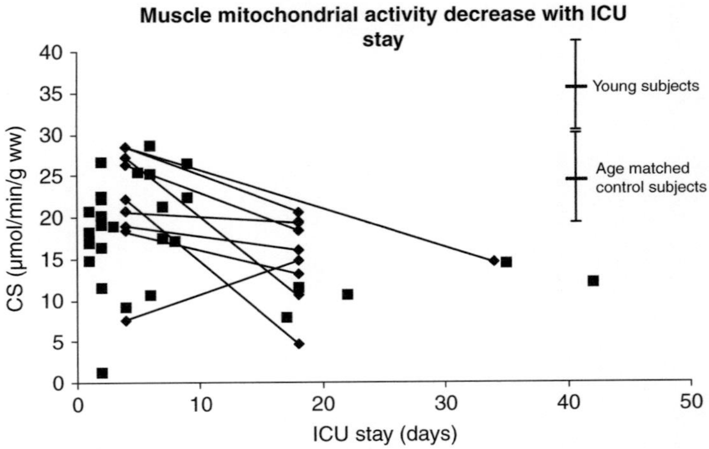

Fig. 4.2 A compilation of citrate synthase (CS) activity measurements in skeletal muscle of critically ill patients treated in the ICU and young and age-matched older healthy controls from different studies analyzed in the same laboratory around the same time and adapted from previous publications [27–29, 51]. CS activities for the critically ill patients are given as individual data in relation to the day of ICU stay, and results from patients that were measured twice are connected with a line. For comparison, mean and 2SD are given for young healthy volunteers (26 ± 3 year; $n = 7$) and to the ICU patient aged-matched health volunteers (65 ± 12 year; $n = 20$)

inflammatory responses to see if a factor can directly influence the mitochondrial function. Isolated human muscle mitochondria showed a slight but nonsignificant decrease in respirational function ex vivo after 30 min incubation with septic or control plasma [34], but other similar experiments show no difference in respirational function (unpublished data). When endothelial cells are incubated with plasma for 4 h, respiration decreases more with septic than with control plasma [35].

In contrast to mitochondria of solid organs, mitochondria of blood cells are more easily accessible and therefore better examined and followed through several stages in patients with severe sepsis and septic shock. Both actual oxygen consumption and CS activity of monocytes progressively increase during the first week in septic patients [36], but monocytes from septic patients have a decreased maximal state 3 respiration ex vivo when compared to monocytes from controls [37, 38]. Platelets, like monocytes, show a temporal increase of mitochondrial respiration [39], and respiration of both platelets and monocytes from healthy volunteers exhibits these changes when exposed to septic plasma [38, 40]. However during a stress insult, immune cells leave the circulation to the place of insult, and the population of cells left in the circulation might not represent the ones that have left. In addition, mitochondria-containing blood cells are very specialized and different in their mitochondrial adaptations [41], and their mitochondrial function in sepsis may not reflect that of muscle or visceral organs [42].

4.5 Mitochondrial Adaptations During Hibernation

Defining hibernation is not easy, and biologists have endless discussion about this. However most agree that it involves periods of depressed metabolic rate and lower body temperatures during several days in the winter season [43]. Shorter and often milder drops in metabolic rate and body temperature, also during the summer period, are called torpor. Metabolic rates drop to about 5–30 % of normal [44]. In larger mammals real hibernation with large drops in body temperature does not occur. For instance, "hibernating" bears decrease their metabolic rate with about 75 % but decrease body temperature only to about 30 °C [43]. Hibernation realizes survival in period with harsh climate and limited food access. In addition to hibernation, other adaptive strategies to survive more stress-related situations, like hypoxia, exist. This is often referred to as metabolic dormancy rather than hibernation [45].

The drop in metabolic rate with hibernation is often preceding a reduction in body temperature, if present. This reduction in metabolic rate is regulated by inhibition of mitochondrial respiration [46]. In the animals that decrease their body temperature, the reduction in mitochondrial respiration, which produces the majority of the body heat, is a logic adjustment. The decreased production of ATP is accompanied by a decreased demand and usage of ATP (e.g., heat production and general transcription and translation), together leading to an adaptive hypometabolic state [47]. Strangely, not many studies have addressed mitochondrial function in hibernating animals. However, the ones that have, in general, show a decreased mitochondrial respiration. For example, in the hibernation squirrel, mitochondrial respiration measured as a decreased state 3 respiration seems to be decreased in the liver, skeletal muscle, and heart muscle but not in the brain [43]. It appears that the main inhibition takes place in complexes III, IV, and V since respiration using succinate as a substrate via complex II is affected to a lesser extent. Although some species show changes in the Krebs cycle enzymes, no clear picture on the effect of hibernation exists nowadays [46].

Most striking is that the changes in mitochondrial respiration in most animals during the start of hibernating or torpor are very fast. During the recovery or arousal periods, the mitochondrial adaptations change back slower but still rather fast. This is also apparent when considering that many hibernating animals have frequent arousal periods with fast recovery of the body temperature and metabolic rates. How these fast changes are regulated is not clear, but the complexes of the electron chain reaction can theoretically be modified by phosphorylation or acetylation. However, no studies seem to be available studying whether these posttranslational modifications are involved in the decreased mitochondria activity during hibernation [43]. Interestingly, a recent study shows that hibernating squirrels have increased expression of PGC-1α, NRF1, and NRF2 in skeletal muscle [48], indicating that the adaptations are on the respiration regulation and do not affect mitochondrial biogenesis and most likely mitochondrial content.

Another change in mitochondria during hibernation is that in several animals, the main substrate for mitochondrial respiration changes from glucose to fatty acids. This results in a respiratory quotient (RQ) of close to 0.7 showing that mainly fatty acids are oxidized. Also direct measurements of glycolytic fluxes show that less glucose is oxidized. This seems to be the result of changes in mRNA and protein levels of several key enzymes including an increase in pyruvate dehydrogenase kinase, directly inhibiting the glycolysis [49]. With this change in substrates, animals can keep metabolism going at a low rate using the body fat reserves.

4.6 Mitochondrial Hibernation During Critical Illness?

As mentioned in the introduction, about a decade ago mitochondrial changes were suggested as a state of hibernation in which the failing organs are reducing their mitochondrial function as a survival strategy [1]. The studies described above shown decreased mitochondrial respiration during both hibernation and organ failure. Also the maintenance of, at least the signal for, mitochondrial biogenesis seems to be present in both situations. Another common characteristic is that in both situations, the recovery of mitochondrial function is relatively fast, or at least faster than can be explained by total new synthesis of mitochondria alone. However, there are also major differences. During hibernation, there are clear decreases in metabolic rates, which are not very common during critical illness, at least not to the levels seen during hibernation. The most striking difference in our view is the fact that patients with organ failure need pharmaceutical or technical support of the failing organs in an ICU to survive. This latter fact speaks against a protective strategy.

Still the hypothesis, or theory, of hibernation during organ failure is intriguing, but the scientific proof for this is weak and largely hypothetical. Maybe the term hibernation is too strong, and we should see this more as a stunning phenomenon as in cardiac failure, a reversible injury with a similar phenotype as hibernation but not protective [50], or metabolic dormancy [45], a strategy to survive metabolic stress by reducing energy production and demands without reducing body temperature.

Mitochondrial hibernation or dormancy will most likely happen in failing organs of some critically ill patients, but the remaining question is whether this is exposing itself as a consequence of mitochondrial damage or an adaptation where cells are intentionally reducing metabolic demands in order to survive. It might also be a strategy that only works in a few and goes over the top and becomes detrimental in other patients. At least, in the acute response to critical illness and stress, an increase in mitochondrial function seems to be favorable for patient's outcome/survival. In the long-term adaptation, we do not know if dormancy/hibernation is a successful adaptation for the survival of patients. As usual, more research is needed before we can even come close to answer these questions. Future clinical studies should discriminate the critically ill survivors from the non-survivors in order to gain knowledge about the mitochondrial adaptation leading to the survival of these patients.

References

1. Brealey D, Singer M (2003) Mitochondrial dysfunction in sepsis. Curr Infect Dis Rep 5(5):365–371
2. Detmer SA, Chan DC (2007) Functions and dysfunctions of mitochondrial dynamics. Nat Rev Mol Cell Biol 8(11):870–879
3. Detmer SA, Chan DC (2007) Complementation between mouse Mfn1 and Mfn2 protects mitochondrial fusion defects caused by CMT2A disease mutations. J Cell Biol 176(4): 405–414
4. Chan DC (2006) Mitochondria: dynamic organelles in disease, aging, and development. Cell 125(7):1241–1252
5. Lemasters JJ, Nieminen AL, Qian T, Trost LC, Elmore SP, Nishimura Y et al (1998) The mitochondrial permeability transition in cell death: a common mechanism in necrosis, apoptosis and autophagy. Biochim Biophys Acta 1366(1–2):177–196
6. Youle RJ, Strasser A (2008) The BCL-2 protein family: opposing activities that mediate cell death. Nat Rev Mol Cell Biol 9(1):47–59
7. Cheng EH, Wei MC, Weiler S, Flavell RA, Mak TW, Lindsten T et al (2001) BCL-2, BCL-X(L) sequester BH3 domain-only molecules preventing BAX- and BAK-mediated mitochondrial apoptosis. Mol Cell 8(3):705–711
8. Kluck RM, Bossy-Wetzel E, Green DR, Newmeyer DD (1997) The release of cytochrome c from mitochondria: a primary site for Bcl-2 regulation of apoptosis. Science 275(5303): 1132–1136
9. Yang J, Liu X, Bhalla K, Kim CN, Ibrado AM, Cai J et al (1997) Prevention of apoptosis by Bcl-2: release of cytochrome c from mitochondria blocked. Science 275(5303):1129–1132
10. Wang X, Yang C, Chai J, Shi Y, Xue D (2002) Mechanisms of AIF-mediated apoptotic DNA degradation in Caenorhabditis elegans. Science 298(5598):1587–1592
11. Larsen S, Nielsen J, Hansen CN, Nielsen LB, Wibrand F, Stride N et al (2012) Biomarkers of mitochondrial content in skeletal muscle of healthy young human subjects. J Physiol 590(Pt 14):3349–3360
12. Fredriksson K, Flaring U, Guillet C, Wernerman J, Rooyackers O (2009) Muscle mitochondrial activity increases rapidly after an endotoxin challenge in human volunteers. Acta Anaesthesiol Scand 53(3):299–304
13. Tonkonogi M, Harris B, Sahlin K (1997) Increased activity of citrate synthase in human skeletal muscle after a single bout of prolonged exercise. Acta Physiol Scand 161(3):435–436
14. Kuznetsov AV, Veksler V, Gellerich FN, Saks V, Margreiter R, Kunz WS (2008) Analysis of mitochondrial function in situ in permeabilized muscle fibers, tissues and cells. Nat Protoc 3(6):965–976
15. Pesta D, Gnaiger E (2012) High-resolution respirometry: OXPHOS protocols for human cells and permeabilized fibers from small biopsies of human muscle. Methods Mol Biol 810: 25–58
16. Spinazzi M, Casarin A, Pertegato V, Salviati L, Angelini C (2012) Assessment of mitochondrial respiratory chain enzymatic activities on tissues and cultured cells. Nat Protoc 7(6): 1235–1246
17. Picard M, Taivassalo T, Gouspillou G, Hepple RT (2011) Mitochondria: isolation, structure and function. J Physiol 589(Pt 18):4413–4421
18. Picard M, Taivassalo T, Ritchie D, Wright KJ, Thomas MM, Romestaing C et al (2011) Mitochondrial structure and function are disrupted by standard isolation methods. PLoS One 6(3):e18317
19. Makrecka-Kuka M, Krumschnabel G, Gnaiger E (2015) High-resolution respirometry for simultaneous measurement of oxygen and hydrogen peroxide fluxes in permeabilized cells, tissue homogenate and isolated mitochondria. Biomolecules 5(3):1319–1338
20. Soderlund K, Hultman E (1986) Effects of delayed freezing on content of phosphagens in human skeletal muscle biopsy samples. J Appl Physiol 61(3):832–835

21. Rooyackers OE, Hesselink MKC, Wagenmakers AJM (1994) Impaired energy metabolism in muscle of zymosan treated rats recovering from critical illness. Clin Nutr 13(Suppl 1):6
22. Lanza IR, Nair KS (2009) Functional assessment of isolated mitochondria in vitro. Methods Enzymol 457:349–372
23. Hamaoka T, Iwane H, Shimomitsu T, Katsumura T, Murase N, Nishio S et al (1996) Noninvasive measures of oxidative metabolism on working human muscles by near-infrared spectroscopy. J Appl Physiol 81(3):1410–1417
24. Jeger V, Djafarzadeh S, Jakob SM, Takala J (2013) Mitochondrial function in sepsis. Eur J Clin Invest 43(5):532–42
25. Singer M (2014) The role of mitochondrial dysfunction in sepsis-induced multi-organ failure. Virulence 5(1):66–72
26. Brealey D, Brand M, Hargreaves I, Heales S, Land J, Smolenski R et al (2002) Association between mitochondrial dysfunction and severity and outcome of septic shock. Lancet 360(9328):219–223
27. Ahlbeck K, Fredriksson K, Rooyackers O, Maback G, Remahl S, Ansved T et al (2009) Signs of critical illness polyneuropathy and myopathy can be seen early in the ICU course. Acta Anaesthesiol Scand 53(6):717–723
28. Fredriksson K, Hammarqvist F, Strigard K, Hultenby K, Ljungqvist O, Wernerman J et al (2006) Derangements in mitochondrial metabolism in intercostal and leg muscle of critically ill patients with sepsis-induced multiple organ failure. Am J Physiol Endocrinol Metab 291(5):E1044–E1050
29. Fredriksson K, Tjader I, Keller P, Petrovic N, Ahlman B, Scheele C et al (2008) Dysregulation of mitochondrial dynamics and the muscle transcriptome in ICU patients suffering from sepsis induced multiple organ failure. PLoS One 3(11):e3686
30. Carre JE, Orban JC, Re L, Felsmann K, Iffert W, Bauer M et al (2010) Survival in critical illness is associated with early activation of mitochondrial biogenesis. Am J Respir Crit Care Med 182(6):745–751
31. Vanhorebeek I, Gunst J, Derde S, Derese I, Boussemaere M, D'Hoore A et al (2012) Mitochondrial fusion, fission, and biogenesis in prolonged critically ill patients. J Clin Endocrinol Metab 97(1):E59–E64
32. Singer M (2007) Mitochondrial function in sepsis: acute phase versus multiple organ failure. Crit Care Med 35(9 Suppl):S441–S448
33. Grip J, Jakobsson T, Hebert C, Klaude M, Sandstrom G, Wernerman J et al (2015) Lactate kinetics and mitochondrial respiration in skeletal muscle of healthy humans under influence of adrenaline. Clin Sci 129(4):375–384
34. Garrabou G, Moren C, Lopez S, Tobias E, Cardellach F, Miro O et al (2012) The effects of sepsis on mitochondria. J Infect Dis 205(3):392–400
35. Boulos M, Astiz ME, Barua RS, Osman M (2003) Impaired mitochondrial function induced by serum from septic shock patients is attenuated by inhibition of nitric oxide synthase and poly(ADP-ribose) synthase. Crit Care Med 31(2):353–358
36. Sjovall F, Morota S, Persson J, Hansson MJ, Elmer E (2013) Patients with sepsis exhibit increased mitochondrial respiratory capacity in peripheral blood immune cells. Crit Care 17(4):R152
37. Japiassu AM, Santiago AP, d'Avila JC, Garcia-Souza LF, Galina A, Castro Faria-Neto HC et al (2011) Bioenergetic failure of human peripheral blood monocytes in patients with septic shock is mediated by reduced F1Fo adenosine-5'-triphosphate synthase activity. Crit Care Med 39(5):1056–1063
38. Belikova I, Lukaszewicz AC, Faivre V, Damoisel C, Singer M, Payen D (2007) Oxygen consumption of human peripheral blood mononuclear cells in severe human sepsis. Crit Care Med 35(12):2702–2708
39. Sjovall F, Hansson MJ, Elmer E (2012) Platelet mitochondrial function in sepsis. Crit Care Med 40(1):357; author reply –8

40. Sjovall F, Morota S, Hansson MJ, Friberg H, Gnaiger E, Elmer E (2010) Temporal increase of platelet mitochondrial respiration is negatively associated with clinical outcome in patients with sepsis. Crit Care 14(6):R214
41. Kramer PA, Ravi S, Chacko B, Johnson MS, Darley-Usmar VM (2014) A review of the mitochondrial and glycolytic metabolism in human platelets and leukocytes: implications for their use as bioenergetic biomarkers. Redox Biol 2:206–210
42. Protti A, Fortunato F, Caspani ML, Pluderi M, Lucchini V, Grimoldi N et al (2014) Mitochondrial changes in platelets are not related to those in skeletal muscle during human septic shock. PLoS One 9(5):e96205
43. Staples JF (2014) Metabolic suppression in mammalian hibernation: the role of mitochondria. J Exp Biol 217(Pt 12):2032–2036
44. Geiser F (2004) Metabolic rate and body temperature reduction during hibernation and daily torpor. Annu Rev Physiol 66:239–274
45. Van Breukelen F, Martin SL (2002) Invited review: molecular adaptations in mammalian hibernators: unique adaptations or generalized responses? J Appl Physiol 92(6):2640–2647
46. Staples JF, Brown JC (2008) Mitochondrial metabolism in hibernation and daily torpor: a review. J Comp Physiol B Biochem Syst Environ Physiol 178(7):811–827
47. Storey KB (2010) Out cold: biochemical regulation of mammalian hibernation – a mini-review. Gerontology 56(2):220–230
48. Xu R, Andres-Mateos E, Mejias R, MacDonald EM, Leinwand LA, Merriman DK et al (2013) Hibernating squirrel muscle activates the endurance exercise pathway despite prolonged immobilization. Exp Neurol 247:392–401
49. Carey HV, Andrews MT, Martin SL (2003) Mammalian hibernation: cellular and molecular responses to depressed metabolism and low temperature. Physiol Rev 83(4):1153–1181
50. Heusch G, Boengler K, Schulz R (2008) Cardioprotection: nitric oxide, protein kinases, and mitochondria. Circulation 118(19):1915–1919
51. Tonkonogi M, Fernstrom M, Walsh B, Ji LL, Rooyackers O, Hammarqvist F et al (2003) Reduced oxidative power but unchanged antioxidative capacity in skeletal muscle from aged humans. Pflugers Archiv Eur J Physiol 446(2):261–269

Chapter 5
Anabolic Resistance

Jean-Paul Thissen

Abstract Muscle atrophy is the hallmark of several catabolic conditions. Whatever the cause, the skeletal muscle loss is associated with comorbidities and poor survival. The mass of the skeletal muscle is maintained normally by equilibrium between protein synthesis and breakdown. Rate of synthesis in particular is positively regulated by nutrition and exercise. Anabolic resistance can be defined as a situation where the skeletal muscle is unable to respond appropriately to these anabolic stimuli by stimulating protein synthesis. Anabolic resistance contributes to muscle mass loss in elderly, during immobilization as well as in response to inflammation and cancer. The mechanisms responsible for this blunted response to anabolic stimuli are still under investigation. Several strategies may serve to compensate for anabolic resistance. Optimization of protein intake, resistance exercise, and anti-inflammatory agents appear promising to override this anabolic resistance and mitigate its consequence, the skeletal muscle mass loss.

5.1 Background

Muscle atrophy is the hallmark of several catabolic conditions. Whatever the cause, the skeletal muscle loss is associated with comorbidities and poor survival [1].

Muscle proteins are in dynamic equilibrium between their respective rates of synthesis and breakdown. A net gain of muscle mass is only possible if muscle protein synthesis [MPS] exceeds muscle protein breakdown [MPB]. Rate of MPS is positively regulated by nutrient availability and physical activity and negatively regulated by disuse, aging, and muscle wasting-related diseases [2].

J.-P. Thissen, MD, PhD
Pôle Endocrinologie, Diabétologie et Nutrition,
Institut de Recherches Expérimentales et Cliniques,
Université Catholique de Louvain,
Avenue Hippocrate 55 bte B1.55.06,
Bruxelles B-1200, Belgium
e-mail: jeanpaul.thissen@uclouvain.be

J.-C. Preiser (ed.), *The Stress Response of Critical Illness: Metabolic and Hormonal Aspects*, DOI 10.1007/978-3-319-27687-8_5

The mass of the skeletal muscle is maintained normally by ingestion of *protein-containing meals*, which results in systemic hyperaminoacidemia. With feeding, MPS is stimulated, and, to a lesser extent, MPB is decreased, causing the protein balance to become positive. During the postprandial period, the balance of muscle protein becomes negative, due to decreased MPS and increased MPB. Therefore, postprandial stimulation of MPS is an important factor in muscle mass maintenance [3].

The stimulation of MPS by protein intake is *transient and dose dependent*. Indeed, increase in MPS after feeding is of finite duration despite enduring substrate availability. MPS increases after an oral protein bolus with a peak at 2 h before returning to baseline levels, despite elevated plasma amino acid (AA) concentrations [4]. Thus, the muscle becomes refractory to persistent elevations of circulating AA concentrations ("muscle full" concept). The relationship between the dose of protein intake and its resulting stimulation of MPS is also well described. With increasing the dose of protein, MPS increases fast to reach a plateau at approximately 20 g of high-quality protein, with higher-protein intake stimulating AA oxidation rather than MPS. In contrast, MPB decreases slightly but continuously with increasing protein intake. Therefore, protein intake higher than known to stimulate MPS maximally might lead to a greater anabolic response via suppression of MPB [5, 6].

While most AAs are contained in proteins, it appears only to be the essential or indispensable AAs (EAAs), which represent 40–50 % of the total AAs of a high-quality protein, that stimulate MPS. Of the EAAs, the branched chain AAs (BCAAs) are primarily responsible for stimulating MPS [7]. In this regard, *leucine* is important as it comprises about one-fifth of EAAs needs, and apart from serving as a substrate, it directly activates the signaling pathway stimulating protein synthesis. Leucine on its own appears to stimulate MPS to nearly the same level as a mixture of AAs [8].

Although *insulin* is of great importance in inhibiting MPB, it plays only a permissive role in stimulating MPS [9]. Although the postprandial rise in circulating insulin might modulate the MPS response through its vasodilatory properties resulting in greater nutritive blood flow to muscle tissue, the basal levels of circulating insulin seem sufficient for maximally stimulating MPS in humans [10]. Systemic administration of insulin alone causes hypoaminoacidemia by inhibiting protein degradation which may in turn inhibit MPS [11]. However, when hypoaminoacidemia is prevented by exogenous AAs replacement, insulin co-administration effectively increases MPS, but this effect is due to the hyperaminoacidemia [12]. The primary effect of insulin on the skeletal muscle is therefore to decrease MPB without a significant effect on MPS [13].

Besides protein intake, *resistance exercise* is a potent stimulator of MPS and appears to synergistically enhance the gain stimulated by feeding. Even though the rate of MPB increases following exercise, the corresponding increase in MPS is three- to fivefold greater [14]. While the feeding-mediated increase in MPS lasts only few hours at most, the resistance exercise-induced MPS is sustained for about 24–48 h. The synergistic effect of resistance exercise and protein ingestion on muscle protein anabolism is well established. Indeed, the effect of protein intake on muscle protein accretion can further be stimulated by prior exercise training [15], thereby permitting muscle hypertrophy when practiced frequently over time. This effect appears to be mediated by an exercise-induced improvement in nutrient-stimulated vasodilatation and nutrient delivery to muscle rather than potentiation of insulin signaling [16]. Food combined to exercise elevates net muscle protein balance for many hours after exercise [17].

5.2 Anabolic Resistance Concept

In many situations, MPS in response to feeding or exercise is blunted. This abnormal response of the skeletal muscle to previously well-established anabolic stimuli is known as anabolic resistance [18, 19]. In these situations, the MPS is refractory to EAA provision, irrespective of the availability of insulin. Therefore, anabolic resistance can be defined as a situation where the skeletal muscle is unable to respond appropriately to anabolic stimuli by stimulating protein synthesis and less importantly by inhibiting proteolysis. Indeed, MPB has a minor role in the protein anabolic response to EAAs [20]. The mechanisms responsible for this blunted response of MPS to anabolic stimuli are still under investigation. However, it is highly probable that alterations in protein digestion, AA absorption, hormonal response, microvascular blood flow, AA uptake into the muscle, and intramuscular signaling may play a role.

5.3 Methodological Considerations

Although the skeletal muscle accounts for 40 % of the body weight and constitutes between 50 and 75 % of all proteins, it represents only 30 % of whole-body protein synthesis. Furthermore, muscle proteins turn over at a rate that is significantly less [about 20-fold] than splanchnic or plasma proteins. Therefore, whole-body protein turnover does not reflect changes which take place into the skeletal muscle [21].

In terms of mechanisms underlying atrophy, the data on rodent and human muscles are difficult to compare for several reasons. Among many, it is worth noting that most of the rodent work has been carried out with young and not adult animals. Moreover, while muscle atrophy in humans mainly involves reduced MPS, increased MPB seems the predominant feature in rodents [22, 23].

Studies focusing on acute changes in MPS cannot predict the net changes in muscle protein balance as opposite changes in MPB may damper the muscle anabolic effect expected based on changes in MPS, especially when long-term changes on the skeletal muscle mass are considered.

Finally, from a functional perspective, changes in muscle function are probably more important than changes in the skeletal muscle mass and should be the most clinically relevant end point to study. This point has not been investigated however in the context of anabolic resistance.

5.4 Clinical Situations of Anabolic Resistance

5.4.1 Aging

Skeletal muscle mass begins to decline in the fourth or fifth decade of life, at a rate of 0.5–1.5 %/year between 50 and 80 years old. The debilitating effects of muscle loss include declines in physical function and quality of life and increases in morbidity and mortality. Loss of muscle mass with aging is thus a major public health concern. The age-related muscle mass wasting is known as sarcopenia. The loss of muscle mass with aging is probably not due to chronic changes in MPS or MPB but to a blunted feeding-induced rise in MPS [24]. Indeed, muscles of the elderly are resistant to normally robust anabolic stimuli. This anabolic resistance may be a key factor in the development and progression of sarcopenia. Elderly are characterized by a resistance to the three main anabolic stimuli (exercise, AAs, and insulin). Indeed, aging reduces the anabolic response to resistance exercise [25, 26], despite equal circulating and muscle AA concentrations. Furthermore, the stimulation of the muscle anabolic signaling pathways and MPS by AA infusion is significantly blunted in elderly [27, 28]. Finally, aging is associated with reduced inhibition of proteolysis in response to insulin [29]. This anabolic resistance may result from gradual decline in physical activity or to low-grade inflammation (cf. infra).

5.4.2 Immobilization

During disuse, the skeletal muscle loss occurs at a rate of 0.5 % of muscle mass per day, which translates in 150 g of muscle tissue lost per day [30]. Prolonged disuse (more than 10 days) leads to a decline in basal and postprandial rates of MPS without apparent changes in muscle MPB, except maybe at the early stage (–5 days) [30, 31]. Protein ingestion or AA infusion, even at high rate, increased MPS less in the immobilized leg than in the control one [30, 32]. Therefore, this anabolic resistance can account for the immobilization-induced muscle atrophy. Older adults are more susceptible than young persons to muscle loss after short-term bed rest [23].

5.4.3 Inflammation

The inflammation associated with sepsis is often responsible for a state of anabolic resistance. In animal models, sepsis blunts the MPS response caused by leucine, exercise, and insulin, the three main anabolic stimuli [33, 34]. The inability of these anabolic stimuli to stimulate muscle protein synthesis during sepsis seems to be related to a defect in signaling to step in translation initiation [34, 35]. This sepsis-induced anabolic resistance in the skeletal muscle results from the cooperative interaction of both cytokines such as TNFα and glucocorticoids [36]. Anabolic resistance in aging may also be related to inflammation, as suggested by the increase in muscle NFkB activity. Indeed, low-grade inflammation as observed in old animals impairs the MPS response to feeding [37].

5.4.4 *Cancer*

Cancer cachexia, a metabolic condition caused by tumor burden, is characterized by muscle atrophy and sometimes fat loss. It is observed in 85 % of cancer patients and is implicated in 25 % of deaths. Cancer patients display reduced postprandial MPS compatible with a state of anabolic resistance. Interestingly, tumor resection is able to restore the normal postprandial MPS response [38]. However, a state of anabolic resistance does not seem to be always observed in cancer patients. Several authors showed indeed that cancer patients and controls show comparable protein anabolism during feeding or AAs ingestion, at least at high dose [39–42]. These observations suggest that a window of anabolic potential exists early on in cachexia development [43]. However, in some of these studies, protein anabolism was assessed at the whole-body level and not at the skeletal muscle level.

5.4.5 *Obesity*

The MPS in response to AAs appears to be negatively correlated to whole-body fat mass and insulin sensitivity [44]. This suggests that insulin resistance caused by lipid excess due to intracellular accumulation of lipid in muscle or to increased free fatty acid availability may lead to anabolic resistance. In animals, chronic lipid accumulation in muscles as observed in high-fat diet-induced obesity is associated with a concomitant reduction of MPS in response to feeding [45]. Muscle ectopic fat deposition may contribute to anabolic resistance through increase in muscle ceramides. Intramuscular accumulation of ceramides has been previously involved in the insulin resistance for glucose metabolism observed in obesity. Interestingly, ceramides are also able to reduce intracellular AAs availability and protein synthesis in muscle cells [46]. The MPS response to exercise is also blunted in obese animals compared to the lean ones [47]. In humans, lipid infusion to cause reduced whole-body glucose disposal impairs the MPS in response to AAs ingestion [48]. This anabolic resistance to AAs caused by lipid infusion is associated with repression of translation initiation. In obese subjects, the net protein anabolic response to insulin was also blunted compared to healthy subjects [49]. Therefore, excess lipid availability can induce insulin resistance of the skeletal muscle glucose metabolism but also anabolic resistance of AA metabolism. This is not unexpected as many conditions of anabolic resistance such as aging, disuse, and critical illness are characterized by the inability of the skeletal glucose metabolism to respond adequately to insulin.

5.4.6 Chronic Kidney Disease

In animal models, acute uremia causes a severe resistance to leucine-induced activation of the MPS [50]. Metabolic acidosis by itself impairs leucine-stimulated MPS [51]. Therefore, acidosis may account for the anabolic resistance and ultimately contribute to the muscle wasting which develops in uremia. In human subjects, besides blunting muscle glucose uptake in response to insulin, chronic renal failure and acidosis interfere with the normal suppression of MPB in response to insulin [52]. This state of insulin resistance is also observed in dialysis patients where it is associated with increased MPB [53].

5.4.7 Other Conditions of Anabolic Resistance

Normobaric hypoxia blunts the increased MPS response to acute resistance exercise [54]. This may contribute to muscle atrophy and blunt the hypertrophic response to resistance exercise in hypoxic conditions.

Glucocorticoids cause the skeletal muscle atrophy by themselves but also by contributing to muscle atrophy observed in many catabolic conditions such as cancer, diabetes, and acute inflammation [55]. Furthermore, glucocorticoids amplify the muscle atrophy caused by immobilization [56].

Most patients who are critically ill combine several causes of anabolic resistance. In addition to the procatabolic hormonal and cytokine milieu, age, immobilization, and hypoxia contribute to a blunted MPS response [18]. Poor delivery of hormones and nutrients caused by compromised microvascular blood flow may also play a role.

5.5 Cellular Mechanisms

Protein synthesis in the skeletal muscle is regulated through a number of signaling pathways that control the mRNA translation. The protein kinase mTORC1 [mechanistic target of rapamycin complex 1] plays a crucial role in this process by serving as a critical point of integration of most of the anabolic stimuli for the skeletal muscle [57]. Furthermore, blocking mTORC1 activity with the rapamycin drug blocks the contraction and the EAAs-mediated increase in MPS [58, 59].

In response to anabolic stimuli, mTORC1 targets and activates downstream kinases such as S6kinase1 (S6K1) or binding proteins like eIF4E-binding protein1

(4E-BP1). The action of mTORC1 and its downstream mediators heightens the efficiency of ribosomal biogenesis and ultimately translation. Indeed, phosphorylation of 4E-BP1 by mTORC1 prevents its association with eIF4E, allowing eIF4E to bind eIF4G to form the active mRNA cap-binding complex, eIF4F. Thus, mTORC1 stimulates mRNA joining to the 43S preinitiation complex [60].

Growth factors such as insulin and IGF-I activate mTORC1 by stimulating the PI3kinase-Akt/PKB pathway. AAs promote mTORC1 signaling independently of changes in growth factors or mechanic load. The mechanism of activation of mTORC1 by AAs, in particular leucine, involves several molecular actors, in particular a family of GTPases called Rags which act as AA sensors. The lysosomal membrane represents the site at which the AA- and growth factor-sensing machineries converge to stimulate mTORC1. Compared with the regulation of mTORC1 signaling by growth factors and AAs, much less is known about the pathway through which resistance exercise stimulates mTORC1 activity. A specific form of PGC-1α, PGC-1α4, which results from alternative promoter usage and splicing of the primary transcript PGC-1α, is preferentially induced in mouse and human muscle during resistance exercise. This isoform specifically induces IGF-I and represses myostatin [61]. Therefore, PGC1α4 may be a major player in the muscle hypertrophy induced by exercise. However, how this factor stimulates MPS activity is still unknown [62].

REDD1 has been recently identified as an inhibitor of mTORC1. Therefore, REDD1 induction by immobilization [63], glucocorticoids [55], hypoxia, or sepsis [33] may limit MPS by inhibiting mTORC1 signaling and contribute to the anabolic resistance observed in these conditions [64]. AMP-activated kinase (AMPK) functions as a fuel sensor. This enzyme plays an important role in regulating the muscle response to negative energy balance. More specifically, it inhibits mTORC1 signaling when cellular ATP levels are decreased and AMP levels increase in response to limited energy availability. Therefore, insufficient energy availability may limit MPS by inhibiting mTORC1 through activation of AMPK.

Many observations support the role of alterations in the mTOR pathway and its downstream effectors in the muscle resistance to anabolic stimuli.

In elderly, the phosphorylation of mTORC1 and its downstream targets, S6K1 and 4E-BP1, is dampened in the skeletal muscle as compared with the young in response to AAs infusion and exercise [25, 28, 65, 66]. Interestingly, this decline in MPS in response to AAs occurs in association with a reduction of AA transporter content [67].

Interestingly, immobilization which causes a decrease in the global rates of MPS has been associated with a decrease [68] as well an increase in mTOR [69] signaling. In the latter case, the mTOR activation might help to alleviate the immobilization-induced decrease in MPS and muscle mass, as blocking mTOR signaling with rapamycin exacerbates the decline in MPS and muscle mass [69]. Nevertheless, in human immobilization studies, decreases in mTOR have not been observed [10].

The inability of the major anabolic stimuli to stimulate MPS during sepsis seems to be related to a defect in signaling to step in translation initiation, with the redistribution of eIF4E from the active eIF4E.eIF4G complex to the inactive eIF4E.4E-BP1 complex [34, 70], impairing the formation of eIF4F.

Muscle ectopic fat deposition may contribute to anabolic resistance through increase in eIF2α activation [71]. The anabolic resistance to AAs caused by lipid infusion is associated with repression of translation initiation at the level of 4E-BP1 [48].

In animal models, acute uremia causes a severe resistance to leucine-induced activation of the MPS [51] and the mTOR anabolic signaling pathway [50]. Metabolic acidosis impairs leucine-stimulated MPS and activation of the signaling downstream of mTOR at the level of S6K1.

5.6 Tissular Mechanisms

5.6.1 Splanchnic Sequestration

About 95 % of the AAs are absorbed through the intestine and released into the portal vein or used by the gut, with only 50–60 % of the ingested dietary protein being released into the systemic circulation. An increase in hepatic/splanchnic uptake of AAs will reduce the amount of AAs available to stimulate the MPS and may blunt the MPS response to protein feeding [72, 73]. This mechanism may therefore contribute to anabolic resistance.

5.6.2 Microvascular Blood Flow Alterations

Nutritive blood flow is a very important determinant of the anabolic response to food. Poor delivery of nutrients at the sites of microvascular perfusion may contribute to anabolic resistance. Changes in MPS induced by insulin are correlated with changes in AA delivery and blood flow. Alterations in microvascular blood flow associated with reduced AA delivery are observed in critically ill patients, after immobilization, and in elderly. This mechanism may therefore contribute to anabolic resistance. However, although resistance exercise enhances muscle microvascular blood flow in older individuals, it does not restore muscle anabolic response to nutrition [74].

5.7 How to Override Anabolic Resistance?

5.7.1 Optimization of Protein Intake

Several nutrition-based strategies may serve to compensate for anabolic resistance. Optimization of protein intake in particular can be applied to maximize the skeletal muscle protein anabolism. The MPS in response to protein intake may be improved by controlling the amount of dietary protein, the nature of the protein, the content in specific AAs, the timing of administration, and the co-ingested macronutrients [3].

In contrast to young adults, in whom postexercise rates of MPS are saturated with 20 g of protein, elderly subjects may need as much as 35–40 g to maximally stimulate MPS [75–79]. Therefore, the elderly may require more protein to acutely increase rates of MPS than the young. This fits with the hypothesis of an increased AA threshold that must be surpassed after protein ingestion to stimulate MPS above rest in elderly [24]. It remains to be determined whether more protein is required to maximize MPS in other situations of anabolic resistance such immobilization and inflammation.

Besides the amount of protein, the nature of the protein ingested may also determine the degree of MPS. The MPS response to a specific protein depends on its digestibility and absorption as well as its AA composition. Both milk and beef ingestion augments the postexercise MPS response, with a stronger stimulation of MPS during the early postprandial stage after milk ingestion [80]. Dairy proteins seem to offer some advantage for muscle anabolism over other protein sources, in particular plant-based soy protein. The two major types of milk protein, casein and whey, markedly stimulate MPS. The more rapidly the protein is digested and absorbed, the greater the postprandial MPS is. Keeping with this, hydrolyzed casein is more potent than intact or micellar casein to stimulate MPS [81]. Whey, a fast digestible soluble protein, increases MPS even more than casein [82]. While casein is converted to a solid clot in the gastric acid environment, whey remains soluble in the stomach, allowing rapid digestion. Differences in anabolic properties of various protein sources are also attributable to differences in AA composition. The higher leucine content of whey protein versus casein may contribute to the greater anabolic properties of whey protein compared to casein. Indeed, there is a good correlation between the rise in circulating leucine concentrations and the postprandial MPS after whey and casein ingestion [83].

Supplementation with BCAAs has been shown to attenuate the loss of muscle mass caused by disuse [84–86] or aging [87]. Supplementation of a suboptimal protein intake with leucine is as effective as a complete protein intake in stimulating postprandial MPS [88]. Leucine-enriched EAAs ingestion after resistance exercise seems to prolong the anabolic response of the skeletal muscle to AAs in older adults [88]. Leucine-rich AA mixtures or proteins appear more efficient than leucine alone to improve muscle mass and performance. However, until now, there is no evidence that chronic free leucine supplementation promotes muscle mass or prevents protein loss during states of anabolic resistance [89, 90]. This may be due to desynchronization between leucine signal and the rise in all AAs, decline in other circulating BCAAs valine, and isoleucine or parallel stimulation of MPB [91].

Finally, the timing of protein intake is an important parameter to consider for optimizing the anabolic response of AAs. The ingestion of protein in the hours just after exercise enhances the MPS. It even seems that this "anabolic window" lasts for at least 24 h following exercise. To reach a near-maximal postprandial MPS response, it is advised to provide 20–25 g dietary protein every 4–5 h and a further 25–40 g protein prior to sleep [30, 92]. Repeated ingestion of 20 g of protein every

3 h during 12 h after a bout of resistance exercise is superior for stimulating MPS than two bolus of 40 g or eight pulses of 10 g [93]. Similarly, emerging evidence suggests that the elderly may need to distribute protein intake evenly throughout the day across three or more daily meals [24], as long as each meal provides enough protein to reach the anabolic threshold (at least 20 g).

It could be suggested that the stimulation of insulin secretion by CHO may enhance the MPS response to protein intake. However, ingestion of CHO with sufficient amounts of protein does not further increase MPS following exercise [94]. Indeed, circulating insulin is more permissive than stimulatory on MPS response [10].

In critically ill patients, there is a lack of data on protein requirements necessary to override the anabolic resistance [95].

5.7.2 Resistance Exercise

Exercise in general appears to depress MPS, whereas MPB is probably increased, causing negative net muscle protein balance. However, the inhibition of MPS that occurs during muscle contraction is rapidly reversed during postexercise recovery. Therefore, positive net balance may be achieved after the exercise when AA availability is increased, thereby raising MPS markedly. Postexercise-increased AA availability is less crucial than insulin for inhibiting MPB.

Resistance exercise is an important countermeasure to disuse atrophy and to age-related declines in the skeletal muscle mass. What is less well understood is how the intensity and the volume of the resistance exercise stimulus are sufficient to result in rises in MPS. Evidence suggests that minimal resistance exercise preserves MPS throughout bed rest [96]. In older adults, frequent high-intensity weight lifting or alternatively low-intensity high-volume weight lifting increases muscle mass.

The synergistic anabolic effect of resistance exercise in combination with EAAs ingestion has been well documented in particular in the elderly. It appears that protein ingestion at doses at least 20 g and perhaps as high as 30–40 g in close proximity to resistance exercise may be able to elicit an anabolic response in the elderly. Resistance training has been shown to sensitize the skeletal muscle to feeding for up to 24 h [15, 97]. Therefore, resistance exercise training combined with appropriately timed protein (likely leucine-rich) ingestion may represent a highly effective treatment strategy to counteract the sarcopenia.

Older adults are more susceptible than young persons to muscle loss after short-term bed rest. Interestingly, exercise rehabilitation has been shown to restore bed rest-induced deficit in lean mass, strength, and nutrient-induced anabolism in older subjects [23].

There are substantial evidence that resistance training increases muscle mass and strength in older adults [98] with improvement in function and performance of activities of daily living [99].

5.7.3 *Anti-inflammatory Agents*

Inflammation has been shown to blunt the anabolic effect of feeding on MPS [100]. Reduction of low-grade inflammation with NSAID restores blunting of postprandial muscle anabolism in old rats and potentiates the exercise-induced increase in muscle mass and strength in humans [101, 102]. Similarly, omega or n-3 fatty acids which exert anti-inflammatory action enhance the sensitivity of MPS to co-infusion of AAs and insulin in older adults [103]. This effect was associated with increased phosphorylation of mTORC1 and S6K1. These observations fit with the hypothesis of an increased anabolic threshold caused by inflammation and an attenuation of anabolic resistance by n-3 fatty acids. It is also possible that n-3 FA have some intrinsic muscle protein anabolic effect, as this stimulation of MPS occurs to the same extent in healthy young subjects where inflammation is probably absent. However, it is not known whether the decrease in the anabolic threshold obtained with anti-inflammatory agents is large enough to preserve muscle mass in the long term in humans.

References

1. Cohen S, Nathan JA, Goldberg AL (2015) Muscle wasting in disease: molecular mechanisms and promising therapies. Nat Rev Drug Discov 14(1):58–74
2. Phillips BE, Hill DS, Atherton PJ (2012) Regulation of muscle protein synthesis in humans. Curr Opin Clin Nutr Metab Care 15(1):58–63
3. Gorissen SH, Remond D, Van Loon LJ (2015) The muscle protein synthetic response to food ingestion. Meat Sci 109:96–100
4. Atherton PJ, Etheridge T, Watt PW, Wilkinson D, Selby A, Rankin D et al (2010) Muscle full effect after oral protein: time-dependent concordance and discordance between human muscle protein synthesis and mTORC1 signaling. Am J Clin Nutr 92(5):1080–1088
5. Dideriksen K, Reitelseder S, Holm L (2013) Influence of amino acids, dietary protein, and physical activity on muscle mass development in humans. Nutrients 5(3):852–876
6. Deutz NE, Wolfe RR (2013) Is there a maximal anabolic response to protein intake with a meal? Clin Nutr 32(2):309–313
7. Kimball SR, Jefferson LS (2006) Signaling pathways and molecular mechanisms through which branched-chain amino acids mediate translational control of protein synthesis. J Nutr 136(1):227S–231S
8. Ham DJ, Caldow MK, Lynch GS, Koopman R (2014) Leucine as a treatment for muscle wasting: a critical review. Clin Nutr 33(6):937–945
9. Svanberg E, Jefferson LS, Lundholm K, Kimball SR (1997) Postprandial stimulation of muscle protein synthesis is independent of changes in insulin. Am J Physiol 272(5 Pt 1): E841–E847
10. Greenhaff PL, Karagounis LG, Peirce N, Simpson EJ, Hazell M, Layfield R et al (2008) Disassociation between the effects of amino acids and insulin on signaling, ubiquitin ligases, and protein turnover in human muscle. Am J Physiol Endocrinol Metab 295(3):E595–E604
11. Barazzoni R, Short KR, Asmann Y, Coenen-Schimke JM, Robinson MM, Nair KS (2012) Insulin fails to enhance mTOR phosphorylation, mitochondrial protein synthesis, and ATP

production in human skeletal muscle without amino acid replacement. Am J Physiol Endocrinol Metab 303(9):E1117–E1125
12. Trommelen J, Groen BB, Hamer HM, de Groot LC, Van Loon LJ (2015) Mechanisms in Endocrinology: exogenous insulin does not increase muscle protein synthesis rate when administered systemically: a systematic review. Eur J Endocrinol 173(1):R25–R34
13. Heslin MJ, Newman E, Wolf RF, Pisters PW, Brennan MF (1992) Effect of hyperinsulinemia on whole body and skeletal muscle leucine carbon kinetics in humans. Am J Physiol 262(6 Pt 1):E911–E918
14. Phillips SM, Tipton KD, Aarsland A, Wolf SE, Wolfe RR (1997) Mixed muscle protein synthesis and breakdown after resistance exercise in humans. Am J Physiol 273(1 Pt 1): E99–E107
15. Biolo G, Tipton KD, Klein S, Wolfe RR (1997) An abundant supply of amino acids enhances the metabolic effect of exercise on muscle protein. Am J Physiol Endocrinol Metab 273(1):E122–E129
16. Timmerman KL, Dhanani S, Glynn EL, Fry CS, Drummond MJ, Jennings K et al (2012) A moderate acute increase in physical activity enhances nutritive flow and the muscle protein anabolic response to mixed nutrient intake in older adults. Am J Clin Nutr 95(6):1403–1412
17. Haran PH, Rivas DA, Fielding RA (2012) Role and potential mechanisms of anabolic resistance in sarcopenia. J Cachexia Sarcopenia Muscle 3(3):157–162
18. Rennie MJ (2009) Anabolic resistance in critically ill patients. Crit Care Med 37(10 Suppl):S398–S399
19. Rennie MJ, Selby A, Atherton P, Smith K, Kumar V, Glover EL et al (2010) Facts, noise and wishful thinking: muscle protein turnover in aging and human disuse atrophy. Scand J Med Sci Sports 20(1):5–9
20. Glynn EL, Fry CS, Drummond MJ, Dreyer HC, Dhanani S, Volpi E et al (2010) Muscle protein breakdown has a minor role in the protein anabolic response to essential amino acid and carbohydrate intake following resistance exercise. Am J Physiol Regul Integr Comp Physiol 299(2):R533–R540
21. Guillet C, Boirie Y, Walrand S (2004) An integrative approach to in-vivo protein synthesis measurement: from whole tissue to specific proteins. Curr Opin Clin Nutr Metab Care 7(5):531–538
22. Bodine SC (2013) Disuse-induced muscle wasting. Int J Biochem Cell Biol 45(10):2200–2208
23. Tanner RE, Brunker LB, Agergaard J, Barrows KM, Briggs RA, Kwon OS et al (2015) Age-related differences in lean mass, protein synthesis and skeletal muscle markers of proteolysis after bed rest and exercise rehabilitation. J Physiol 593(18):4259–4273
24. Breen L, Phillips SM (2011) Skeletal muscle protein metabolism in the elderly: interventions to counteract the 'anabolic resistance' of ageing. Nutr Metab [Lond] 8:68
25. Kumar V, Selby A, Rankin D, Patel R, Atherton P, Hildebrandt W et al (2009) Age-related differences in the dose-response relationship of muscle protein synthesis to resistance exercise in young and old men. J Physiol 587(Pt 1):211–217
26. Durham WJ, Casperson SL, Dillon EL, Keske MA, Paddon-Jones D, Sanford AP et al (2010) Age-related anabolic resistance after endurance-type exercise in healthy humans. FASEB J 24(10):4117–4127
27. Volpi E, Mittendorfer B, Rasmussen BB, Wolfe RR (2000) The response of muscle protein anabolism to combined hyperaminoacidemia and glucose-induced hyperinsulinemia is impaired in the elderly. J Clin Endocrinol Metab 85(12):4481–4490
28. Cuthbertson D, Smith K, Babraj J, Leese G, Waddell T, Atherton P et al (2005) Anabolic signaling deficits underlie amino acid resistance of wasting, aging muscle. FASEB J 19(3): 422–424
29. Wilkes EA, Selby AL, Atherton PJ, Patel R, Rankin D, Smith K et al (2009) Blunting of insulin inhibition of proteolysis in legs of older subjects may contribute to age-related sarcopenia. Am J Clin Nutr 90(5):1343–1350
30. Wall BT, Snijders T, Senden JM, Ottenbros CL, Gijsen AP, Verdijk LB et al (2013) Disuse impairs the muscle protein synthetic response to protein ingestion in healthy men. J Clin Endocrinol Metab 98(12):4872–4881

31. Breen L, Stokes KA, Churchward-Venne TA, Moore DR, Baker SK, Smith K et al (2013) Two weeks of reduced activity decreases leg lean mass and induces "anabolic resistance" of myofibrillar protein synthesis in healthy elderly. J Clin Endocrinol Metab 98(6):2604–2612
32. Glover EI, Phillips SM, Oates BR, Tang JE, Tarnopolsky MA, Selby A et al (2008) Immobilization induces anabolic resistance in human myofibrillar protein synthesis with low and high dose amino acid infusion. J Physiol 586(Pt 24):6049–6061
33. Steiner JL, Lang CH (2015) Sepsis attenuates the anabolic response to skeletal muscle contraction. Shock 43(4):344–351
34. Vary TC, Jefferson LS, Kimball SR (2001) Insulin fails to stimulate muscle protein synthesis in sepsis despite unimpaired signaling to 4E-BP1 and S6K1. Am J Physiol Endocrinol Metab 281(5):E1045–E1053
35. Lang CH, Frost RA (2004) Differential effect of sepsis on ability of leucine and IGF-I to stimulate muscle translation initiation. Am J Physiol Endocrinol Metab 287(4):E721–E730
36. Lang CH, Frost RA (2006) Glucocorticoids and TNFalpha interact cooperatively to mediate sepsis-induced leucine resistance in skeletal muscle. Mol Med 12(11–12):291–299
37. Balage M, Averous J, Remond D, Bos C, Pujos-Guillot E, Papet I et al (2010) Presence of low-grade inflammation impaired postprandial stimulation of muscle protein synthesis in old rats. J Nutr Biochem 21(4):325–331
38. Williams JP, Phillips BE, Smith K, Atherton PJ, Rankin D, Selby AL et al (2012) Effect of tumor burden and subsequent surgical resection on skeletal muscle mass and protein turnover in colorectal cancer patients. Am J Clin Nutr 96(5):1064–1070
39. Deutz NE, Safar A, Schutzler S, Memelink R, Ferrando A, Spencer H et al (2011) Muscle protein synthesis in cancer patients can be stimulated with a specially formulated medical food. Clin Nutr 30(6):759–768
40. Winter A, Macadams J, Chevalier S (2012) Normal protein anabolic response to hyperaminoacidemia in insulin-resistant patients with lung cancer cachexia. Clin Nutr 31(5):765–773
41. Engelen MP, Safar AM, Bartter T, Koeman F, Deutz NE (2015) High anabolic potential of essential amino acid mixtures in advanced nonsmall cell lung cancer. Ann Oncol 26(9): 1960–1966
42. van Dijk DP, van de Poll MC, Moses AG, Preston T, Olde Damink SW, Rensen SS et al (2015) Effects of oral meal feeding on whole body protein breakdown and protein synthesis in cachectic pancreatic cancer patients. J Cachexia Sarcopenia Muscle 6(3):212–221
43. Prado CM, Sawyer MB, Ghosh S, Lieffers JR, Esfandiari N, Antoun S et al (2013) Central tenet of cancer cachexia therapy: do patients with advanced cancer have exploitable anabolic potential? Am J Clin Nutr 98(4):1012–1019
44. Guillet C, Delcourt I, Rance M, Giraudet C, Walrand S, Bedu M et al (2009) Changes in basal and insulin and amino acid response of whole body and skeletal muscle proteins in obese men. J Clin Endocrinol Metab 94(8):3044–3050
45. Masgrau A, Mishellany-Dutour A, Murakami H, Beaufrere AM, Walrand S, Giraudet C et al (2012) Time-course changes of muscle protein synthesis associated with obesity-induced lipotoxicity. J Physiol 590(Pt 20):5199–5210
46. Hyde R, Hajduch E, Powell DJ, Taylor PM, Hundal HS (2005) Ceramide down-regulates System A amino acid transport and protein synthesis in rat skeletal muscle cells. FASEB J 19(3):461–463
47. Nilsson MI, Dobson JP, Greene NP, Wiggs MP, Shimkus KL, Wudeck EV et al (2013) Abnormal protein turnover and anabolic resistance to exercise in sarcopenic obesity. FASEB J 27(10):3905–3916
48. Stephens FB, Chee C, Wall BT, Murton AJ, Shannon CE, Van Loon LJ et al (2015) Lipid-induced insulin resistance is associated with an impaired skeletal muscle protein synthetic response to amino acid ingestion in healthy young men. Diabetes 64(5):1615–1620
49. Murphy J, Chevalier S, Gougeon R, Goulet ED, Morais JA (2015) Effect of obesity and type 2 diabetes on protein anabolic response to insulin in elderly women. Exp Gerontol 69: 20–26
50. McIntire KL, Chen Y, Sood S, Rabkin R (2014) Acute uremia suppresses leucine-induced signal transduction in skeletal muscle. Kidney Int 85(2):374–382

51. Sood S, Chen Y, McIntire K, Rabkin R (2014) Acute acidosis attenuates leucine stimulated signal transduction and protein synthesis in rat skeletal muscle. Am J Nephrol 40(4): 362–370
52. Garibotto G, Sofia A, Russo R, Paoletti E, Bonanni A, Parodi EL et al (2015) Insulin sensitivity of muscle protein metabolism is altered in patients with chronic kidney disease and metabolic acidosis. Kidney Int 88(6):1419–1426
53. Siew ED, Ikizler TA (2010) Insulin resistance and protein energy metabolism in patients with advanced chronic kidney disease. Semin Dial 23(4):378–382
54. Etheridge T, Atherton PJ, Wilkinson D, Selby A, Rankin D, Webborn N et al (2011) Effects of hypoxia on muscle protein synthesis and anabolic signaling at rest and in response to acute resistance exercise. Am J Physiol Endocrinol Metab 301(4):E697–E702
55. Schakman O, Kalista S, Barbe C, Loumaye A, Thissen JP (2013) Glucocorticoid-induced skeletal muscle atrophy. Int J Biochem Cell Biol 45(10):2163–2172
56. Paddon-Jones D, Sheffield-Moore M, Cree MG, Hewlings SJ, Aarsland A, Wolfe RR et al (2006) Atrophy and impaired muscle protein synthesis during prolonged inactivity and stress. J Clin Endocrinol Metab 91(12):4836–4841
57. Zheng X, Liang Y, He Q, Yao R, Bao W, Bao L et al (2014) Current models of mammalian target of rapamycin complex 1 [mTORC1] activation by growth factors and amino acids. Int J Mol Sci 15(11):20753–20769
58. Drummond MJ, Dreyer HC, Fry CS, Glynn EL, Rasmussen BB (2009) Nutritional and contractile regulation of human skeletal muscle protein synthesis and mTORC1 signaling. J Appl Physiol [1985] 106(4):1374–1384
59. Dickinson JM, Fry CS, Drummond MJ, Gundermann DM, Walker DK, Glynn EL et al (2011) Mammalian target of rapamycin complex 1 activation is required for the stimulation of human skeletal muscle protein synthesis by essential amino acids. J Nutr 141(5):856–862
60. Kimball SR, Jefferson LS (2010) Control of translation initiation through integration of signals generated by hormones, nutrients, and exercise. J Biol Chem 285(38):29027–29032
61. Ruas JL, White JP, Rao RR, Kleiner S, Brannan KT, Harrison BC et al (2012) A PGC-1alpha isoform induced by resistance training regulates skeletal muscle hypertrophy. Cell 151(6): 1319–1331
62. Marcotte GR, West DW, Baar K (2015) The molecular basis for load-induced skeletal muscle hypertrophy. Calcif Tissue Int 96(3):196–210
63. Kelleher AR, Kimball SR, Dennis MD, Schilder RJ, Jefferson LS (2013) The mTORC1 signaling repressors REDD1/2 are rapidly induced and activation of p70S6K1 by leucine is defective in skeletal muscle of an immobilized rat hindlimb. Am J Physiol Endocrinol Metab 304(2):E229–E236
64. Gordon BS, Williamson DL, Lang CH, Jefferson LS, Kimball SR (2015) Nutrient-induced stimulation of protein synthesis in mouse skeletal muscle is limited by the mTORC1 repressor REDD1. J Nutr 145(4):708–713
65. Guillet C, Zangarelli A, Mishellany A, Rousset P, Sornet C, Dardevet D et al (2004) Mitochondrial and sarcoplasmic proteins, but not myosin heavy chain, are sensitive to leucine supplementation in old rat skeletal muscle. Exp Gerontol 39(5):745–751
66. Rivas DA, Morris EP, Haran PH, Pasha EP, Morais MS, Dolnikowski GG et al (2012) Increased ceramide content and NFkappaB signaling may contribute to the attenuation of anabolic signaling after resistance exercise in aged males. J Appl Physiol [1985] 113(11):1727–1736
67. Drummond MJ, Dickinson JM, Fry CS, Walker DK, Gundermann DM, Reidy PT et al (2012) Bed rest impairs skeletal muscle amino acid transporter expression, mTORC1 signaling, and protein synthesis in response to essential amino acids in older adults. Am J Physiol Endocrinol Metab 302(9):E1113–E1122
68. Bodine SC, Stitt TN, Gonzalez M, Kline WO, Stover GL, Bauerlein R et al (2001) Akt/mTOR pathway is a crucial regulator of skeletal muscle hypertrophy and can prevent muscle atrophy *in vivo*. Nat Cell Biol 3(11):1014–1019
69. You JS, Anderson GB, Dooley MS, Hornberger TA (2015) The role of mTOR signaling in the regulation of protein synthesis and muscle mass during immobilization in mice. Dis Model Mech 8(9):1059–1069

70. Lang CH, Frost RA, Vary TC (2007) Regulation of muscle protein synthesis during sepsis and inflammation. Am J Physiol Endocrinol Metab 293(2):E453–E459
71. Tardif N, Salles J, Guillet C, Tordjman J, Reggio S, Landrier JF et al (2014) Muscle ectopic fat deposition contributes to anabolic resistance in obese sarcopenic old rats through eIF2alpha activation. Aging Cell 13(6):1001–1011
72. Boirie Y, Gachon P, Beaufrere B (1997) Splanchnic and whole-body leucine kinetics in young and elderly men. Am J Clin Nutr 65(2):489–495
73. Gorissen SH, Burd NA, Hamer HM, Gijsen AP, Groen BB, Van Loon LJ (2014) Carbohydrate coingestion delays dietary protein digestion and absorption but does not modulate postprandial muscle protein accretion. J Clin Endocrinol Metab 99(6):2250–2258
74. Phillips BE, Atherton PJ, Varadhan K, Limb MC, Wilkinson DJ, Sjoberg KA et al (2015) The effects of resistance exercise training on macro- and micro-circulatory responses to feeding and skeletal muscle protein anabolism in older men. J Physiol 593(12):2721–2734
75. Pennings B, Groen B, de Lange A, Gijsen AP, Zorenc AH, Senden JM et al (2012) Amino acid absorption and subsequent muscle protein accretion following graded intakes of whey protein in elderly men. Am J Physiol Endocrinol Metab 302(8):E992–E999
76. Yang Y, Churchward-Venne TA, Burd NA, Breen L, Tarnopolsky MA, Phillips SM (2012) Myofibrillar protein synthesis following ingestion of soy protein isolate at rest and after resistance exercise in elderly men. Nutr Metab [Lond] 9(1):57
77. Yang Y, Breen L, Burd NA, Hector AJ, Churchward-Venne TA, Josse AR et al (2012) Resistance exercise enhances myofibrillar protein synthesis with graded intakes of whey protein in older men. Br J Nutr 108(10):1780–1788
78. Witard OC, Jackman SR, Breen L, Smith K, Selby A, Tipton KD (2014) Myofibrillar muscle protein synthesis rates subsequent to a meal in response to increasing doses of whey protein at rest and after resistance exercise. Am J Clin Nutr 99(1):86–95
79. Witard OC, Cocke TL, Ferrando AA, Wolfe RR, Tipton KD (2014) Increased net muscle protein balance in response to simultaneous and separate ingestion of carbohydrate and essential amino acids following resistance exercise. Appl Physiol Nutr Metab 39(3):329–339
80. Burd NA, Gorissen SH, van Vliet S, Snijders T, Van Loon LJ (2015) Differences in postprandial protein handling after beef compared with milk ingestion during postexercise recovery: a randomized controlled trial. Am J Clin Nutr 102(4):828–836
81. Koopman R, Crombach N, Gijsen AP, Walrand S, Fauquant J, Kies AK et al (2009) Ingestion of a protein hydrolysate is accompanied by an accelerated in vivo digestion and absorption rate when compared with its intact protein. Am J Clin Nutr 90(1):106–115
82. Walrand S, Gryson C, Salles J, Giraudet C, Migne C, Bonhomme C et al (2015) Fast-digestive protein supplement for ten days overcomes muscle anabolic resistance in healthy elderly men. Clin Nutr (in press)
83. Pennings B, Boirie Y, Senden JM, Gijsen AP, Kuipers H, Van Loon LJ (2011) Whey protein stimulates postprandial muscle protein accretion more effectively than do casein and casein hydrolysate in older men. Am J Clin Nutr 93(5):997–1005
84. Stein TP, Schluter MD, Leskiw MJ, Boden G (1999) Attenuation of the protein wasting associated with bed rest by branched-chain amino acids. Nutrition 15(9):656–660
85. Paddon-Jones D, Sheffield-Moore M, Urban RJ, Sanford AP, Aarsland A, Wolfe RR et al (2004) Essential amino acid and carbohydrate supplementation ameliorates muscle protein loss in humans during 28 days bedrest. J Clin Endocrinol Metab 89(9):4351–4358
86. Paddon-Jones D (2006) Interplay of stress and physical inactivity on muscle loss: nutritional countermeasures. J Nutr 136(8):2123–2126
87. Fiatarone MA, O'Neill EF, Ryan ND, Clements KM, Solares GR, Nelson ME et al (1994) Exercise training and nutritional supplementation for physical frailty in very elderly people. N Engl J Med 330(25):1769–1775
88. Ferrando AA, Paddon-Jones D, Wolfe RR (2006) Bed rest and myopathies. Curr Opin Clin Nutr Metab Care 9(4):410–415
89. Verhoeven S, Vanschoonbeek K, Verdijk LB, Koopman R, Wodzig WK, Dendale P et al (2009) Long-term leucine supplementation does not increase muscle mass or strength in healthy elderly men. Am J Clin Nutr 89(5):1468–1475

90. Balage M, Dardevet D (2010) Long-term effects of leucine supplementation on body composition. Curr Opin Clin Nutr Metab Care 13(3):265–270
91. Dardevet D, Remond D, Peyron MA, Papet I, Savary-Auzeloux I, Mosoni L (2012) Muscle wasting and resistance of muscle anabolism: the "anabolic threshold concept" for adapted nutritional strategies during sarcopenia. ScientificWorldJournal 2012:269531
92. Groen BB, Res PT, Pennings B, Hertle E, Senden JM, Saris WH et al (2012) Intragastric protein administration stimulates overnight muscle protein synthesis in elderly men. Am J Physiol Endocrinol Metab 302(1):E52–E60
93. Areta JL, Burke LM, Ross ML, Camera DM, West DW, Broad EM et al (2013) Timing and distribution of protein ingestion during prolonged recovery from resistance exercise alters myofibrillar protein synthesis. J Physiol 591(Pt 9):2319–2331
94. Koopman R, Beelen M, Stellingwerff T, Pennings B, Saris WH, Kies AK et al (2007) Coingestion of carbohydrate with protein does not further augment postexercise muscle protein synthesis. Am J Physiol Endocrinol Metab 293(3):E833–E842
95. Weijs PJ, Cynober L, Delegge M, Kreymann G, Wernerman J, Wolfe RR (2014) Proteins and amino acids are fundamental to optimal nutrition support in critically ill patients. Crit Care 18(6):591
96. Ferrando AA, Paddon-Jones D, Wolfe RR (2002) Alterations in protein metabolism during space flight and inactivity. Nutrition 18(10):837–841
97. Devries MC, Phillips SM (2015) Supplemental protein in support of muscle mass and health: advantage whey. J Food Sci 80(Suppl 1):A8–A15
98. Hagerman FC, Walsh SJ, Staron RS, Hikida RS, Gilders RM, Murray TF et al (2000) Effects of high-intensity resistance training on untrained older men. I. Strength, cardiovascular, and metabolic responses. J Gerontol A Biol Sci Med Sci 55(7):B336–B346
99. Little JP, Phillips SM (2009) Resistance exercise and nutrition to counteract muscle wasting. Appl Physiol Nutr Metab 34(5):817–828
100. Costamagna D, Costelli P, Sampaolesi M, Penna F (2015) Role of inflammation in muscle homeostasis and myogenesis. Mediators Inflamm 2015:805172
101. Rieu I, Magne H, Savary-Auzeloux I, Averous J, Bos C, Peyron MA et al (2009) Reduction of low grade inflammation restores blunting of postprandial muscle anabolism and limits sarcopenia in old rats. J Physiol 587(Pt 22):5483–5492
102. Trappe TA, Carroll CC, Dickinson JM, LeMoine JK, Haus JM, Sullivan BE et al (2011) Influence of acetaminophen and ibuprofen on skeletal muscle adaptations to resistance exercise in older adults. Am J Physiol Regul Integr Comp Physiol 300(3):R655–R662
103. Smith GI, Atherton P, Reeds DN, Mohammed BS, Rankin D, Rennie MJ et al (2011) Dietary omega-3 fatty acid supplementation increases the rate of muscle protein synthesis in older adults: a randomized controlled trial. Am J Clin Nutr 93(2):402–412

Chapter 6
Use of Lipids as Energy Substrates

Philip C. Calder and Pierre Singer

Abstract Complex lipids and their fatty acid components have important biological activities and are involved in the regulation of many metabolic and physiological processes. Fatty acids are important energy sources and upon complete β-oxidation yield more energy per mole and per carbon atom than glucose. Fatty acid β-oxidation occurs mainly in the mitochondria, and there are specific mechanisms for transporting fatty acids from the cytosol to the mitochondrial matrix to enable their oxidation. Ensuring fatty acid availability for oxidation reduces the need for glucose provision. Fatty acids in foods and in formulas used for nutrition support are esterified into triacylglycerols. There are specific mechanisms for releasing fatty acids from triacylglycerols provided orally and for taking these up into enterocytes. These involve coordinated physical, chemical and enzymatic activities operating from the mouth to the small intestine. In healthy people these processes are very efficient, but they can be disrupted by injury, illness or disease, including critical illness, meaning that fatty acid availability can be decreased in these situations. The products of triacylglycerol digestion and absorption ultimately appear in the bloodstream as triacylglycerols in lipoproteins called chylomicrons. Fatty acids are removed from chylomicrons by the action of lipoprotein lipase, which is promoted by insulin, and can be stored in adipose tissue following their re-esterification into triacylglycerols. In stress states or times of limited glucose availability, fatty acids are released from stored triacylglycerols and appear in the bloodstream as non-esterified fatty acids. These are the substrates for β-oxidation and energy generation. Lipid emulsions used in intravenous nutrition support are metabolised similarly to chylomicrons, but they need to acquire proteins from native lipoproteins to enable

P.C. Calder (✉)
Human Development and Health Academic Unit, Faculty of Medicine,
University of Southampton, Southampton, UK

NIHR Southampton Biomedical Research Centre,
University Hospital Southampton NHS Foundation Trust and University of Southampton,
Southampton, UK
e-mail: pcc@soton.ac.uk

P. Singer
Institute for Nutrition Research, Rabin Medical Center, Beilinson Hospital,
Petah Tikva, Israel

J.-C. Preiser (ed.), *The Stress Response of Critical Illness: Metabolic and Hormonal Aspects*, DOI 10.1007/978-3-319-27687-8_6

this to happen. ESPEN guidelines recommend intravenous lipid infusion in critically ill patients where enteral feeding is not possible. However, excess rates of lipid infusion can lead to hypertriacylglycerolemia and can disrupt organ function, and therefore the rate of lipid infusion needs to be controlled and limited. The critically ill patient displays alterations in lipid metabolism and lipid utilisation that result from insulin resistance, the stress response, inflammation and nutrition support. Fatty acids are the preferred fuel in critical illness, and there is an increase in whole body fat oxidation. However, fatty acid availability may be in excess of needs, and fatty acids not oxidised may be incorporated into triacylglycerols in the liver resulting in hepatic steatosis and hypertriacylglycerolemia, which may be promoted by lipid infusion and by impaired triacylglycerol clearance. Whether these events happen or not is determined by the specific state of the individual critically ill patient. Because the fatty acid components of triacylglycerols are biologically active, the precise composition of lipid used in artificial nutrition support of critically ill patients may affect metabolic, physiological and clinical outcomes.

6.1 Lipids and Fatty Acids

The terminology of lipids can be confusing. The terms 'fat' and 'lipid' are often used interchangeably. This is not inappropriate, but the terms may be context dependent. Usually lipids are compounds that are insoluble in aqueous solution but soluble in organic solvent. Lipids may be simple or complex in structure, and they may be associated with one another or with non-lipid structures. Their insolubility in aqueous solution poses challenges for the transportation of lipids in the bloodstream. The most common complex lipids encountered in the diet, in the bloodstream and in cells and tissues are triacylglycerols (sometimes called triglycerides), phospholipids and cholesteryl esters [3]. These are each composed of fatty acids esterified to a 'backbone'. In triacylglycerols and phospholipids, the backbone is glycerol, while in cholesteryl esters it is cholesterol. Quantitatively triacylglycerols make up the bulk of dietary fat, comprising at least 90 % of the fat in most diets. Triacylglycerols represent a mechanism for storage of fatty acids, for example, in adipose tissue, and for transporting fatty acids in the bloodstream. Phospholipids and similar complex lipids are important structural and functional components of all cell membranes, and they are also involved in lipid transport in the bloodstream, as are cholesteryl esters. Cholesterol itself is also a membrane component and is an important biosynthetic precursor, for example, of steroid hormones, bile acids and vitamin D. Some phospholipids and derivatives of phospholipids (e.g. lysophosphatidylcholine, platelet activating factor and ceramides), some derivatives of triacylglycerols (e.g. diacylglycerols) and some fatty acids and derivatives of fatty acids (e.g. prostaglandins and thromboxanes) are very important intracellular and extracellular signalling molecules involved in regulating many cellular responses and many physiological processes. A variety of fatty acids may be present in triacylglycerols, phospholipids and their derivatives and in cholesteryl esters, and the fatty acid 'makeup' (called fatty acid composition) of these complex lipids influences their physical properties and may also influence their functions. In turn, the fatty acids that are released from complex lipids by hydrolytic enzymes called lipases have biological activities that are related to their structures [6]. There is quite a diversity of fatty acids (mainly as components of complex lipids) within foods, formulas used for nutrition support, the bloodstream, adipose tissue stores and cell membranes [7]. These fatty acids may differ according to hydrocarbon chain length, number of double bonds in the hydrocarbon chain (if any), the position of the bond(s) and the configuration around the double bond (*cis* or *trans*). The most abundant fatty acids in the human diet and in the human body have straight hydrocarbon chains of an even number of carbon atoms, although odd-chain fatty acids do exist. Fatty acid hydrocarbon chain lengths vary from 2 to 30, and based upon chain length, fatty acids are classified as short chain (2–6 carbon atoms), medium chain (8–12 carbon atoms) and long chain (14 or more carbon atoms); sometimes, fatty acids of 20 or more carbon atoms are referred to as very long chain. Fatty acids are also classified according to the degree of unsaturation (i.e. the number of double bonds in the hydrocarbon chain). Fatty acids containing double bonds in the hydrocarbon chain are called unsaturated fatty acids; a fatty acid containing two or more double bonds is called a polyunsaturated fatty acid or PUFA. Saturated fatty acids do not contain double bonds in the hydrocarbon chain. Fatty acids have systematic names that are based upon their structural characteristics; many also have widely used common names, and there is also a commonly used systematic nomenclature that describes the key structural characteristics of the fatty acid. Most commonly occurring unsaturated fatty acids contain *cis* rather than *trans* double bonds, although the latter do occur in fatty acids ruminant fats (e.g. cow's milk), in plant lipids and in some seed oils, and they may also be introduced by exposure of *cis* unsaturated fatty acids to high temperatures such as when oils are used for deep fat frying.

As well as coming from the diet, many fatty acids can be synthesised de novo from non-fat sources like glucose and amino acids [3, 7, 15]. Exceptions to this are linoleic and alpha-linolenic acids, which cannot be synthesised in animals due to lack of the relevant desaturase enzymes. Because these two fatty acids have specific metabolic and functional roles, they must be consumed in the diet and so are consequently known as essential fatty acids.

6.2 The Handling of Dietary Lipids

As indicated above, the bulk of dietary fat (and dietary fatty acids) is in the form of triacylglycerols. For those fatty acids to be assimilated into the body, the triacylglycerols need to by hydrolysed in the gut lumen. Although the process of digestion (hydrolysis) mainly occurs in the upper small intestine, earlier events occurring in the mouth (chewing, mixing with saliva) and stomach (acidification, churning) are important. Once in the small intestine, 'oil' droplets composed of triacylglycerols are emulsified by bile salts released from the gall bladder via the bile duct, and this enables the enzyme pancreatic lipase to hydrolyse fatty acids from the first and third carbons of the glycerol backbone of the triacylglycerol releasing the two free fatty acids and a 2-monocylglycerol. Those products are taken up into the enterocytes. From here, medium-chain fatty acids pass directly into the hepatic portal vein and are transported directly to the liver for metabolism. In contrast, long-chain fatty acids are re-esterified into triacylglycerols within the enterocytes. It is evident that effective digestion and absorption of dietary fat require the coordinated action of the mouth, stomach, liver, gall bladder and bile duct, pancreas and enterocytes. Normally these processes are very efficient, and studies with stable isotopes have demonstrated that healthy adult subjects are able to digest and absorb at least 95 % of dietary fat [20, 21, 23]. However, dysfunction or absence of any of the key components involved in lipid digestion or absorption through injury or illness will result in impaired digestion and absorption of fat [24].

The triacylglycerols formed within enterocytes are packaged into large structures called chylomicrons with the hydrophobic triacylglycerols in the core coated by a monolayer of amphipathic phospholipids. Chylomicrons are a type of lipoprotein. Certain proteins, called apoproteins, are embedded in the coat of the chylomicron, and these have a role in targeting the chylomicron for metabolism once it enters the bloodstream. The chylomicron first enters the lymphatic system making its way into the bloodstream at the thoracic duct's connection with the left subclavian vein. Once in the bloodstream, chylomicrons receive apoproteins from other lipoproteins, for example, apoprotein-C2 from high-density lipoprotein. This enhances the ability of the chylomicron to act as a substrate for lipoprotein lipase. In the fed state, the activity of this enzyme is enhanced in adipose tissue by the action of insulin. Lipoprotein lipase hydrolyses fatty acids from chylomicron triacylglycerols. The main fate of these fatty acids is uptake into adipocytes and re-esterification into triacylglycerols for storage. The triacylglycerol-depleted chylomicron remnant is ultimately cleared by the liver. Therefore in the period after fat is consumed in the diet, there is an increase in chylomicron and triacylglycerol concentrations in the bloodstream as uptake from the gut exceeds removal from the bloodstream. However, after several hours, the concentrations of chylomicrons and triacylglycerols decline as the chylomicrons and chylomicron remnants are cleared. The clearance will be impaired in insulin-resistant states because the activity of lipoprotein lipase may be lower.

6.3 The Handling of Intravenous Lipids

In some individuals, the gut may be damaged through injury or surgery, or one or more of the organs required for digestion of dietary triacylglycerols or absorption of the products of this digestion may be absent, damaged or functioning poorly due to injury, illness or disease. In this case, triacylglycerols provided orally or directly into the gastrointestinal tract will not be efficiently assimilated, and steatorrhoea will ensue. In order to avoid this and to provide fatty acids to the individual, intravenous infusion of lipids can be used. A number of emulsified lipids are available commercially for this purpose. These lipids are based upon naturally occurring oils, with the component fatty acids being esterified into triacylglycerols forming the core of the lipid emulsion which is surrounded by a phospholipid monolayer. In this regard, the lipid emulsion resembles a chylomicron. However, the emulsion, as infused, does not contain proteins. Instead, the emulsion particles acquire proteins from lipoproteins within the circulation, ultimately forming structures that are similar to chylomicrons and which are metabolised in a similar way. The rate of infusion of a lipid emulsion must be carefully controlled in order not to exceed the ability of the recipient to clear the lipid, which will influenced by the individuals physiology and pathology. Clearly one indicator of impaired ability to clear an infused lipid emulsion will be an elevation of blood triacylglycerol concentrations above what might be expected. Interestingly the fatty acid composition of an infused lipid emulsion, which is determined by the oils used to produce the emulsion, affects the metabolism and rate of clearance of the emulsion. This has been studied in both experiential animals and humans. Hultin et al. [19] demonstrated in rats that a lipid emulsion containing medium-chain fatty acids in addition to long-chain fatty acids was cleared more quickly than one that just contained long-chain fatty acids. Simoens et al. [27] demonstrated this same phenomenon in dogs, while Richelle et al. [26] reported more rapid clearance of a physical mixture of oils rich in medium-chain and long-chain fatty acids compared with an oil rich in long-chain fatty acids alone in humans. Later Simoens et al. [28] reported faster clearance of an emulsion blended from soybean oil, medium-chain triglycerides and fish oil (in a ratio of 5:4:1) compared to one blended from soybean oil and medium-chain triglycerides. Such differences in clearance rate are important in terms of preventing hypertriacylglycerolaemia, but they also represent altered abilities of emulsions of different composition to deliver bioactive fatty acids to target tissues.

6.4 Fatty Acid Release from Stored Triacylglycerols

Fatty acids are important metabolic and bioactive components of triacylglycerols [6]. As indicated above, lipases are enzymes that hydrolyse fatty acids from acylglycerols, and the roles of pancreatic lipase in hydrolysing fatty acids from dietary triacylglycerols and of lipoprotein lipase in hydrolysing fatty acids from circulating triacylglcerols were described. The main site of fatty acid storage is adipose tissue where they are esterified into triacylglycerols that form large droplets within the adipocytes. Lipase enzymes are required to release these fatty acids in order that they can be utilised. Hormone-sensitive lipase acts on the surface of the triacylglycerol droplet stored in the adipocyte to release the stored fatty acids. These can then be delivered to the circulation as 'free' fatty acids (or more correctly as non-esterified fatty acids which are non-covalently bound to albumin) from where they are made available to tissues. As its name suggests, hormone-sensitive lipase is regulated by various hormones, including adrenaline, noradrenaline, glucagon and insulin. Insulin acts to inhibit its activity, while adrenaline and glucagon increase its activity. Therefore, through its concerted actions on the activities of lipoprotein lipase and hormone-sensitive lipase, insulin acts to make fatty acids from circulating lipoproteins available for storage in adipose tissue and to retain those fatty acids held there in stored triacylglycerols. In insulin-resistant states, circulating triacylglycerols will be less well cleared by lipoprotein lipase meaning that their concentration in the bloodstream may become elevated, while fatty acids will be less well retained in triacylglycerols in adipose tissue meaning that the blood concentration of non-esterified fatty acids will also become elevated [15]. In contrast to what is seen with insulin, an increase in adrenaline or noradrenaline concentration, as seen in many stress situations, enhances the activity of hormone-sensitive lipase, thus promoting release of non-esterified fatty acids from adipose tissue. Thus, physiological stress in an insulin-resistant individual creates a scenario that results in significant disturbances in lipid homeostasis. Several inflammatory cytokines interfere with insulin signalling and create an insulin-resistant state [13, 18, 32]. Hence, local inflammation in adipose tissue can lead to efflux of non-esterified fatty acids which can lead to metabolic abnormalities in other tissues [13, 25].

6.5 Fatty Acids as Energy Sources

Fatty acids represent important energy sources and provide an alternative to glucose as a fuel [7, 15]. β-Oxidation is the major metabolic pathway by which energy is released from fatty acids. The rate of fatty acid β-oxidation is partly controlled by the intracellular concentration of 'free' (i.e. unesterified) fatty acids, which in turn is determined by their concentration in the blood, so that a rise in the concentration of circulating non-esterified fatty acids increases fatty acid oxidation in the tissues that can use them (most aerobic tissues but not the brain). Non-esterified fatty acids become important energy sources during times of metabolic stress and when carbohydrate supply is limiting. Prior to β-oxidation, the fatty acid substrate is converted to its coenzyme A (CoA) thioester derivative in a reaction catalysed by a cytosolic acyl-CoA synthase, of which there are several with different substrate specificities according to fatty acid chain length:

$$\text{Fatty acid} + \text{ATP} + \text{CoA} \rightarrow \text{Acyl-CoA} + \text{AMP} + \text{PPi}$$

Fatty acid β-oxidation occurs in the mitochondrial matrix, and therefore, the fatty acid substrate (fatty acyl-CoA) needs to be transported across the outer and inner mitochondrial membranes that are not permeable to fatty acids or fatty acyl-CoAs with a hydrocarbon chain longer than 12 carbons. Shorter-chain fatty acids can cross both the outer and the inner mitochondrial membranes. However, medium- and long-chain acyl-CoAs require a special transport mechanism to cross the

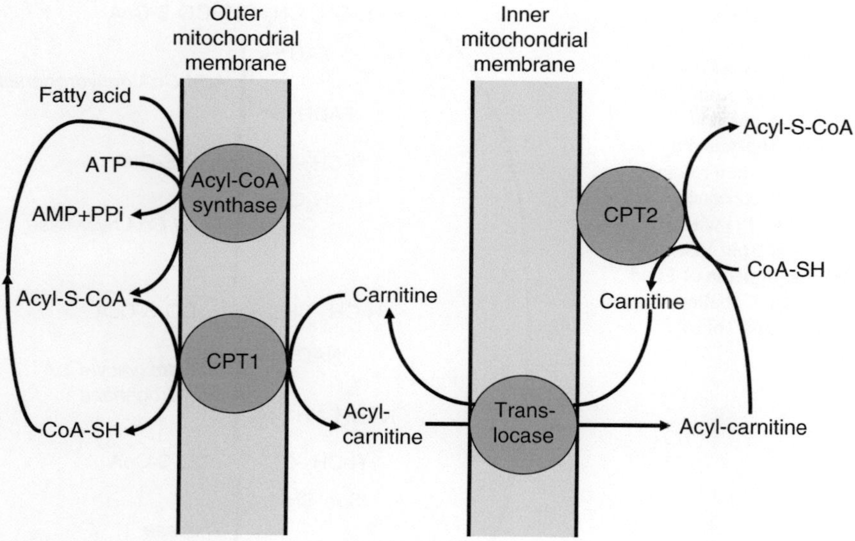

Fig. 6.1 The carnitine palmitoyltransferase (CPT) system for transport of fatty acyl-CoA across the mitochondrial membranes into the matrix prior to β-oxidation (Reproduced from Calder [7] with permission from Elsevier from Encylopedia of Food and Health (Caballero B, Finglas P, and Toldrá F (eds.))

mitochondrial membranes. Translocation of these is a carnitine-dependent process involving the coordinate action of isoforms of carnitine palmitoyltransferase (CPT) on the mitochondrial outer and inner membranes. CPT1 forms the fatty acylcarnitine at the outer mitochondrial membrane, and this is then transported to the intramembrane space via porin (Fig. 6.1). The fatty acylcarnitine is transported through the inner mitochondrial membrane via acylcarnitine translocases in exchange for free carnitine. Once across the inner mitochondrial membrane, the fatty acyl-CoA is reformed by CPT2. CPT1 is the rate-limiting step for mitochondrial β-oxidation. It is inhibited by malonyl-CoA, and thus, conditions that promote malonyl-CoA synthesis (e.g. the fed state since the enzyme that forms malonyl-CoA acetyl-CoA carboxylase is promoted by insulin) suppress fatty acid β-oxidation. Conversely, conditions that promote a decline in malonyl-CoA concentrations (e.g. fasting, starvation, exercise and insulin resistance) will act to promote fatty acid β-oxidation.

Fatty acid β-oxidation itself involves the progressive removal of two-carbon units, as acetyl-CoA, from the carboxyl end of the fatty acyl-CoA substrate in a series of four reactions that act sequentially and repeatedly (Fig. 6.2). Each round of the cycle generates $FADH_2$ and NADH in addition to acetyl-CoA and an acyl chain that is two carbons shorter than the original. The latter re-enters the cycle. Thus, complete β-oxidation of palmitoyl-CoA will generate eight acetyl-CoA, seven $FADH_2$ and seven NADH molecules:

$$\text{Palmitoyl-CoA} + 7\text{CoA} + 7\text{FAD} + 7\text{NAD}^+ + 7\text{H}_2\text{O} \rightarrow 8\ \text{Acetyl-CoA} + 7\text{FADH}_2 + 7\text{NADH} + 7\text{H}^+$$

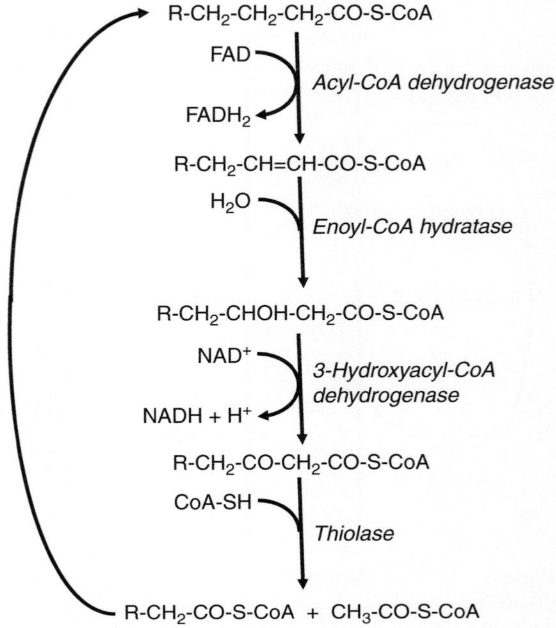

Fig. 6.2 The pathway of β-oxidation of fatty acyl-CoA. Each cycle of four reactions produces acetyl-CoA and an acyl-CoA shortened by two carbons that then re-enters the cycle (Reproduced from Calder [7] with permission from Elsevier from Encylopedia of Food and Health (Caballero B, Finglas P, and Toldrá F (eds.))

The acetyl-CoA produced by β-oxidation is normally oxidised in the citric acid (Krebs) cycle, while the $FADH_2$ and NADH pass their electrons to the mitochondrial electron transport chain. Hence, fatty acid β-oxidation generates a large amount of ATP per mole of fatty acid and per mole of fatty acid carbon oxidised:

$$\text{Palmitoyl-CoA} + 23O_2 + 131\text{Pi} + 131\text{ADP} \rightarrow \text{CoA} + 131\text{ATP} + 16CO_2 + 146H_2O$$

Because the activation of palmitate to palmitoyl-CoA consumes two ATP equivalents, the net gain per molecule of palmitic acid oxidised is 129 ATP. This is equivalent to approximately 37 kJ or 9 kcal of energy per gram of fatty acid oxidised, over twice the energy yield for carbohydrate or amino acid oxidation.

Entry of acetyl-CoA into the citric acid (Krebs) cycle releases CoA, and this is needed to maintain β-oxidation. This entry of acetyl-CoA requires a supply of oxaloacetate for it to condense to, so producing citrate (the 'first' reaction of the cycle catalysed by citrate synthase). The supply of oxaloacetate comes from pyruvate via the enzyme pyruvate carboxylase. Pyruvate carboxylase is activated by acetyl-CoA, which indicates a lack of oxaloacetate. In turn, the pyruvate is produced by glycolysis. Thus, some glucose metabolism is required to support continued fatty acid β-oxidation. The conversion of pyruvate to oxaloacetate is a type of anaplerotic reaction, and, because of this requirement for some glucose metabolism to support fatty acid β-oxidation, it is said that 'fats burn in the flame of carbohydrates'.

A second β-oxidation system occurs in peroxisomes. Fatty acid transport into peroxisomes involves the CPT system, with similar enzymes to mitochondrial CPT2 and regulation via malonyl-CoA. Compared with mitochondrial oxidation,

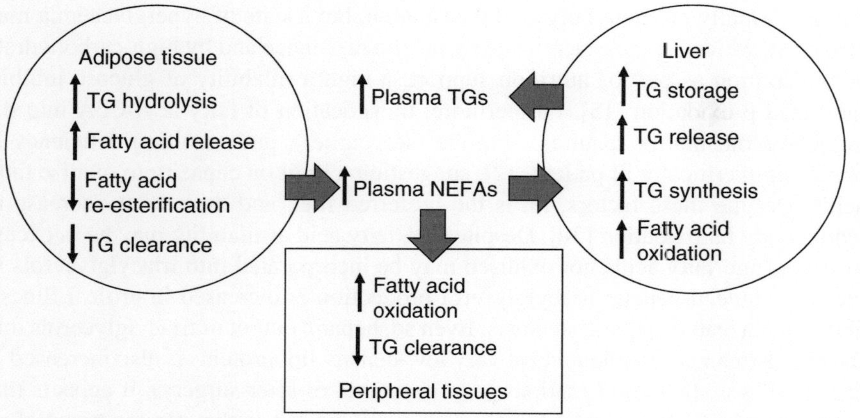

Fig. 6.3 Summary of the changes in fatty acid metabolism in critical illness. Under the influence of stress hormones, inflammation and insulin resistance, adipose tissue hydrolyses stored triacylglycerols (TGs) releasing non-esterified fatty acids (NEFAs) into the circulation. Higher plasma NEFA concentrations promote fatty acid β-oxidation by the liver and peripheral tissues. NEFA supply to the liver can exceed the requirements of β-oxidation, so that the non-oxidised fatty acids are incorporated into TGs, some of which may be stored in the liver and some released into the circulation as very low-density lipoproteins. Clearance of circulating TGs by adipose tissue and by peripheral tissues may be impaired so that plasma TG concentrations become elevated

peroxisomal β-oxidation has a much broader substrate specificity and is especially active towards very long-chain fatty acids and also towards many fatty acids with less common structural features and fatty acid derivatives and more complex lipids. Acyl-CoA oxidase is an important enzyme involved in catalysing the first step of peroxisomal β-oxidation.

6.6 The Situation in the Critically Ill Patient

6.6.1 Altered Lipid Uptake and Metabolism in Critical Illness

Lipid absorption from the gastrointestinal tract is impeded in the critically ill patient: a recent study showed a 50 % reduction in absorption of long-chain fatty acids in mechanically ventilated critically ill patients compared with healthy controls [1]. It is not clear which component or components of triacylglycerol digestion and absorption are impaired in critical illness, but deficits in bile secretion, pancreatic function and enterocyte absorptive capacity are all possible.

The critically ill patient displays alterations in lipid metabolism and lipid utilisation that result from insulin resistance, the stress response, inflammation and nutrition support (Fig. 6.3). Overall, there is a stimulation of catabolic pathways and of energy expenditure [17, 30]. There is hydrolysis of stored triacylglycerols and increased appearance of non-esterified fatty acids in the bloodstream. This would normally promote fatty acid β-oxidation, but a state of hyperglycaemia may also exist, which can be exacerbated by insulin resistance and by high-carbohydrate administration as part of nutrition support; a high availability of glucose inhibits fatty acid β-oxidation [15]. Furthermore, translocation of fatty acyl-CoA into the mitochondrial matrix requires carnitine (see earlier), and carnitine deficiency is prevalent in critically ill patients [2], suggesting a limit on capacity to oxidise fatty acids. Despite these factors, fat is the preferred fuel, and there is an increase in whole body fat oxidation [30]. Despite this, fatty acid availability may be in excess of needs, and fatty acids not oxidised may be incorporated into triacylglycerols in the liver. Indeed hepatic triacylglycerol production is increased in critical illness, and this can lead to hepatic steatosis. Even so, hepatic output of triacylglycerols into the bloodstream as components of very low-density lipoproteins is also increased in critical illness. In some situations (e.g. in trauma or after surgery), it appears that clearance of circulating triacylglycerols is not impaired so that plasma triacylglycerol concentrations are not excessively elevated. However, in some conditions, like sepsis, inflammation-induced insulin resistance means clearance of circulating triacylglycerols is impaired, and hypertriacylglycerolaemia results. Thus, in some patients a situation of hyperglycaemia, hypertriacylglycerolaemia and high non-esterified fatty acid concentrations may be created. It is important to keep in mind that lipoproteins including very low-density lipoproteins can bind endotoxin and target it for degradation in liver parenchymal cells. Thus, a rise in very low-density lipoprotein concentration may be, in part, a protective mechanism. Plasma cholesterol concentration is decreased in stress conditions with concentrations of both low-density lipoproteins and high-density lipoproteins being decreased [11]. This decrease occurs despite increased hepatic cholesterol production. The decreased high-density lipoprotein concentration appears to be the result of increased catabolism, while the decreased low-density lipoprotein concentration may be due to increased sequestration and retention in sub-endothelial spaces of the vasculature. Septic intensive care unit patients with low concentrations of high-density lipoprotein or low-density lipoprotein had a higher risk of mortality than those with higher concentrations of these lipoproteins [12, 22]. The composition of lipoproteins is also changed in stress conditions, and this might change their metabolism and properties.

6.6.2 Lipid Metabolism in the Critically Ill Patient Receiving Intravenous Nutrition Support

ESPEN guidelines recommend administering intravenous lipid emulsions on a daily basis in critically ill patients both to prevent essential fatty acid deficiency and to provide an energy source to allow a lower carbohydrate load, decreasing insulin requirements [29]. Although infusion of lipid emulsions can result in hypertriacylglycerolaemia, this is not always seen in the critically ill. For example, Druml et al. [14] reported that patients with sepsis and those with sepsis and liver failure had a lower plasma triacylglycerol response than seen in healthy controls when infused with a lipid emulsion at identical rates. Furthermore, the pharmacokinetics of triacylglycerol elimination were similar between the three groups, and lipid oxidation was increased by the same amount in all three groups [14]. Tappy et al. [31] compared isoenergetic glucose-based (70 % glucose, 15 % lipid, 15 % amino acids) or lipid-based (15 % glucose, 70 % lipid, 15 % amino acids) parenteral nutrition on respiratory gas exchange in critically ill patients. They found that CO_2 exchange was lower with lipid-rich than glucose-rich nutrition support, which suggests pulmonary advantage of the former. These authors also confirmed a switch away from glucose oxidation towards lipid (i.e. fatty acid) oxidation when lipid is the predominant substrate being infused. In accord with this, Caresta et al. [10] showed a reduction in respiratory quotient, indicating increased fatty acid oxidation, when lipid was infused into infants and children with systemic inflammatory response syndrome and sepsis. Taken together, these studies suggest that intravenous lipid emulsions can be metabolised efficiently in critically ill patients, that there may be metabolic advantages from lipid (less need for glucose and so less risk for hyperglycaemia) and that there may be pulmonary advantages from lipid (less CO_2 production). However, the key to these advantages is the lipid infusion rate. A too high rate will overload the ability to handle the infused triacylglycerols resulting in fat accumulation in many sites with a resulting impairment of leukocyte, platelet, pulmonary and hepatic function and to further metabolic and clinical disturbances. Thus, lipid infusion and metabolism need tight control to allow for safe and efficient administration in critically ill patients [16].

Because the fatty acid components of infused triacylglycerols are biologically active [6], the precise composition of a lipid emulsion may affect metabolic, physiological and clinical outcomes. This is discussed in detail elsewhere [4, 5, 9]. There is some evidence that the fatty acid composition of infused lipid can affect infection rate, liver function, ventilation requirement and length of hospital stay, but without effect on mortality [4, 5, 8, 9].

6.7 Summary and Conclusions

Complex lipids and their fatty acid components have important biological activities and are involved in the regulation of many metabolic and physiological processes [3, 6, 7, 15]. Fatty acids are important energy sources and upon complete β-oxidation yield more energy per mole and per carbon atom than glucose. Fatty acid β-oxidation occurs mainly in the mitochondria, and there are specific mechanisms for transporting fatty acids from the cytosol to the mitochondrial matrix to enable their oxidation. Ensuring fatty acid availability for oxidation reduces the need for glucose provision. Thus, providing fatty acids is a key strategy to reduce the need for glucose and insulin in patients receiving artificial nutrition support, particularly intravenous. Fatty acids in foods and in formulas used for nutrition support are esterified into triacylglycerols. There are specific mechanisms for releasing fatty acids from triacylglycerols provided orally and for taking these up into enterocytes. These involve coordinated physical, chemical and enzymatic activities operating from the mouth to the small intestine. In healthy people these processes are very efficient, but they can be disrupted by injury, illness or disease meaning that fatty acid availability can be decreased in these situations. For example, lipid absorption from the gastrointestinal tract is impeded in the critically ill patient.

The products of triacylglycerol digestion and absorption ultimately appear in the bloodstream as triacylglycerol components of lipoproteins called chylomicrons. Fatty acids are removed from chylomicrons by the action of lipoprotein lipase, which is promoted by insulin, and can be stored in adipose tissue following their re-esterification into triacylglycerols. In stress states or times of limited glucose availability, fatty acids are released from stored triacylglycerols and appear in the bloodstream as non-esterified fatty acids. These are the substrates for oxidation and energy generation. Lipid emulsions used in intravenous nutrition support are metabolised similarly to chylomicrons, but they need to acquire apoproteins from native lipoproteins to enable this to happen. ESPEN guidelines recommend intravenous lipid infusion in critically ill patients where enteral feeding is not possible. However, excess rates of lipid infusion can lead to hypertriacylglycerolaemia and can disrupt organ function, and therefore the rate of lipid infusion needs to be controlled and limited. The critically ill patient displays alterations in lipid metabolism and lipid utilisation that result from insulin resistance, the stress response, inflammation and nutrition support (Fig. 6.3). Fatty acids are the preferred fuel in critical illness, and there is an increase in whole body fat oxidation. However, fatty acid availability may be in excess of needs, and fatty acids not oxidised may be incorporated into triacylglycerols in the liver resulting in hepatic steatosis and hypertriacylglycerolaemia, which may be promoted by lipid infusion and by impaired triacylglycerol clearance. In some situations (e.g. in trauma or after surgery), it appears that clearance of circulating triacylglycerols is not impaired so that plasma triacylglycerol concentrations are not excessively elevated. However, in some conditions, like sepsis, inflammation-induced insulin resistance means clearance of circulating triacylglycerols can be impaired and hypertriacylglycerolaemia can occur. In such situations, control of the rate of lipid infusion is important to avert adverse consequences while still gaining the metabolic and functional advantages of lipid [16]. Finally, because the fatty acid components of triacylglycerols are biologically active [6], the precise composition of lipid used in artificial nutrition support of critically ill patients may affect metabolic, physiological and clinical outcomes [4, 5, 8, 9].

References

1. Abdelhamid YA, Cousins CE, Sim JA, Bellon MS, Nguyen NQ, Horowitz M, Chapman MJ, Deane AM (2015) Effect of critical illness on triglyceride absorption. J Parenter Enteral Nutr 39:966–972
2. Bonafe L, Berger M, Que YA, Mechanick JJ (2014) Carnitine deficiency in chronic critical illness. Curr Opin Clin Nutr Metab Care 179:200–209

3. Burdge GC, Calder PC (2015) Introduction to fatty acids and lipids. World Rev Nutr Diet 112:1–16
4. Calder PC (2010) Rationale and use of n-3 fatty acids in artificial nutrition. Proc Nutr Soc 69:565–573
5. Calder PC (2013) Lipids for intravenous nutrition in hospitalised adult patients: a multiple choice of options. Proc Nutr Soc 72:263–276
6. Calder PC (2015) Functional roles of fatty acids and their effects on human health. J Parenter Enteral Nutr 39:18S–32S
7. Calder PC (2016) Fatty acids: metabolism. In: Caballero B, Finglas P, Toldrá F (eds) The encyclopedia of food and health, vol 2. Academic, Oxford, pp 632–644
8. Calder PC, Deckelbaum RJ (2013) Intravenous fish oil in hospitalized adult patients: reviewing the reviews. Curr Opin Clin Nutr Metab Care 16:119–123
9. Calder PC, Jensen GL, Koletzko BV, Singer P, Wanten GJ (2010) Lipid emulsions in parenteral nutrition of intensive care patients: current thinking and future directions. Intensive Care Med 36:735–749
10. Caresta E, Pierro A, Chowdhury M, Peters MJ, Piastra M, Eaton S (2007) Oxidation of intravenous lipid in infants and children with systemic inflammatory response syndrome and sepsis. Pediatr Res 61:228–232
11. Carpentier YA, Scruel O (2002) Changes in the concentration and composition of plasma lipoproteins during the acute phase response. Curr Opin Clin Nutr Metab Care 5:153–158
12. Chien JY, Jih-Shuin J, Chong-Jen Y, Pan-Chyr Y (2005) Low serum level of high-density lipoprotein cholesterol is a poor prognostic factor for severe sepsis. Crit Care Med 33: 1688–1693
13. de Luca C, Olefsky JM (2006) Stressed out about obesity and insulin resistance. Nat Med 12:41–42
14. Druml W, Fischer M, Ratheiser K (1998) Use of intravenous lipids in critically ill patients with sepsis without and with hepatic failure. J Parenter Enteral Nutr 22:217–223
15. Frayn KN (2010) Metabolic regulation: a human perspective. Wiley-Blackwell, Chichester
16. Green P, Theilla M, Singer P (2016) Lipid metabolism in critical illness. Curr Opin Clin Nutr Metab Care 19:111–115
17. Hill AG, Hill GL (1998) Metabolic response to severe injury. Br J Surg 85:884–890
18. Hotamisligil GS, Shargill NS, Spiegelman BM (1993) Adipose expression of tumor necrosis factor-alpha: direct role in obesity-linked insulin resistance. Science 259:87–91
19. Hultin M, Mullertz A, Zundel MA, Olivecronna G, Hansen TT, Deckelbaum RJ, Carpentier YA, Olivecronna T (1994) Metabolism of emulsions containing medium- and long-chain triglycerides or interesterified triglycerides. J Lipid Res 35:1850–1860
20. Jones AE, Stolinski M, Smith RD, Murphy JL, Wootton SA (1999) Effect of fatty acid chain length and saturation on the gastrointestinal handling and metabolic disposal of dietary fatty acids in women. Br J Nutr 81:37–43
21. Jones PJ, Pencharz PB, Clandinin MT (1985) Whole body oxidation of dietary fatty acids: implications for energy utilization. Am J Clin Nutr 42:769–777
22. Lekkou A, Mouzaki A, Siagris D, Ravani I, Gogos CA (2014) Serum lipid profile, cytokine production, and clinical outcome in patients with severe sepsis. J Crit Care 29:723–727
23. Murphy JL, Jones A, Brookes S, Wootton SA (1995) The gastrointestinal handling and metabolism of [1-^{13}C]palmitic acid in healthy women. Lipids 30:291–298
24. Murphy JL, Laiho KM, Jones AE, Wootton SA (1998) Metabolic handling of 13C labelled tripalmitin in healthy controls and patients with cystic fibrosis. Arch Dis Child 79:44–47
25. Olefsky JM, Glass CK (2010) Macrophages, inflammation, and insulin resistance. Annu Rev Physiol 72:219–246
26. Richelle M, Deckelbaum RJ, Vanweyenberg V, Carpentier YA (1997) Lipoprotein metabolism during and after a 6-h infusion of MCT/LCT vs LCT emulsion in man. Clin Nutr 16:119–123
27. Simoens C, Deckelbaum RJ, Carpentier YA (2004) Metabolism of defined structured triglyceride particles compared to mixtures of medium and long chain triglycerides intravenously infused in dogs. Clin Nutr 23:665–672

28. Simoens CM, Deckelbaum RJ, Massaut JJ, Carpentier YA (2008) Inclusion of 10% fish oil in mixed medium-chain triacylglycerol-long-chain triacylglycerol emulsions increases plasma triacylglycerol clearance and induces rapid eicosapentaenoic acid (20:5n-3) incorporation into blood cell phospholipids. Am J Clin Nutr 88:282–288
29. Singer P, Berger MM, Van den Berghe G, Biolo G, Calder P, Forbes A, Griffiths R, Kreyman G, Leverve X, Pichard C (2009) ESPEN guidelines on parenteral nutrition: intensive care. Clin Nutr 28:387–400
30. Tappy L, Chiolero R (2007) Substrate utilization in sepsis and multiple organ failure. Crit Care Med 35:S531–S534
31. Tappy L, Schwarz J-M, Schneiter P, Cayeux C, Revelly J-P, Fagerquist C, Jequier E, Chiolero R (1998) Effects of isoenergetic glucose-based or lipid-based parenteral nutrition on glucose metabolism, de novo lipogenesis, and respiratory gas exchanges in critically ill patients. Crit Care Med 26:860–867
32. Tilg H, Moschen AR (2006) Adipocytokines: mediators linking adipose tissue, inflammation and immunity. Nat Rev Immunol 6:772–783

Chapter 7
The Stress Response of Critical Illness: Metabolic and Hormonal Aspects

Luc Tappy

Abstract Stress responses are essentially elicited by conditions threatening animal's survival, and elicit coordinated adaptation with the immediate goal of prevent death. Although it was initially proposed that all stressors elicited stereotyped neuro-endocrine responses, it is now well recognized that there are important variations in the pattern of responses according to specific stressors. Hypovolemia or low blood pressure essentially activates sympathetic nervous centres, resulting in arteriolar constriction and increased systemic vascular resistance. Hypoglycemia and mental stress in addition activate the release of liver glycogen stores through activation of both the sympathetic nervous system and the hypothalamo-pituitary axis.

Critically ill patients are typically submitted to various stressors simultaneously. The relative importance of cardiogenic shock, hemodynamic alterations due to sepsis, and catabolic responses varies according to their initial condition and their responses to treatment. They often present initially with prominent hemodynamic disorders and activation of the sympaho-adrenal system. This phase is usually transient in survivorsis followed by increased energy expenditure (associated or not with fever) and a high turnover of energy substrate. The stress responses to critical illness have strong impact on blood glucose homeostasis, and invariably lead to increased blood glucose concentrations. Increased blood glucose in the consequence of a marked stimulation of endogenous glucose production, mainly secondary to enhanced hepatic gluconeogenesis, and to decreased glucose transport in insulin-dependent tissues such as skeletal muscle and adipose tissue.

L. Tappy, MD
Department of Physiology, University of Lausanne School of Biology and Medicine, Lausanne, Switzerland
e-mail: Luc.Tappy@unil.ch

J.-C. Preiser (ed.), *The Stress Response of Critical Illness: Metabolic and Hormonal Aspects*, DOI 10.1007/978-3-319-27687-8_7

7.1 Introduction: What Is Stress?

Stress is one of the most frequently used words nowadays, but its actual meaning is not well defined. In everyday life, people often talk of stress to refer to conditions as various as having to deal with an adverse environment at work, having to face a work overload, being anxious before playing a sport game, or giving a public performance, etc. In physiology and medicine, its use is somewhat more focused to refer to conditions representing a threat to the organism or disturbing the composition of the internal milieu. However, there is neither a universal definition of stress nor an agreement among scientist regarding its physiological functions.

Much of the present research was initiated in the 1950s when Selye reported that mice showed the same set of acute reactions, composed of adrenal hypertrophy, acute gastrointestinal ulcers, and thymus atrophy, when exposed to experimental injuries as varied as bleeding, infection, trauma, surgery, burns, etc. [1]. This led to the concept that pathological conditions threatening the individual's survival were associated with unspecific, stereotyped answers, referred to as stress responses. In this context, stress can be defined as being the set of involuntary, reflex physiological responses to "the fact of being ill." It was subsequently recognized that these answers were mediated by both the autonomic nervous system and the endocrine system and aimed primarily at maintaining hemodynamics and cells' energy production. The concept of stereotyped stress answers is now recognized to be an oversimplification, and one may recognize several patterns of stress responses which vary according to the initial stimulus or stressor. These various patterns most likely appeared progressively during evolution, involve different brain structures, and have different functional purposes [28].

Stress responses are essentially elicited by conditions threatening the animal's survival and elicit coordinated adaptation with the immediate goal of preventing death [28]. As their simplest expression, such survival responses will be activated when substrate supply to tissues becomes insufficient to ensure energy production. In humans and other warm-blooded animals, this can acutely occur when access to oxygen is impaired (breathing oxygen-devoid air, acute respiratory failure), when arterial circulation to organs is impaired (massive hemorrhage, cardiac failure, arterial collapse), or when oxygen transport in the blood is deficient (severe anemia, hemolysis). This may also occur when blood energy substrate levels become abnormally low, as during hypoglycemia. Given the absolute need of oxygen delivery to the brain and to vital organs, animals have evolved with efficient structures allowing to detect a low arterial pressure (baroreceptors located in the arterial system) and arterial hypoxia and its accompanying hypercapnia (carotid and aortic bodies, central respiratory chemoreceptors). In case of an injury resulting in acute hemorrhage, low cardiac output, and tissue hypoxia, activation of these sensors elicits immediate response to ensure that a sufficient amount of oxygen is delivered to the brain (Fig. 7.1).

Of importance, cells need a constant supply of ATP in order to achieve their specialized function. Their energy turnover will increase in proportion to their

Fig. 7.1 Overview of stress responses and adaptive hemodynamic changes to low blood volume and low cardiac output

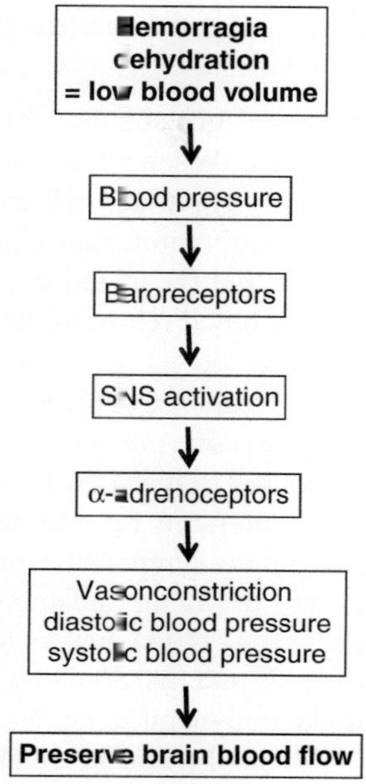

activity (i.e., mechanical work in skeletal muscle, metabolic processes in the liver, synthesis and secretion of cytokines and antibodies in immune cells, etc.) and will vary according to physiological conditions. Increased ATP will be signaled by physiological local mechanisms such as changes in intracellular physicochemical properties during muscle contraction and to interorgan information conveyed by the nervous and endocrine systems. Stimulation of ATP use in response to a physiological stimulation (e.g., voluntary muscle contraction) will result in increased intracellular ADP, which will secondarily stimulate energy substrate catabolism and oxidative phosphorylation [2]. The energy metabolism of any organ therefore depends primarily of its physiological workload. It however depends also on adequate energy substrate and oxygen availability and hence on adequate levels of energy substrate and oxygen in blood and on adequate local blood flow [3]. These are generally not limiting in resting conditions but may become so during exercise in pathological conditions such as myocardial infarction or hemorrhagic shock.

7.2 Main Stressors and Patterns of Stress Responses

Although it was initially proposed that all stressors elicited a set of stereotyped neuroendocrine response, it is now well recognized that there are important variations in the pattern of responses according to specific stressors [4, 5]. In a very schematic and simplified way, one may identify some of the specific responses elicited by a few "basic" stressors:

7.2.1 Low Cardiac Blood Flow

A low oxygen and nutrient delivery represents a threat for any organ or tissue of the organism. When a low cardiac output and systemic arterial flow causes generalized lack of oxygen and substrates, it represents an acute threat for survival and elicits accordingly immediate corrective responses. Whatever the initial cause for low cardiac output (heart failure, severe hemorrhage, or massive venodilation decreasing venous blood return to the heart), it invariably results in a decreased arterial blood pressure.

The response to acute hemorrhage can be assessed clinically by applying a lower body negative pressure, thus decreasing venous blood return to the heart. The stress responses to lower body negative pressure rest essentially on the detection of low blood pressure by arterial baroreceptors and elicit a reflex activation of alpha-adrenergic sympathetic nerves targeted to arterioles of most organs and tissues except the brain and the heart [6]. It thus limits the drop of blood pressure by decreasing blood flow to nonessential organs. There is little activation of the adrenal medulla and hypothalamo-pituitary axis in this setting, and the effects are primarily on hemodynamics, i.e., increased diastolic blood pressure.

Metabolic effects are also observed as a consequence of compromised hemodynamics in critically ill patients; they are mainly secondary to low blood flow to organs and tissue and can include a decreased whole-body energy expenditure and muscle insulin resistance [7].

7.2.2 Low-Energy Substrate Availability

The healthy human organism has sufficient endogenous energy stores to meet its global energy requirements even when not fed over several days. Most of it is stored as fat in subcutaneous adipose tissue, while glycogen stores are limited to a few 100 g, mainly in the liver and skeletal muscle. Since the brain, unless other organs, essentially relies on glucose oxidation for energy production, the human organism has developed tight regulatory mechanisms to ensure a constant blood glucose supply. Given the absolute requirements of brain for glucose, there is no surprise that an abnormal drop in blood glucose elicits immediate stress responses (Fig. 7.2). These are initiated by activation of nervous (hypothalamic) cells which have glucose-sensing properties due to the presence of GLUT2 transporter and of glucokinase, both characterized by a high Km for glucose. Activation of these cells by low blood glucose stimulates the adrenal medulla to release epinephrine and increases the secretion of cortisol. Hypoglycemia also stimulates the release of glucagon and growth hormone. The effects of increased blood levels of these hormones result in the release of blood glucose from the liver [8, 9]. Simultaneously, the increase in fatty acids released from adipose tissue [10] and direct diabetogenic effects of adrenaline and growth hormones [11] decrease insulin sensitivity, thus sparing glucose to restore normoglycemia and fuel the brain. Beside these compensatory metabolic effects, activation of the sympathetic nervous system also increases heart rate and blood pressure, while epinephrine exerts inotropic effects to increase cardiac output.

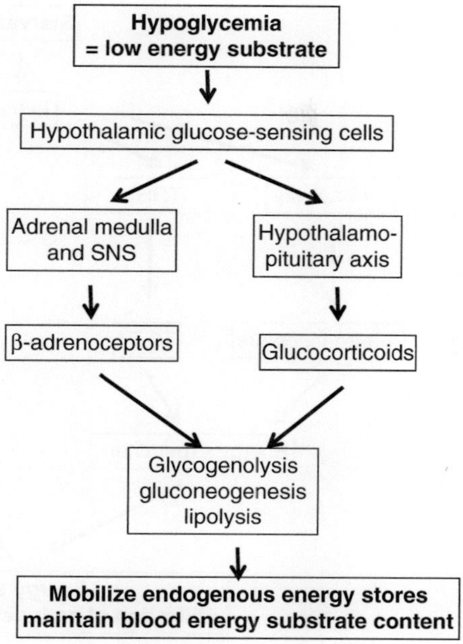

Fig. 7.2 Overview of metabolic adaptations to hypoglycemia

7.2.3 *Starvation*

Failure to feed oneself, if long-lasting, represents an important threat to the organism. In spite of sufficient energy stores to survive and meet daily energy requirements for several weeks, the organism has limited stores of liver glycogen which can be released as blood glucose. In the initial hours of fasting, a low insulin secretion and a release of glucagon, cortisol, epinephrine, and growth hormones stimulate hepatic glycogenolysis and gluconeogenesis. Hepatic glycogen stores are however exhausted in less than 24 h fasting, and the organism thereafter has to rely entirely on gluconeogenesis from amino acids to produce glucose. Knowing the brain consumes about 125 g glucose daily, this would correspond to the breakdown of about 250 g protein daily and would rapidly exhaust protein stores if no further adaptations occurred. Specific adaptations to starvation (Fig. 7.3) include stimulation of adipose lipolysis and of hepatic ketogenesis by glucagon, cortisol, growth hormone, and epinephrine [12]. The increased blood ketone bodies' concentration in turn stimulates the expression of monocarboxylate transporters on neuron membranes and increases ketone bodies' utilization by neurons, thus sparing glucose utilization endogenous protein breakdown [13]. In addition adaptations aimed at reducing energy needs are initiated by an inhibition of leptin secretion by adipocytes. The ensuing low blood leptin levels stimulate the expression of the orexigenic neuropeptide Y (NPY) in the hypothalamus, which produces the feeling of hunger and triggers food-seeking behavior but also decreases sympathetic nervous system activity and increases cortisol secretion. Low leptin concentrations also inhibit thyroid hormone secretion and the hypophyso-gonadal axis. Decreased sympathetic activity, low thyroid hormone, and prevention of energy requiring pregnancies all aim at reducing energy requirements to face potentially long-lasting starvation [14].

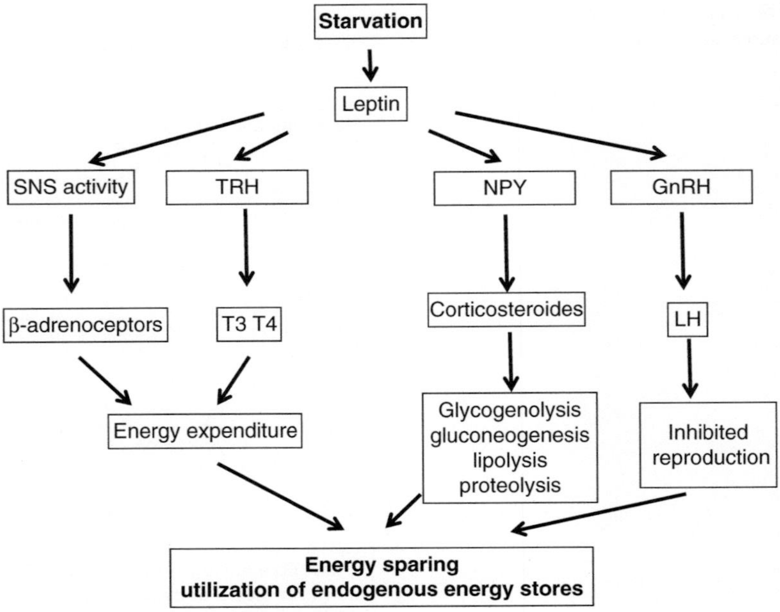

Fig. 7.3 Neuroendocrine and metabolic responses to starvation

7.2.4 Escaping Predators

In wild animals, most injuries occur as a consequence of being attacked by a predator (and being fortunate enough to be only wounded instead of being killed and eaten). Injury may result in hemorrhagic shock and impaired functional abilities, including impaired ability to feed oneself. They will eventually be effective to support life on a short-term basis, but long-term survival will depend on successful healing processes, reparation of initial injuries, and resuming food intake. The best chances to survive a predator would be to avoid being eaten or hurt, however. This is best done by outrunning the predator. In case it is not possible, the only remaining option is to oppose it by strength and defeat it. In this setting, survival will eventually depend on the muscle function and hence on both oxygen and substrate supply to muscle. Interestingly, stress responses have developed to support this "fight or flight" reaction (Fig. 7.4) [15]. These stress responses anticipate any actual injury and depend on advanced cognitive functions, which are mainly carried out by the mesolimbic system. They can be elicited in animals and humans by various procedures usually referred to as mental stress: immobilization for animals, complex mental mathematics or speaking in front of an audience for humans, etc. [16–18].

Mental stress (Fig. 7.4) involves the simultaneous activation of the hypothalamo-pituitary-adrenal axis, the adrenal medulla, and the sympathetic nervous system. One major effect is to boost the cardiovascular system in order to maintain brain blood flow but at the same time increase muscle blood flow. Chronotropic and inotropic effects of epinephrine are responsible for an increased cardiac output. In addi-

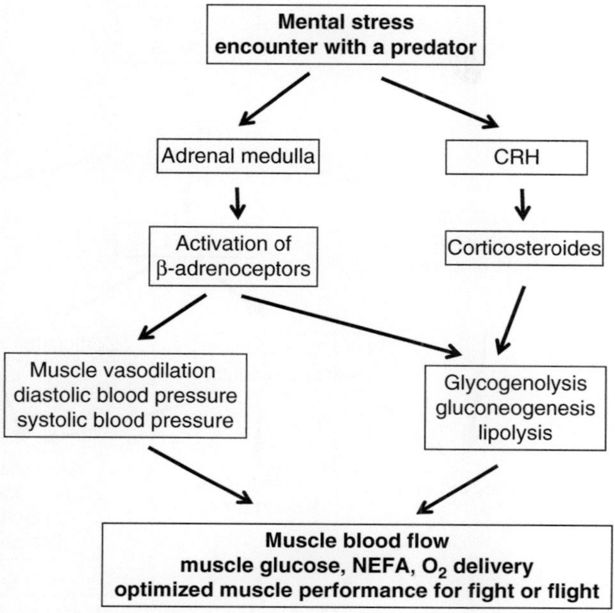

Fig. 7.4 Overview of metabolic and hemodynamic responses to mental stress

tion, activation of beta-adrenergic sympathetic nerve fibers targeted to skeletal muscle produce muscle vasodilation, decrease peripheral insulin resistance, and thus increase muscle blood flow. These vasodilatory sympathetic nerve fibers have different properties than those activated by hemorrhage or low blood pressure, which caused peripheral vasoconstriction and increased systemic vascular resistances [16–18]. The other major effect of mental stress is to stimulate the mobilization of energy stores. Epinephrine and cortisol stimulate hepatic glycogenolysis, gluconeogenesis, and hepatic glucose production, thus increasing blood glucose levels [19]. Epinephrine also activates adipose tissue lipolysis and increases blood NEFA concentrations. Together, the hemodynamic and metabolic effects of mental stress increase the delivery of both energy substrate and oxygen to skeletal muscle [16].

7.2.5 *Infection and Inflammation as Stressors*

Circulatory shock and hypoxia are clearly acute, life-threatening conditions which elicit strong, immediate counter-regulatory responses. They are not the sole conditions which threaten homeostasis and may be seen as stressors, however, and numerous conditions (hydro-electrolytic disorders, endocrine dysfunctions, tumors, and many others) will also elicit various regulatory responses. Of special interest for critical care patients, bacterial and viral infections are common conditions which may represent a major threat to homeostasis. Infection also invariably results in the lysis of host cells and in areas of necrosis in infected organs, which will require healing and repair at a later stage [20]. In a similar way, traumatic injury can cause

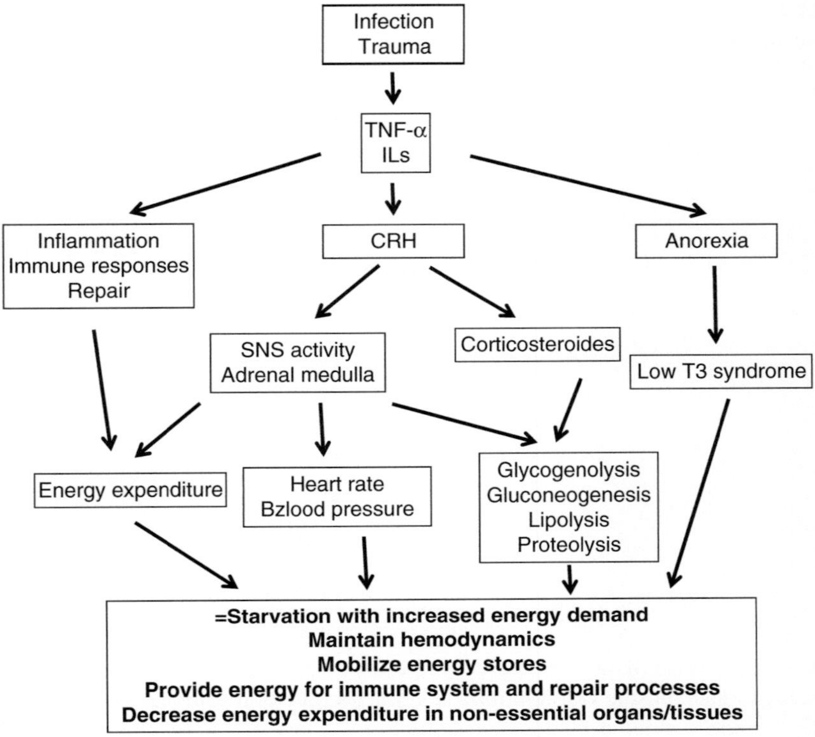

Fig. 7.5 Mixed metabolic alterations observed in critically ill patients

the necrosis of tissues which require healing. In response to these specific needs, activation of immune cells by microbial antigens or endotoxin triggers the chain release of cytokines (TNF-alpha, IL-1, IL-2, IL-6), which orchestrate the differentiation, proliferation, and coordinate actions of lymphocytes and macrophages [20, 21]. Cytokines also orchestrate the metabolic adaptations needed for eradication of microbial agents and for tissue repair. Schematically, TNF-alpha is one of the earlier cytokines produced during severe infection or injury. It is responsible for anorexia and fever on one hand, for chain activation of other cytokines, and for initiation of immune responses and repair (Fig. 7.5). In contrast with starvation, anorexia is not associated with energy-sparing adaptations, since metabolic rate increases in response to fever and since immune cells and repair mechanisms require energy and amino acids. This may be explained by the fact that inflammation-associated anorexia is not associated with activation of NPY in the hypothalamus. Instead, TNF-alpha directly induces anorexia while simultaneously activating the hypothalamo-pituitary axis by triggering the release of the hypothalamic corticotropin-releasing hormone (CRH) [22].

Metabolic effects of inflammation paradoxically include both anorexia and an increased energy expenditure. Metabolic effects of TNF-alpha and IL-1, together with the other cytokines and inflammatory mediators, contribute to face this challenge by impairing insulin-mediated glucose utilization in skeletal muscle, thus sparing blood glucose for the central nervous system and immune cells. The latter are characterized by an important glycolytic metabolism, at the origin of an increased glucose-lactate cycling. Simultaneously, the activation of the hypothalamo-pituitary-adrenal axis and of the sympathoadrenal system also is responsible for increased lipolysis and proteolysis (the latter occurring mainly in skeletal muscle) [22–24].

7.3 Stress Responses in Critically Ill Patients

For what regards stress responses and metabolic adaptations, critically ill patients as encountered in our present intensive care units represent a special population of subjects who have been or are submitted to many stressors simultaneously. In many regards, they do not fit in a physiological categorization, however, since responses to severe injury merely represent the best way to temporarily deal with severe threats. In this setting, anorexia prevents digestive organs' energy and oxygen consumption, and cytokines and stress hormones operate a massive mobilization of endogenous energy stores to provide energy to the brain for its survival and to immune cells for repair mechanisms. In that, it represents a paradoxical condition of starvation associated with increased energy and protein needs, which cannot be normally sustained in the long term, as the lean body mass is rapidly eroded. The spontaneous evolution of such patients would be either a rapid recovery resulting in recovery or death. The presence of critically ill patients in intensive care units for sometimes several weeks is clearly the consequence of medical and nursing progresses but faces us with a condition which may be called "pathological starvation," i.e., continuous endogenous protein breakdown together with a resistance to normal energy-sparing mechanisms and to anabolic factors. This leads to loss of lean body mass, enteral or parenteral nutrition at times inefficient, increased stay in ICU, and delayed recovery.

Critically ill patients are usually exposed to all of the abovementioned basic stressors at some time during their course. The relative importance of cardiogenic shock, hemodynamic alterations due to sepsis, and catabolic responses varies according to their initial condition and their responses to treatment. Typically patients with severe initial injuries (polytrauma patients, burn patients) and patients after cardiac surgery initially have prominent hemodynamic disorders. In such patients, blood flow is the main limiting factor and activation of the sympathoadrenal system is prominent. Energy expenditure is usually not increased and may even be low in some patients. This phase, often referred to as the "ebb phase" [25], is usually transient in survivors. In contrast, patients without prominent hemodynamic failure are characterized by increased energy expenditure (associated or not with fever) and a high turnover of energy substrate. This condition often follows the "ebb phase" after resuscitation of hemodynamically compromised patients and is often referred to as the "flow phase" [25]. It is characterized by insulin resistance as a consequence of endogenous cortisol and epinephrine and of endogenous and sometimes of exogenous drugs [25, 26].

The stress responses to critical illness have strong impact on blood glucose homeostasis and invariably lead to increased blood glucose concentrations.

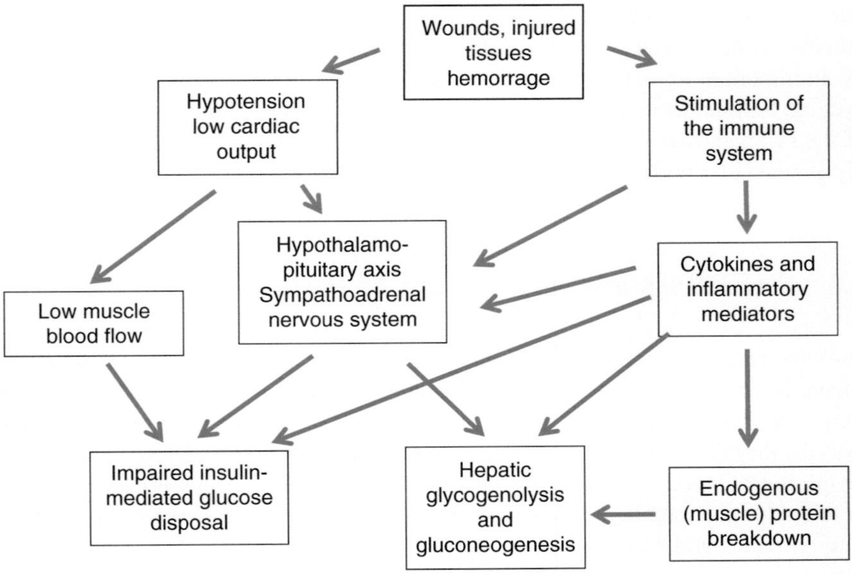

Fig. 7.6 Metabolic adaptations to critical illness. Injury, inflammation, and hemodynamic alterations secondary to the primary illness elicit a secretion of stress hormones, cytokines, and inflammatory mediators. These in turn stimulate endogenous protein breakdown and impair glucose homeostasis

Increased blood glucose is the consequence of a marked stimulation of endogenous glucose production, mainly secondary to enhanced hepatic gluconeogenesis, and to decreased glucose transport in insulin-dependent tissues such skeletal muscle and adipose tissue. These metabolic changes are secondary to both stress hormone release and to inflammatory mediators and to hemodynamic factors, as depicted in Fig. 7.6. In critical illnesses, inflammation can be severe and stimulation of stress hormone release can be massive, resulting at times to markedly elevated blood glucose concentrations [27]. This corresponds to a change from normal glucose homeostasis, which may be presented as "pathological" (i.e., stress-induced diabetes) but may also be seen as a "normal" deviation from normal homeostatic set points: in this perspective, an increase in blood glucose occurs as part of an "allostatic response" to allow beneficial effects of high blood glucose in this particular setting [28]. Hyperglycemia in critically ill patients may therefore exert simultaneous beneficial and deleterious effects, as depicted in Fig. 7.7. On one hand, it ensures that blood glucose remain available to the brain; this is a high priority in critical illness since metabolic responses to inflammation prevent the normal metabolic adaptations to fasting. In addition, hyperglycemia together with insulin resistance stimulates non-insulin-dependent glucose transport in inflammatory cells, which mainly rely on glycolytic metabolism. This effect is instrumental in providing a constant energy supply to support immune responses and repair mechanism. On the other hand, metabolic adaptations to critical illness may have adverse effects since high

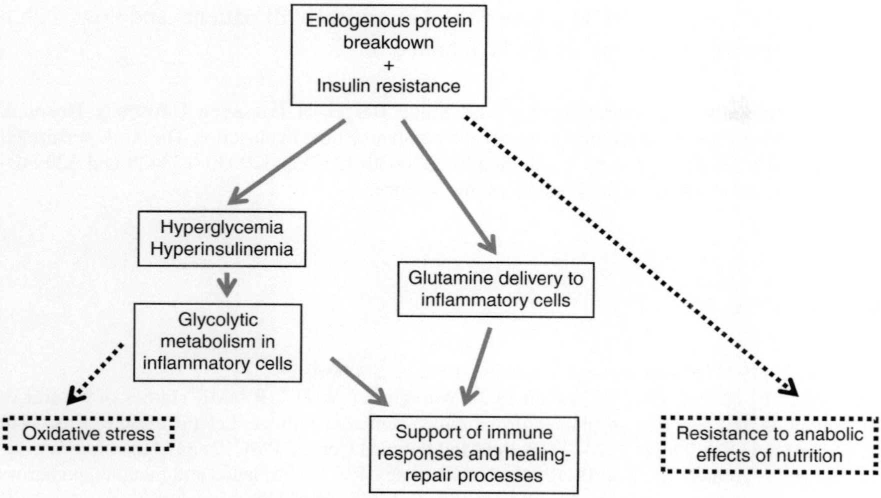

Fig. 7.7 Potentially beneficial (*solid lines*) and deleterious (*dotted lines*) effects of metabolic adaptations to critical illness

blood glucose can induce oxidative damages, while insulin resistance and high levels of stress hormones may lead to a state of "resistance to the anabolic effects of nutrition" [29].

7.4 Conclusion

Humans have developed various patterns of stress responses, each of them suited to adapt to specific life-threatening situations. Stress responses certainly have many beneficial effects which improve the immediate outcome of patients with severe acute illnesses, at least until they gain medical attention. However, once patients have been admitted to the intensive care units and receive hemodynamic and nutritional support, continuing stress responses may also have significant adverse effects. Stress invariably results in a coordinated release of endogenous energy stores. This enhances the odds of survival in acutely injured subjects unable to feed themselves but results in some degree of "resistance" to enteral or parenteral nutrition. One of the foremost consequences of stress responses is the development of hyperglycemia, which may in the long term have adverse effects on patients' outcome, presumably due to oxidative damages induced by hyperglycemia. The control of hyperglycemia has thus become one of the major metabolic issues in critically ill patients and has been reported to dramatically improve patients' outcome [30]. However, it has also been observed that attempts to achieve a tight, "physiological" blood glucose control were associated with an increased risk of hyperglycemia and adverse outcomes [31]. It remains yet to be determined which would be an "optimal" blood glucose level in critically ill patients and how such a blood glucose level can practically be attained.

Acknowledgments The author thanks Prof. Mette Berger of Lausanne University Hospital, Lausanne, Switzerland, for having reviewed and commented the manuscript. The work performed in the author's laboratory has by grants number 320030–135782, 320030–138428 and 32003B-156167 from the Swiss National Foundation for Science.

References

1. Selye H (1971) Hormones and resistance. J Pharm Sci 60:1–28
2. Chance B, Eleff S, Bank W, Leigh JS Jr, Warnell R (1982) 31P NMR studies of control of mitochondrial function in phosphofructokinase-deficient human skeletal muscle. Proc Natl Acad Sci U S A 79(24):7714–7718, PubMed Pubmed Central PMCID: 347418
3. Turner N, Hulbert AJ, Else PL (2006) Limits to physical performance and metabolism across species. Curr Opin Clin Nutr Metab Care 9(6):691–696, PubMed
4. Seematter G, Binnert C, Martin JL, Tappy L (2004) Relationship between stress, inflammation and metabolism. Curr Opin Clin Nutr Metab Care 7(2):169–173, PubMed
5. Esler M (2010) The 2009 Carl Ludwig Lecture: pathophysiology of the human sympathetic nervous system in cardiovascular diseases: the transition from mechanisms to medical management. JAP 108(2):227–237, PubMed Epub 2009/11/27. eng
6. Ryan KL, Rickards CA, Hinojosa-Laborde C, Cooke WH, Convertino VA (2012) Sympathetic responses to central hypovolemia: new insights from microneurographic recordings. Front Physiol 3:110, PubMed Pubmed Central PMCID: 3337468
7. Puhakka K, Rasanen J, Leijala M, Peltola K (1994) Oxygen consumption following pediatric cardiac surgery. J Cardiothorac Vasc Anesth 8(6):642–648, PubMed
8. Guenat E, Seematter G, Philippe J, Temler E, Jequier E, Tappy L (2000) Counterregulatory responses to hypoglycemia in patients with glucokinase gene mutations. Diabetes Metab 26(5):377–384, PubMed Epub 2000/12/19. eng
9. Postic C, Shiota M, Magnuson MA (2001) Cell-specific roles of glucokinase in glucose homeostasis. RPHR 56:195–217, PubMed Epub 2001/03/10. eng
10. Boden G (1997) Role of fatty acids in the pathogenesis of insulin resistance and NIDDM. Diabetes 46(1):3–10, PubMed
11. Shamoon H, Hendler R, Sherwin RS (1981) Synergistic interactions among antiinsulin hormones in the pathogenesis of stress hyperglycemia in humans. JCEM 52:1235–1241
12. Cahill GF (1970) Starvation in man. NEJM 282:668–675
13. Schutkowski A, Wege N, Stangl GI, Konig B (2014) Tissue-specific expression of monocarboxylate transporters during fasting in mice. PLoS One 9(11):e112118, PubMed Pubmed Central PMCID: 4229183
14. Ahima RS, Prabakaran D, Mantzoros C, Qu D, Lowwel B, Maratos-Flier E et al (1996) Role of leptin in the neuroendocrine response to fasting. Nature 382:250–252
15. Jansen AS, Nguyen XV, Karpitskiy V, Mettenleiter TC, Loewy AD (1995) Central command neurons of the sympathetic nervous system: basis of the fight-or-flight response. Science 270(5236):644–646, PubMed
16. Seematter G, Guenat E, Schneiter P, Cayeux C, Jéquier E, Tappy L (2000) Effects of mental stress on insulin-mediated glucose metabolism and energy expenditure in lean and obese women. AJP 279:E799–E805
17. Moan A, Hoieggen A, Nordby G, Os I, Eide I, Kjeldsen SE (1995) Mental stress increases glucose uptake during hyperinsulinemia: associations with sympathetic and cardiovascular responsiveness. Metab Clin Exp 44(10):1303–1307

18. Linde B, Hjemdahl P, Freyschuss U, Juhlin-Dannfelt A (1989) Adipose tissue and skeletal muscle blood flow during mental stress. AJP 256(1 Pt 1):E12–E18
19. Jern S (1991) Effects of acute carbohydrate administration on central and peripheral hemodynamic responses to mental stress. Hypertension 18(6):790–797, PubMed
20. Kadhim HJ, Duchateau J, Sebire G (2008) Cytokines and brain injury: invited review. J Intensive Care Med 23(4):236–249, PubMed
21. Surbatovic M, Veljovic M, Jevdjic J, Popovic N, Djordjevic D, Radakovic S (2013) Immunoinflammatory response in critically ill patients: severe sepsis and/or trauma. Mediators Inflamm 2013:362793, PubMed Pubmed Central PMCID: 3859159
22. McMinn JE, Baskin DG, Schwartz MW (2000) Neuroendocrine mechanisms regulating food intake and body weight. Obes Rev 1(1):37–46, PubMed
23. Michie HR, Sherman ML, Spriggs DR, Rounds J, Christie M, Wilmore DW (1989) Chronic TNF infusion causes anorexia but not accelerated nitrogen loss. Ann Surg 209(1):19–24, PubMed Pubmed Central PMCID: 1493883
24. Lang CH, Dobrescu C, Bagby GJ (1992) Tumor necrosis factor impairs insulin action on peripheral glucose disposal and hepatic glucose output. Endocrinology 130(1):43–52, PubMed
25. Wilmore DW, Aulick LH, Mason AD, Pruitt BA (1977) Influence of the burn wound on local and systemic responses to injury. AS 186:444–456
26. Ruttimann Y, Schutz Y, Jéquier E, Lemarchand T, Chioléro R (1991) Thermogenic and metabolic effects of dopamine in healthy men. CCM 19:1030–1036
27. Tappy L, Chiolero R (2007) Substrate utilization in sepsis and multiple organ failure. Crit Care Med 35(9 Suppl):S531–S534, PubMed
28. McEwen BS (2007) Physiology and neurobiology of stress and adaptation: central role of the brain. Physiol Rev 87(3):873–904, PubMed
29. Ling PR, Smith RJ, Bistrian BR (2007) Acute effects of hyperglycemia and hyperinsulinemia on hepatic oxidative stress and the systemic inflammatory response in rats. Crit Care Med 35(2):555–560, PubMed
30. Van den Berghe G, Wouters P, Weekers F, Verwaest C, Bruyninckx F, Schetz M et al (2001) Intensive insulin therapy in the critically ill patients. N Engl J Med 345:1359–1367
31. Investigators N-SS, Finfer S, Chittock DR, Su SY, Blair D, Foster D et al (2009) Intensive versus conventional glucose control in critically ill patients. N Engl J Med 360(13):1283–1297, PubMed

Chapter 8
Stress Hyperglycemia

Jean-Charles Preiser, Aurélie Thooft, and Rafael Machado Tironi

Abstract The understanding and management of stress hyperglycemia has dramatically changed since 2001. In addition to the development of insulin resistance, stress hyperglycemia is characterised by a poorly inhibitable endogenous production of glucose leading to a severe hyperglycemia. The toxicity of hyperglycemia have been supported by numerous association studies, which reported strong correlations between the magnitude of hyperglycemia and poor outcome. However, tight glycemic control by intensive insulin therapy has not been improved outcomes in most interventional studies and is currently not recommended.

Before 2001, the hyperglycemia found in most critically ill patients was considered as a component of the stress response [1]. Current understanding was completely changed by the publication of the first Leuven study article in 2001 [2]. This investigation compared an intensive insulin regimen targeting a blood glucose level within the 80–110 mg/dL range with a "conventional" management cohort in which blood glucose was treated only when above 200 mg/dL. Van den Berghe and colleagues found a 4 % decrease in the absolute mortality of critically ill patients randomized to intensive insulin therapy. These unexpectedly impressive results triggered a huge wave of enthusiasm. Recommendations to implement tight glucose control in intensive care units (ICUs) were rapidly issued by several healthcare agencies (the Joint Commission on Accreditation of Healthcare Organization, the Institute for Healthcare Improvement, and the Volunteer Hospital Organization). Simultaneously, several different teams tried to reproduce the results and to examine the underlying mechanisms of the findings of the Leuven team. Overall, the results

J.-C. Preiser, MD, PhD (✉) • A. Thooft, MD • R.M. Tironi, MD
Department of Intensive Care, Erasme University Hospital, Université libre de Bruxelles, 808 route de Lennik, Brussels B-1070, Belgium
e-mail: Jean-Charles.Preiser@erasme.ulb.ac.be

J.-C. Preiser (ed.), *The Stress Response of Critical Illness: Metabolic and Hormonal Aspects*, DOI 10.1007/978-3-319-27687-8_8

of the Leuven study have not been reproduced [3–11]. Nonetheless, these follow-up studies have given rise to several controversies, shed light on the pathophysiology of stress hyperglycemia, and raised important but as yet unanswered questions for the physicians taking care of critically ill patients, including the optimal value of blood glucose, the risks associated with hypoglycemia, and the categories of patient might benefit from tight glucose control by intensive insulin therapy.

8.1 Pathophysiology

It has long been recognized that critically ill patients tend to be hyperglycemic [1]. For many years, this was attributed to stress and was believed to be a part of the adaptive host response to critical illness and designed to provide high amounts of glucose to white blood cells and other obligatory glucose users. Because the blood supply to injured tissue often has been interrupted or diminished, delivery is primarily through mass action across the intracellular matrix. Thus, hyperglycemia was believed to be a biomarker of the severity of illness. The Leuven studies [2, 3] started with the hypothesis that hyperglycemia was not just a biomarker. Rather, these investigators postulated that elevations in serum glucose contributed to the pathophysiology of critical illness. This proposal spawned the current field of investigation.

The physiology behind "stress hyperglycemia" is very different from type II diabetes (Table 8.1). In type II diabetes, the cause of hyperglycemia is a combination of insulin resistance and defective secretion of insulin by pancreatic β-cells. During stress

Table 8.1 Main differences between type II diabetes and stress hyperglycemia

	Diabetes	Stress hyperglycemia
Etiology	Combination of lifestyle and genetic factors	Secondary to trauma, surgery or acute illness
Glycosylated hemoglobin	Elevated if poorly controlled	Normal
Pathogenetic mechanisms	Insulin resistance Defective secretion of insulin (by pancreatic â-cells)	Interaction of regulatory hormones, cytokines Production of glucose by the liver Insulin resistance (IMGU tissues)
Causes of hypoglycemic episodes	Oral medications Insulin	Insulin therapy Interruption of carbohydrates infusion Severe sepsis, liver failure, adrenal insufficiency
Complications	Micro- and macroangiopathy (renal, cardiac, ocular, cerebral, and neurological)	Rather: *complications* related to 1° condition causing dysglycemia
Evolution	Chronic Not curable	Can disappear after resolution of acute illness Higher risk to develop type 2 diabetes
Treatment	Lifestyle Oral medications Insulin (added to oral medication when insufficient)	Treatment of underlying cause Insulin therapy

hyperglycemia, complex interactions between counter-regulatory hormones and cytokines lead to an excessive and non-inhibitable production of glucose associated with insulin resistance of the tissues where glucose uptake is insulin dependent (IMGU), perhaps as an adaptive response needed to promote survival during the acute phase [10, 11]. Indeed, this highly complex interplay is largely variable over time [1, 13].

The stress-related increase in hepatic output of glucose results from glycogenolysis and gluconeogenesis. Glycogenolysis is primarily triggered by catecholamines and perpetuated under the influence of epinephrine and cortisol. Gluconeogenesis is triggered to a larger extent by glucagon than by epinephrine and cortisol. Among the numerous inflammatory mediators released in the acutely ill, tumor necrosis factor-α (TNF-α) might promote gluconeogenesis by stimulating glucagon production. The increase in peripheral resistance is characterized by the inability of skeletal muscles and adipocytes to take up glucose, related to an alteration of insulin signaling and with a downregulation of type 4 glucose transporters (GLUT-4).

An increased glucose reabsorption or a decreased renal glucose clearance has also been reported and likely contribute to hyperglycemia in acute conditions [15]. In the postoperative patient, the surgical stress itself is an important trigger, via the induction of insulin resistance under the influence of cytokines and counter-regulatory hormones. The degree of insulin resistance has been related to the magnitude and the duration of the surgical stress. The avoidance of hypothermia, excessive blood losses, prolonged preoperative fasting period, and prolonged immobilization synergize to reduce perioperative insulin resistance.

8.2 Toxicity

In experimental conditions, concentrations of glucose higher than 300 mg/dL are clearly deleterious. New insights into the cellular mechanisms of glucose toxicity suggest a link among glucose, cytopathic hypoxia, and the production of reactive oxygen and nitrogen species [10, 13, 14]. However, the optimal blood glucose target is undefined yet and could differ according to the underlying condition, including the preexistence and the control of diabetes. Likewise, the ultimate proof that hyperglycemia is an independent risk factor for poor outcome in critically ill patients is lacking. Importantly, insulin exerts effects other than the promotion of glucose metabolism and utilization. These include vasodilatory, anti-inflammatory, and anti-apoptotic activities that can be viewed as a homeostatic control mechanism limiting some of the processes that occur in inflammation and other potentially injurious responses. The non-glycemic effects of insulin might also explain some of the beneficial effects of intensive insulin therapy.

In stress conditions, an overall massive glucose overload happens in organs where glucose uptake is not regulated by insulin, usually quoted as NIMGU (*non-insulin-mediated glucose uptake*) tissues under the influence of pro-inflammatory mediators, counter-regulatory hormones, and hypoxia [10]. Hence, a wide range of tissues, including hepatocytes, endothelial cells, neurons, nephrons, and immune cells, may be susceptible to enhanced glucose toxicity as a result of acute illness.

Several deleterious effects have been associated with these high glucose concentrations in cells [1, 12]. Damages to mitochondrial proteins occur, and the formation of reactive oxygen species (ROS) is increased as a consequence of the shift from glycolysis toward accessory metabolic pathways (pentose phosphate, hexosamines, polyols) [13]. Other effects of excess glucose concentrations include the exacerbation of inflammatory pathways, decreased complement activity, modifications in the innate immune system, impairment in endothelial and hepatic mitochondrial functions, abolishment of the ischemic preconditioning, and protein glycosylation. Acute complications attributed to stress hyperglycemia include renal failure, increased susceptibility to infections and polyneuropathy, and impaired microcirculation [1].

8.3 Clinical Associations Between Hyperglycemia and Poor Outcome

Quite consistently, retrospective studies performed on large cohorts of different categories of critically ill patients reported poorer outcome of patients who experienced dysglycemic events. However, the strength of the relationship between markers of dysglycemia and outcome is variable according to the diabetic status. Overall, admission hyperglycemia was found as an independent marker of mortality and morbidity [16–20].

After cardiac surgery, the occurrence of hyperglycemia 180 mg/dl was consistently and independently associated with a significant increase in both deep sternal wound infections and mortality [20–22].

Comparing the relationship between dysglycemia and outcome in diabetic and nondiabetic critically ill patients yielded interesting and consistent differences. Several studies consistently reported a flatter relationship or J-shaped curve between BG and mortality in diabetic than in nondiabetic patients [23–28].

8.4 Conclusions

A consistent and clear association between hyperglycemia and poor outcome is present in critically ill patients. These findings support the current recommendation of liberal glucose control by insulin, namely, in view of the risks associated with tighter therapeutic strategies [29–31]. The use of consistent indices of the three domains of dysglycemia (hyperglycemia, hypoglycemia, and high glycemic variability) is required to delineate the optimal BG target in different categories of patients, the logistical requirements for a safe and reliable glucose control, and to assess technical advances that could improve the quality and safety of glucose control [32].

References

1. Dungan KM, Braithwaite SS, Preiser JC (2009) Stress hyperglycaemia. Lancet 23: 1798–1807
2. Van den Berghe G, Wouters P, Weekers F et al (2001) Intensive insulin therapy in the critically ill patients. N Engl J Med 345:1359–1367
3. Van den Berghe G, Wilmer A, Hermans G et al (2006) Intensive insulin therapy in the medical ICU. N Engl J Med 3545:449–461
4. Arabi YM, Dabbagh OC, Tamin HM et al (2008) Intensive versus conventional insulin therapy: a randomized controlled trial in medical and surgical critically ill patients. Crit Care Med 36:3190–3197
5. De la Rosa GC, Donado JH, Restrepo AH et al (2008) Strict glycaemic control in patients hospitalized in a mixed medical and surgical intensive care unit: a randomized clinical trial. Crit Care 12:R120
6. Brunkhorst FM, Engel C, Bloos F et al (2008) Intensive insulin therapy and pentastarch resuscitation in severe sepsis? N Engl J Med 358:125–139
7. Preiser JC, Devos P, Ruiz-Santana S et al (2009) A prospective randomised multi-centre controlled trial on tight glucose control by intensive insulin therapy in adult intensive care units: the Glucontrol study. Intensive Care Med 35:1738–1748
8. NICE-SUGAR Study Investigators, Finfer S, Chittock DR et al (2009) Intensive versus conventional glucose control in critically ill patients. N Engl J Med 360:1283–1297
9. Marik P, Preiser JC (2010) Toward understanding tight glycemic control in the ICU: a systematic review and metaanalysis. Chest 137:544–551
10. Lena D, Kalfon P, Preiser JC, Ichai C (2011) Glycemic control in the intensive care unit and during the postoperative period. Anesthesiology 114:438–444
11. Marik PE, Bellomo R (2013) Stress hyperglycemia: an essential survival response! Crit Care 17:305
12. Preiser JC, Ichai C, Orban JC, Groeneveld AB (2014) Metabolic response to the stress of critical illness. Br J Anaesth 113:945–954
13. Brownlee M (2001) Biochemistry and molecular cell biology of diabetic complications. Nature 414:813–820
14. Bagry HS, Raghavendran S, Carli F, Phil M (2008) Metabolic syndrome and insulin resistance. Perioperative considerations. Anesthesiology 108:506–523
15. Sicardi SZ, Rodhe P, Hahn G (2006) Progressive decrease in glucose clearance during surgery. Acta Anaesthesiol Scand 50:848–854
16. Krinsley JS (2004) Effect of an intensive glucose management protocol on the mortality of critically ill adult patients. Mayo Clin Proc 79:992–1000
17. Finney SJ, Zekveld C, Elia A, Evans TW (2003) Glucose control and mortality in critically ill patients. JAMA 290:2041–2047
18. Falciglia M, Freyberg RW, Almenoff PL, D'Alessio DA, Render ML (2009) Hyperglycemia-related mortality in critically ill patients varies with admission diagnosis. Crit Care Med 37:1–9
19. Badawi O, Waite MD, Fuhrman SA, Zuckerman IH (2012) Association between intensive care unit-acquired dysglycemia and in-hospital mortality. Crit Care Med 40:3180–3188
20. Furnary AP, YingSing W (2006) Eliminating the diabetic disadvantage: the Portland Diabetic Project. Semin Thor Cardiovasc Surg 18:302–308
21. D'Alessandro C, Leprince P, Golmard JL et al (2007) Strict glycemic control reduces EuroSCORE expected mortality in diabetic patients undergoing myocardial revascularization. J Thorac Cardiovasc Surg 134:29–37
22. Ouattara A, Lecompte P, Le Manach Y et al (2005) Poor intraoperative blood glucose control is associated with a worsened hospital outcome after cardiac surgery in diabetic patients. Anesthesiology 103:687–694

23. Krinsley JS, Preiser JC (2015) Time in blood glucose range 70 to 140 mg/dl >80% is strongly associated with increased survival in non-diabetic critically ill adults. Crit Care 19:179
24. Egi M, Bellomo R, Stachowski E, French CJ, Hart GK, Hegarty C, Bailey M (2008) Blood glucose concentration and outcome of critical illness: the impact of diabetes. Crit Care Med 36:2249–2255
25. Rady MY, Johnson DJ, Patel BM, Larson JS, Helmers RA (2005) Influence of individual characteristics on outcome of glycemic control in intensive care unit patients with or without diabetes mellitus. Mayo Clin Proc 80:1558–1567
26. Kosiborod M, Rathore SS, Inzucchi SE, Masoudi FA, Wang Y, Havranek EP, Krumholz HM (2005) Admission glucose and mortality in elderly patients hospitalized with acute myocardial infarction: implications for patients with and without recognized diabetes. Circulation 111:3078–3086
27. Van den Berghe G, Wilmer A, Milants I et al (2006) Intensive insulin therapy in mixed medical/surgical intensive care units: benefit versus harm. Diabetes 55:3151–3159
28. Plummer MP, Bellomo R, Cousins CE et al (2014) Dysglycaemia in the critically ill and the interaction of chronic and acute glycaemia with mortality. Intensive Care Med 40:973–980
29. Moghissi SE, Korythowski MT, DiNardo M et al (2009) American Association of clinical endocrinologists and American Diabetes Association consensus statement on inpatient glycaemic control. Endocr Pract 15:1–17
30. Ichai C, Preiser JC, on behalf of the Steering Committee, the Expert panel (2010) International recommendations for glucose control in adult non diabetic critically ill patients. Crit Care 14:R166
31. Jacobi J, Bircher N, Krinsley J et al (2012) Guidelines for the use of an insulin infusion for the management of hyperglycemia in critically ill patients. Crit Care Med 40:3251–3276
32. Finfer S, Wernerman J, Preiser JC et al (2013) Clinical review: consensus recommendations on measurement of blood glucose and reporting glycemic control in critically ill adults. Crit Care 17:229

Chapter 9
Protein Metabolism

Åke Norberg, Felix Liebau, and Jan Wernerman

Abstract Protein metabolism is a core part of metabolism in particular in critical illness. Overall the critically ill subject has an elevated protein turnover to meet the demand associated with critical illness. Regulating mechanisms are incompletely understood, which make recommendations on nutrition support or other therapeutic efforts difficult. The alterations of protein metabolism in critical illness are not uniform between individual tissues, which make global nutrition protocols difficult to evaluate. Recent advances in isotopic techniques to assess protein turnovers in the whole body as well as in individual tissues or even proteins together with advances in imaging will give opportunities to better understand the mechanisms and consequently give more evidence-based recommendation over optimal care.

9.1 Background

Critical illness is associated with loss of lean body mass. In particular sarcopenia is a characteristic feature of long-standing critical illness [1–3]. This is often obvious at bedside, but in addition it has been extensively documented in terms of negative nitrogen balance and loss of muscle tissue [4–6]. The loss of both muscle proteins

---

Å. Norberg, MD, PhD • F. Liebau, MD • J. Wernerman, MD, PhD (✉)
Department of Anesthesiology and Intensive Care Medicine, Karolinska University Hospital Huddinge and Karolinska Institute, Stockholm, Sweden
e-mail: jan.wernerman@karolinska.se

J.-C. Preiser (ed.), *The Stress Response of Critical Illness: Metabolic and Hormonal Aspects*, DOI 10.1007/978-3-319-27687-8_9

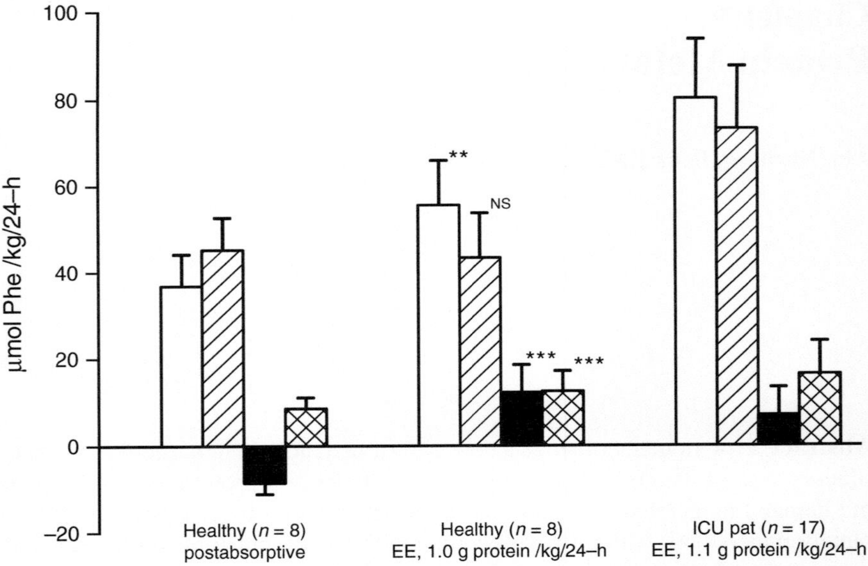

Fig. 9.1 Whole body protein turnover in healthy individuals in the postabsorptive state and in the IV-fed state, together with IV-fed critically ill patients. All kinetic measurements made by isotopic labeled phenylalanine. *Open bars* represent protein synthesis, *hatched bars* protein degradation, *filled bars* protein balance, and finally *cross-hatched bars* protein oxidation. For the healthy subjects, statistical comparisons of paired measurements were made as indicated, where ** represents $P<0.001$ and *** $P<0.0001$. Between healthy subjects and patients, no formal comparisons were made, but the higher levels of both synthesis rate and degradation rate are obvious. In addition the protein balance for the patients is not different from zero (Combined data from [7, 13] with permission)

and of muscle mass is in rough terms proportional to the severity of critical illness [2]. When it comes to nutrition support, the major target of this intervention may be defined as to minimize the loss of lean body mass.

A loss of body proteins corresponds to an imbalance between synthesis and degradation of proteins. On the whole body level, this is reflected by a negative whole body nitrogen balance. This balance, however, is extremely unevenly distributed between organs and tissues and even between singular proteins in a given tissue. This means that protein metabolism in the critically ill may be discussed on a whole body level, on an organ level, or on the level of individual proteins.

Besides the loss of lean body mass, the most characteristic feature of protein metabolism in the critically ill is the elevated whole body protein turnover as illustrated in Fig. 9.1 [7]. As compared to healthy individuals, both de novo synthesis rate and degradation rate are doubled. The net protein balance is, as illustrated, not different from zero in the fed state of critical illness, but as pointed out above this is very different between tissues. For contractile proteins in skeletal muscle, there is clearly a negative balance [8].

9.2 Techniques of Assessment

9.2.1 Nitrogen Balance

The classic technique to evaluate protein metabolism is by whole body nitrogen balance. In healthy subjects this may be done by monitoring intake and collecting and analyzing excretions. In addition there is a small insensible nitrogen loss. In a weight stable subject adapted to a standardized nutrition intake (in terms of caloric and protein intake), the nitrogen balance technique allows for comparisons between different isocaloric or isonitrogenous products. Comparisons between nutrition products differing in protein and caloric content is much more complicated and must be accompanied by sufficient time periods for adaptation to the different intake levels [9]. Furthermore, studying malnourished or catabolic subjects add concerns over comparability between groups of subjects.

9.2.2 Imaging

Recent developments of imaging techniques have made ultrasound and radiology techniques more useful in estimating muscle mass and lean body mass [10]. Single-slice CT scans on the level L3 for estimation of muscle mass are reported to give good prediction of outcomes in critical illness [11]. Simultaneously temporal patterns of thigh muscle thickness estimated by transcutaneous ultrasound give information over development of sarcopenia and have illustrated the severity of disease as a determinant of degree of sarcopenia [2, 3]. Possible limitations lie in reproducibility of measurements and sensitivity when different treatments are compared in the critically ill. Neutron activation analysis is often regarded as the gold standard to follow changes in lean body mass in critical illness. A number of studies from New Zeeland have been instrumental in expanding our knowledge of the temporal development of depletion associated with critical illness, including the effects of feeding and overfeeding [4, 6]. The obvious limitation of the technique is its sparse availability and logistic challenge in applying the technique for body mass diagnostics only in critically ill subjects.

9.2.3 Isotopic Tracer Techniques

The use of isotopic studies to assess and monitor protein turnover opens up opportunities to study protein de novo synthesis and protein degradation simultaneously. Applications may be on the whole body level as well as on the tissue level or for individual proteins [12]. Just as for nitrogen balance studies, the presence of metabolic as well as isotopic steady states is a necessary prerequisite for reliable results.

In contrast to nitrogen balance, the time patterns of steady states may be much shorter and therefore more practical. Whole body measurements, as illustrated in Fig. 9.1, may be performed when steady state periods of just 3–4 h exist. Results of comparisons between such short periods may be difficult to interpret, which calls for caution. Then it is advisable to predefine criteria for comparability between time-points of interest. In addition to quantification of synthesis rate and degradation rate, measurement of whole body turnover rate also enables determination of amino acid oxidation [7]. As proteins may not be stored in the human body in the way adipose tissue may store a surplus of energy intake, a possibility to measure the amount of protein oxidized will reflect the fraction of protein intake that is not utilized in protein turnover, but has to be eliminated as an increase in oxidation, which may be interpreted as a metabolic burden of overnutrition. Figure 9.2 illustrates how an increase of protein intake from 0.53 g/kg/24 h to 1.06 g/kg/24 h increase whole body net protein balance in head trauma patients without increasing protein oxidation [13].

The demand for a metabolic steady state also includes a steady state of nutrition intake. When parenteral nutrition is given, this can usually be controlled, but as the

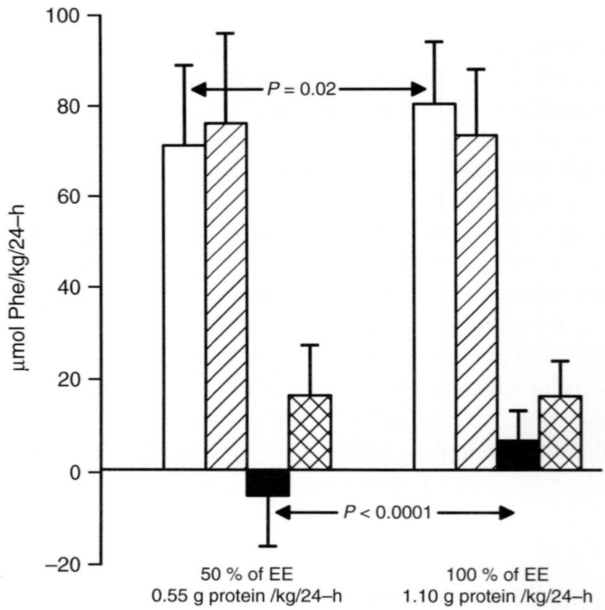

Fig. 9.2 Whole body protein turnover in IV-fed critically ill patients ($n=17$) with traumatic brain injury or subarachnoid bleedings. All kinetic measurements made by isotopic labeled phenylalanine. *Open bars* represent protein synthesis, *hatched bars* protein degradation, *filled bars* protein balance, and finally *cross-hatched bars* protein oxidation. Hypocaloric feeding combined with low protein intake gave a lower protein synthesis rate and a less favorable protein balance. It is noteworthy that the protein oxidation does not increase by doubling protein intake in this level of intake (Data from [13] with permission)

majority of critically ill patients are fed enterally, both a steady state of enteral intake and a steady state of first pass elimination through the splanchnic organs have to be documented. At measurements of whole body turnover, sampling is done in the central compartment (plasma), which necessitates documentation of the constancy of this first pass elimination during the measurement period. This may be done by adding an isotopic tracer to the enteral feeding given and assess its appearance in plasma [14].

9.3 Tissues and Individual Proteins

The overview of techniques above reflects the whole body situation, but it is in principle also applicable to individual tissues or proteins. Balance techniques may be used for individual organs or tissues. For example, urinary excretion of 3-methylhistidine has been widely used to study degradation of contractile proteins [15]. If quantified, this may be interpreted as the degradation rate of skeletal muscle proteins. The background is the irreversible (in man) posttranslational modification of histidine in contractile proteins. Furthermore, the arteriovenous balance of 3-methylhistidine may also be analyzed across muscle tissue [16]. A limb, most often the leg, is then postulated to represent muscle tissue. The use of 3-methyl-histidine is, however, associated with a number of underlying assumptions, and also the fact that only degradation is reflected is another limitation.

Arteriovenous balances also including measurements of blood flow may be used to study balances of a wide variety of substances across organs or tissues. In the area of protein metabolism, amino acid balances are frequently applied [17]. Besides skeletal muscle, the liver, kidney, brain, and lungs are examples of tissues where this approach has been used. A necessary prerequisite is that the tissue studied is supplied and drained by accessible blood vessels, and if concentration differences are small, a high precision in concentration determinations is necessary. The obvious limitation in plain balances is that it is not possible to discriminate between what is attributable to synthesis and degradation, respectively.

A further development of arteriovenous balance techniques is to also include isotopic labels [18]. This carries the possibility to quantitatively asses both synthesis and degradation at the same time. With a constant infusion of an isotopically labeled amino acid, the rate of appearance from a given tissue will correspond to the degradation rate, while the rate of disappearance will correspond to the synthesis rate. A critical assumption is the isotopic enrichment of the labeled amino acid in the immediate precursor pool for incorporation of amino acids into protein. A snapshot of the intracellular pool may be obtained by adding tissue biopsies. If biopsies are included, a 3-pool model is established, otherwise a 2-pool model [8].

Isotopically labeled amino acids are also widely used to assess de novo protein synthesis, when the incorporation rate of the labeled amino acid into proteins is measured. This may be applied to mixed tissue proteins or fraction of proteins or individual proteins [19, 20]. If proteins are in a solid organ, tissue biopsies are required. If it is circulating proteins or proteins in circulating cells, blood sampling will be sufficient [21, 22]. Just as for the calculation of synthesis rate from the rate of disappearance requires an estimate of the isotopic enrichment in the precursor pool for protein synthesis, correct estimation of the precursor pool in these calculated synthesis rates is critical. In particular when metabolic steady states are not obvious, which, for example, may be the case after feeding, erroneous precursor enrichment estimates may introduce considerable uncertainty.

9.4 Protein Synthesis Rates

The elevation in whole body protein synthesis rate seen in the critically ill, as illustrated in Fig. 9.1, is mainly attributable to high synthesis rates in the liver and in immune cells [21, 22]. Also for export proteins such as albumin, often referred to as a negative acute phase reactant due to its low plasma concentration, there is an increase in synthesis rate [23]. In parallel to the increase in synthesis rate of proteins in the liver and in immune cells, remaining tissues are found to have synthesis rates not different from what is seen in healthy subjects. This is particularly true for skeletal muscle, which related to the large size of the tissue make up a substantial portion of whole body protein synthesis [8]. Also when muscle proteins are subgrouped into contractile and mitochondrial proteins, for all groups a similar level of synthesis rates is seen both for the critically ill and for healthy subjects [24]. As critically ill patients are a very heterogeneous group of individuals, there is a large interindividual scatter, but in principle there are no tissues so far studied that expose a decrease in protein synthesis rate in critical illness.

9.5 Protein Degradation Rates

Breakdown of proteins is less well studied, related to the methodological difficulties described above. The whole body increase in degradation rate is to a large extent attributable to the elevated rate of protein degradation in skeletal muscle [25]. This is also in accord with the negative protein balance seen in muscle and the pronounced sarcopenia. Just as for synthesis rates, the degradation rates are similar in between different subgroups of proteins in muscle. From small case series of critically ill subjects, muscle protein degradation rate may be threefold higher than normal [8]. This may not cover the entire doubling of whole body degradation rate reported, but at least a major portion thereof. Very little information over degradation rates on the tissue level is available from other organs, and therefore it is hard to know whether or not degradation rates in the rest of the body also increase or stay unaltered. Indirectly the balance equation of, for example, albumin with a low, but constant over time, plasma albumin concentration combined with an elevated synthesis rate indicates an increase also in degradation rate. However, this has so far not been objectively measured.

A challenging question is the role of autophagy in critical illness. In protein degradation there are three principally different tracks for degradation: (i) cytoplasmic free enzymes, (ii) the proteasome system, and (iii) the lysosomal system. The latter system is also named autophagy. All systems are stimulated in the critically ill, but in particular the lysosomal system [8, 26]. Efforts to decrease or to attenuate the development of sarcopenia by preventing degradation may result in a decrease of lysosomal activity or in other words a decrease in autophagia. Simultaneously it is hypothesized that autophagia is a necessary mechanism to overcome critical illness and to recover [27]. If so, to attenuate autophagia may not at all be a good thing. Further studies in this field will be necessary to fully comprehend these mechanisms.

9.6 Interfering with Protein Metabolism

The close connection between lean body mass and outcomes has fostered hypothesis that actions to attenuate the loss of lean body mass may be a good strategy to improve outcomes. There are at least four strategies to try to obtain this: (i) source control, (ii) nutrition, (iii) pharmacology, and (iv) mobilization.

9.6.1 Source Control

This is clearly the least controversial part. Source control may be to stop bleeding, to control infections, to stabilize fractures, to control pain, etc. This is also the main strategy in any critically ill patient. Although it is not evidence based that the clinical improvement associated with source control also is accompanied by an increased lean body mass, there is at least a temporal coincidence.

9.6.2 Nutrition

In malnourished but otherwise healthy subjects, adequate nutrition is necessary (but not sufficient) to increase lean body mass. In non-malnourished and healthy adults, an increase in lean body mass can only be achieved by simultaneous physical activity and adequate nutrition in combination. This is, however, not a constant finding. Subjects respond very differently in terms of lean body mass to an increase in physical activity. Also the type of physical activity may be of importance. In critically ill subjects, the response to feeding in terms of alterations in lean body mass is not sufficiently explored. Although all critically ill subjects are catabolic in the sense that they develop sarcopenia, differences in nutrition status may be crucial for the response to feeding. In this context the temporal aspect is very important. The response to nutrition may differ in the early and late phases of critical illness. The autophagy hypothesis alluded to above may be an example of such a temporal factor.

The relation between lean body mass and outcomes does not immediately imply that preservation or attenuation of lean body mass will affect outcomes. So far it is reasonably well evidenced that caloric substitution will give a lower whole body protein loss as compared to no caloric substitution, but it is not evidenced that it will affect outcomes. If the caloric substitution turns into an over-substitution, this is associated with harm. The possible association with protein metabolism is not clear, but an attenuation of autophagy may be a suggestion. Lately the provision of protein nutrition has attained a large interest. The recommendation of a protein intake of 0.8 g/kg/24 h (together with a normocaloric energy intake) given for healthy subjects has been hypothesized to be far too low for the critically ill [28, 29]. The evidence for this hypothesis, however, is not very strong. No prospective randomized studies with outcome parameters but merely observational case series exist [9]. Nevertheless, recommendations from nutritional societies suggest a higher intake as compared to the WHO recommendations for the healthy [30, 31], 1.2–1.5 g/kg/24 h, together with a normocaloric intake is recommended by both ESPEN and ASPEN [32–34].

The use of isotopic labeling to assess whole body protein turnover offers the possibility to assess the short-term effect of an increased protein intake on protein balance and on protein oxidation. Figure 9.3 depicts data from such short-term studies in the early phase of critical illness, illustrating a clear relationship between protein intake and protein balance [14]. This must, however, be interpreted with caution. It is a short-term observation, very few observations above an intake of 1.8 g/kg/24 h are included, and studied subjects are all in the early phase of critical illness. Beyond

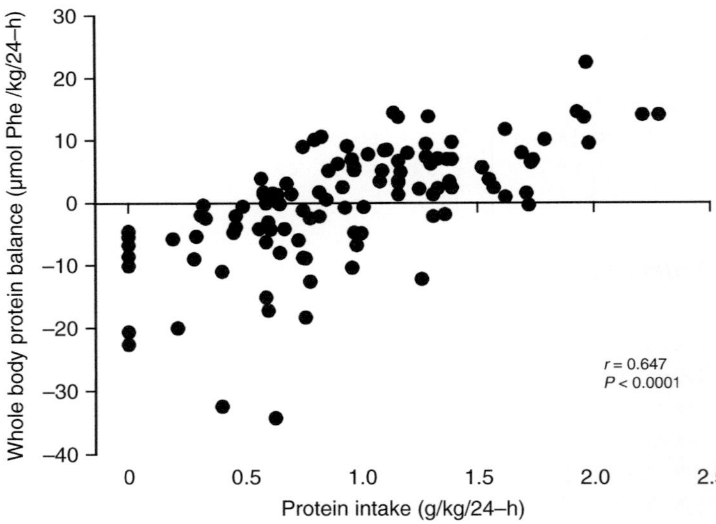

Fig. 9.3 Observations ($n = 112$) of whole body protein balance in relation to protein intake for critically ill patients ($n = 39$) given variable amounts of energy and protein (amino acids). Whole body protein balance was assessed by measurements of isotopic labeled phenylalanine. The statistical correlation seen is suggestive of a positive whole protein balance on the protein intake level suggested by the ESPEN guidelines (Combined data from [7, 13, 14] with permission)

that the relations between a positive protein balance, lean body mass, and outcome all remain to be established.

9.6.3 *Pharmacology*

On the side of the rather confusing hypotheses around pharmaco-nutrition, there have been efforts to interfere with protein metabolism by pharmacological agents. The well-known example of growth hormone supplementation illustrated that although a stimulating effect on skeletal muscle combined with protein synthesis rate could be demonstrated in critically ill patients [35], a prospective randomized blinded trial showed an increase in mortality in the growth hormone-treated group of patients [36]. This experience clearly illustrates the necessity to understand the underlying mechanisms before starting large-scale trials. In addition there are small studies exploring high insulin doses [37], testosterone [38], anabolic steroids [39], as well as beta-blockers [40]. The experience of multi-supplemented formulas under the heading of pharmaco-nutrition has so far not contributed to a better outcome and should preferably be better investigated before being recommended.

9.6.4 *Mobilization*

There has been a discussion over the relative contributions to sarcopenia from critical illness itself (general inflammation) and the immobilization that also accompanies critical illness. Studies of immobilized healthy subjects indicate an initial delay in the development of sarcopenia [41]. Long-term immobilization on the other hand is associated with considerable loss of muscle mass [42]. In critically ill patients, efforts to prevent muscle wasting by activity have attained a lot of interest [43]. Presented studies are most often case series, and the absence of blinding is common. In addition selection of patients by extensive exclusion criteria is also common. In the context of protein metabolism, there are no reports over physical mobilization or training and protein turnover, although this is an area where reports of beneficial effects from muscle contractions during critical illness are emerging [44].

9.7 Conclusions

Protein metabolism is a core part of metabolism in particular in critical illness. Overall the critically ill subject has an elevated protein turnover to meet the demand associated with critical illness. Regulating mechanisms are incompletely understood, which make recommendations on nutrition support or other therapeutic efforts difficult. The alterations of protein metabolism in critical illness are not uniform between individual tissues, which make global nutrition protocols difficult to evaluate. Recent advances in isotopic techniques to assess protein turnovers in the whole body as well as in individual tissues or even proteins together with advances in imaging will give opportunities to better understand the mechanisms and consequently give more evidence-based recommendation over optimal care.

References

1. Gamrin L, Essen P, Forsberg AM, Hultman E, Wernerman J (1996) A descriptive study of skeletal muscle metabolism in critically ill patients: free amino acids, energy-rich phosphates, protein, nucleic acids, fat, water, and electrolytes. Crit Care Med 24(4):575–583
2. Puthucheary ZA, Rawal J, McPhail M, Connolly B, Ratnayake G, Chan P, Hopkinson NS, Padhke R, Dew T, Sidhu PS et al (2013) Acute skeletal muscle wasting in critical illness. JAMA 310(15):1591–1600
3. Reid CL, Campbell IT, Little RA (2004) Muscle wasting and energy balance in critical illness. Clin Nutr 23(2):273–280
4. Ishibashi N, Plank LD, Sando K, Hill GL (1998) Optimal protein requirements during the first 2 weeks after the onset of critical illness. Crit Care Med 26(9):1529–1535
5. Larsson J, Lennmarken C, Martensson J, Sandstedt S, Vinnars E (1990) Nitrogen requirements in severely injured patients. Br J Surg 77(4):413–416
6. Streat SJ, Beddoe AH, Hill GL (1987) Aggressive nutritional support does not prevent protein loss despite fat gain in septic intensive care patients. J Trauma 27(3):262–266
7. Rooyackers O, Kouchek-Zadeh R, Tjader I, Norberg A, Klaude M, Wernerman J (2015) Whole body protein turnover in critically ill patients with multiple organ failure. Clin Nutr 34(1):95–100
8. Klaude M, Mori M, Tjader I, Gustafsson T, Wernerman J, Rooyackers O (2012) Protein metabolism and gene expression in skeletal muscle of critically ill patients with sepsis. Clin Sci (Lond) 122(3):133–142
9. Rooyackers O, Werneman J (2015) Protein intake in critical illness. In: Vincent J-L (ed) Annual update in intensive care and emergency medicine 2015. Springer, Berlin, pp 459–468. DOI 10.1007/978-3-319-13761-2_23
10. Rooyackers O, Wernerman J (2014) Imaging opens possibilities both to target and to evaluate nutrition in critical illness. Crit Care 18(3):144
11. Weijs PJ, Looijaard WG, Dekker IM, Stapel SN, Girbes AR, Oudemans-van Straaten HM, Beishuizen A (2014) Low skeletal muscle area is a risk factor for mortality in mechanically ventilated critically ill patients. Crit Care 18(1):R12
12. Wolfe RR, Goodenough RD, Wolfe MH (1983) Isotopic approaches to the estimation of protein requirements in burn patients. Adv Shock Res 9:81–98
13. Berg A, Rooyackers O, Bellander BM, Wernerman J (2013) Whole body protein kinetics during hypocaloric and normocaloric feeding in critically ill patients. Crit Care 17(4):R158
14. Liebau F, Sundstrom M, van Loon LJ, Wernerman J, Rooyackers O (2015) Short term amino acid infusion improves protein balance in critically ill patients. Crit Care 19(1):844
15. Young VR, Havenberg LN, Bilmazes C, Munro HN (1973) Potential use of 3-methylhistidine excretion as an index of progressive reduction in muscle protein catabolism during starvation. Metabolism 23(2):1429–1436
16. Vesali RF, Klaude M, Thunblad L, Rooyackers OE, Wernerman J (2004) Contractile protein breakdown in human leg skeletal muscle as estimated by [2H3]-3-methylhistidine: a new method. Metabolism 53(8):1076–1080
17. Wernerman J, Vinnars E (1987) The effect of trauma and surgery on interorgan fluxes of amino acids in man. Clin Sci (Lond) 73(2):129–133

18. Biolo G, Maggi SP, Williams BD, Tipton KD, Wolfe RR (1995) Increased rates of muscle protein turnover and amino acid transport after resistance exercise in humans. Am J Physiol 268(3 Pt 1):E514–E520
19. Barle H, Nyberg B, Essen P, Andersson K, McNurlan MA, Wernerman J, Garlick PJ (1997) The synthesis rates of total liver protein and plasma albumin determined simultaneously in vivo in humans. Hepatology 25(1):154–158
20. Garlick PJ, Wernerman J, McNurlan MA, Essen P, Lobley GE, Milne E, Calder GA, Vinnars E (1989) Measurement of the rate of protein synthesis in muscle of postabsorptive young men by injection of a 'flooding dose' of [1-13C]leucine. Clin Sci (Lond) 77(3):329–336
21. Ballmer PE, McNurlan MA, Milne E, Heys SD, Buchan V, Calder AG, Garlick PJ (1990) Measurement of albumin synthesis in humans: a new approach employing stable isotopes. Am J Physiol 259(6 Pt 1):E797–E803
22. Januszkiewicz J, Klaude M, Loré K, Andersson J, Ringdén O, Rooyackers O, Wernerman J (2005) In vivo protein synthesis in immune cells of ICU patients. Clin Nutr 24:575
23. Essen P, McNurlan MA, Gamrin L, Hunter K, Calder G, Garlick PJ, Wernerman J (1998) Tissue protein synthesis rates in critically ill patients. Crit Care Med 26(1):92–100
24. Fredriksson K, Tjader I, Keller P, Petrovic N, Ahlman B, Scheele C, Wernerman J, Timmons JA, Rooyackers O (2008) Dysregulation of mitochondrial dynamics and the muscle transcriptome in ICU patients suffering from sepsis induced multiple organ failure. PLoS One 3(11):e3686
25. Biolo G, Fleming RY, Maggi SP, Nguyen TT, Herndon DN, Wolfe RR (2002) Inverse regulation of protein turnover and amino acid transport in skeletal muscle of hypercatabolic patients. J Clin Endocrinol Metab 87(7):3378–3384
26. Biolo G, Bosutti A, Iscra F, Toigo G, Gullo A, Guarnieri G (2000) Contribution of the ubiquitin-proteasome pathway to overall muscle proteolysis in hypercatabolic patients. Metabolism 49(6):689–691
27. Casaer MP, Van den Berghe G (2014) Nutrition in the acute phase of critical illness. N Engl J Med 370(13):1227–1236
28. Hoffer LJ, Bistrian BR (2012) Appropriate protein provision in critical illness: a systematic and narrative review. Am J Clin Nutr 96(3):591–600
29. Sauerwein HP, Serlie MJ (2010) Optimal nutrition and its potential effect on survival in critically ill patients. Neth J Med 68(3):119–122
30. Stein J, Boehles HJ, Blumenstein I, Goeters C, Schulz R, Working Group for Developing the Guidelines for Parenteral Nutrition of The German Association for Nutritional Medicine (2009) Amino acids – guidelines on parenteral nutrition, Chapter 4. GMS German medical science. 7:Doc24
31. World Health Organization (2007) Protein and amino acid requirements in human nutrition. WHO Technical Report Series, p 935
32. Kreymann KG, Berger MM, Deutz NE, Hiesmayr M, Jolliet P, Kazandjiev G, Nitenberg G, van den Berghe G, Wernerman J, Ebner C et al (2006) ESPEN guidelines on enteral nutrition: intensive care. Clin Nutr 25(2):210–223
33. Singer P, Berger MM, Van den Berghe G, Biolo G, Calder P, Forbes A, Griffiths R, Kreyman G, Leverve X, Pichard C (2009) ESPEN guidelines on parenteral nutrition: intensive care. Clin Nutr 28(4):387–400
34. Martindale RG, McClave SA, Vanek VW, McCarthy M, Roberts P, Taylor B, Ochoa JB, Napolitano L, Cresci G, American College of Critical Care M et al (2009) Guidelines for the provision and assessment of nutrition support therapy in the adult critically ill patient: society of Critical Care Medicine and American Society for parenteral and enteral nutrition: executive summary. Crit Care Med 37(5):1757–1761
35. Gamrin L, Essen P, Hultman E, McNurlan MA, Garlick PJ, Wernerman J (2000) Protein-sparing effect in skeletal muscle of growth hormone treatment in critically ill patients. Ann Surg 231(4):577–586
36. Takala J, Ruokonen E, Webster NR, Nielsen MS, Zandstra DF, Vundelinckx G, Hinds CJ (1999) Increased mortality associated with growth hormone treatment in critically ill adults. N Engl J Med 341(11):785–792

37. Gore DC, Wolf SE, Sanford AP, Herndon DN, Wolfe RR (2004) Extremity hyperinsulinemia stimulates muscle protein synthesis in severely injured patients. Am J Physiol Endocrinol Metab 286(4):E529–E534
38. Ferrando AA, Raj D, Wolfe RR (2005) Amino acid control of muscle protein turnover in renal disease. J Ren Nutr Off J Counc Ren Nutr Natl Kidney Found 15(1):34–38
39. Jiang ZM, Wilmore DW, Liu W, Liu YW (2000) Growth factors in clinical practice. World J Surg 24(12):1514–1518
40. Gauglitz GG, Williams FN, Herndon DN, Jeschke MG (2011) Burns: where are we standing with propranolol, oxandrolone, recombinant human growth hormone, and the new incretin analogs? Curr Opin Clin Nutr Metab Care 14(2):176–181
41. Schonheyder F, Heilskov NS, Olesen K (1954) Isotopic studies on the mechanism of negative nitrogen balance produced by immobilization. Scand J Clin Lab Invest 6(3):178–188
42. Dalla Libera L, Ravara B, Gobbo V, Tarricone E, Vitadello M, Biolo G, Vescovo G, Gorza L (2009) A transient antioxidant stress response accompanies the onset of disuse atrophy in human skeletal muscle. J Appl Physiol 107(2):549–557
43. Winkelman C (2007) Inactivity and inflammation in the critically ill patient. Crit Care Clin 23(1):21–34
44. Weber-Carstens S, Schneider J, Wollersheim T, Assmann A, Bierbrauer J, Marg A, Al Hasani H, Chadt A, Wenzel K, Koch S et al (2013) Critical illness myopathy and GLUT4: significance of insulin and muscle contraction. Am J Respir Crit Care Med 187(4):387–396

Chapter 10
Micronutrients

Mette M. Berger

Abstract The status of 11 trace elements and 13 vitamins, collectively named micronutrients, is challenged in several critical care conditions. Inflammation and oxidative stress cause redistribution of micronutrients to organs involved in synthesis and immunity resulting in significant drops of plasma concentrations even in absence of real deficits. Nevertheless these changes alter the organism's capacity to respond to circulating stressors, and participate in worsening organ function in patients dependent on intensive care. Only one vitamin deficiency may be critical during the first 48 hours: Thiamine. Other alterations will result in later consequences in conditions characterized by the combination of a strong inflammation and of losses of biological fluids. The properties, risks and potential for intervention of the essential micronutrients are discussed, mainly regarding their immune, antioxidant and wound healing properties. The place in metabolism of carnitine and choline, actually missing in parenteral nutrition, is addressed.

Micronutrient is the collective name for trace elements and vitamins: both categories of substances are required for substrate metabolism, antioxidant and immune defences. They have no proper energetic value. Micronutrients are present in minute amounts and small changes will result in important changes in their distribution in the body [1]. Tables 10.1 and 10.2 summarise some aspects of their physiology and usual requirements: this knowledge only partially addresses the issues encountered during acute and chronic critical illness.

Oxidative stress and inflammatory response belong to the standardised body's answer to infection of any origin and severity or of any acute injury. Production of

M.M. Berger
Service de Médecine Intensive Adulte et Brûlés, University Hospital CHUV, Lausanne CH 1011, Switzerland
e-mail: Mette.Berger@chuv.ch

J.-C. Preiser (ed.), *The Stress Response of Critical Illness: Metabolic and Hormonal Aspects*, DOI 10.1007/978-3-319-27687-8_10

Table 10.1 Essential trace element in adults

Trace elements	Body stores	Location in the body	DRI	Parenteral nutrition recommendations
Cu – copper	100 mg	Liver, enzymes	0.9 mg	0.3–0.5 mg (5–8 umol) 1.3 mg (20 umol) in major burns and GI losses
Se – selenium	6–20 mg	Liver, kidney > muscle, bone, blood	55 mcg	30–70 mcg (0.4–0.84 umol)
Zn – zinc	1.4–2.3 g	Bone > genitalia, skin, liver, kidney, muscle, pancreas	11 mg	2.5–5 mg (38–76 umol) plus 2.5–4 mg (38–62 umol) in catabolic states but not >30 mg in ICU
Fe – iron	3 g (female) – 4 g (male)	Liver, spleen > Hb, myoglobin, cytochromes	8 mg	0 to 1.0–1.2 mg (18–20 umol)
Mn – manganese	12–16 mg	Mitochondria (liver, bone, kidney, pancreas, small intestine)	2.3 mg	0–55 mcg (1 mmol max)
Mo – molybdenum	9–16 mg	Mitochondria (same as Mn)	45 mcg	100–200 mcg (1.0–2.1 umol)
Cr – chromium	4–6 mg	Spleen, heart, kidney	35 mcg	10–15 mcg (0.2–0.3 umol) 20 mg (0.4 umol) in ICU
F – fluoride	<1 mg	Bone, teeth	4 mg	0.95 mg (50 umol)
I – iodide	20–50 mg	60 % thyroid > muscle, ovaries, blood	15 mcg	70 mcg (0.6 umol)
Co – cobalt	<1 mg	Blood	None	None
V – vanadium	20–25 mg	Throughout, stored in fat tissue	None	None

Adapted from [62, 63]
DRI dietary reference intake

reactive oxygen species (ROS) is a normal phenomenon that is amplified as soon as inflammation is activated. But the ROS production may overwhelm the endogenous antioxidant defences and reinforce inflammation. Pro-inflammatory mediators (such as TNF-a, IL-1, IL-6, bradykinins, leukotrienes, prostaglandins) are released in amounts proportional to the severity of the condition [2]. They may contribute to the development of multisystem organ dysfunction and even failure, when uncontrolled by the anti-inflammatory defence mechanisms and mediators (e.g., IL-4, IL-10, etc). After the initial hyper-inflammatory state, cytokine levels generally return to normal, a passage of hypo-inflammatory status being possible [3].

Micronutrients are very sensitive to circulating cytokines and other biomarkers of inflammation, which divert them from the circulating compartment to specific tissues and organs, reducing the blood concentrations. Insufficiency of the endogenous defences may result from deficiency or suboptimal status prior to disease or to this redistribution. This is particularly the case with the micronutrients involved in antioxidant defences such as selenium, zinc, ascorbic acid and α-tocopherol. Indeed Se and Zn concentrations below reference ranges during criti-

Table 10.2 Essential vitamins

Vitamins [13]	Units	EN recommended min-max	PN recommended dose	Absorption site	Main location
A – retinol	ug	700–3600	1000	Duodenum, upper jejunum	Various target organs
D – cholecalciferol	ug	10–50	5	Small intestine	Lymph, kidneys, adrenals, bones, intestines
E – alpha-tocopherol	mg	10–60	10	Small intestine	Lymph, all tissues
K – phylloquinone	ug	70–400	150	Small intestine, colon	Lymph
B1 – thiamine	mg	1.2–10	3	Small intestine	Heart, brain, kidney, liver, skeletal muscle
B2 – riboflavin	mg	1.6–10	3.6	Small intestine	All tissues, little storage
B3 – niacin (PP)	mg	18–60	40	Throughout gastrointestinal tract	All tissues, particularly liver
B5 – pantothenic acid	mg		4–7	Throughout gastrointestinal tract	All tissues
B6 – pyridoxine	*mg*	1.6–10	4	Throughout gastrointestinal tract	Brain liver kidneys
B8 – biotin (H)	mg	15–150	60	Throughout gastrointestinal tract	Liver, brain
B9 – folic acid	μg	200–1000	400	Small intestine	Liver tissues
B12 – cobalamin	*mg*	1.4–14	50	Ileum	Liver, heart, kidney, spleen, brain
C – ascorbic acid	mg	45–440	100	Intestine	Plasma, body cells

Adapted from [62, 63]

cal illness are associated with increased oxidative stress and elevated inflammatory biomarkers, particularly in patients with sepsis [4]. Several trace elements and vitamins will exhibit blood concentrations below reference ranges even in the absence of a true deficiency state: Fe, Se, Zn and vitamin concentrations are heavily altered. Suboptimal Se and Zn status in turn worsens oxidative stress [5]. This was recently confirmed in 114 critically ill patients: elevated CRP and low Se, Zn and albumin values were a constant finding [4], as it was in 800 non-critically ill patients referred for nutritional assessment.

In the intensive care unit (ICU), micronutrient prescription is generally confined to parenteral nutrition (PN). The below text will describe conditions in which this concept is insufficient to address the patient's requirements.

10.1 Which Micronutrients Matter in Critically Ill Patients?

In patients staying less than 4 days in the ICU and in absence of pre-existing deficiency, there is little time for micronutrient problems to develop or become source of concern, with one major exception: acute thiamine deficiency in the context of the refeeding syndrome which develops in a few hours upon re-administration of carbohydrates in patients who have not been fed for a few days [6] (see below Sect. 10.10.5).

But several acute conditions requiring ICU treatment are characterised by major micronutrient alterations, which have been identified as contributors to the worsening of their condition: they are generally characterised by the combination of a strong inflammation and of losses of biological fluids such as major burns and multiple trauma, patients on continuous renal replacement therapy, acute pancreatitis, and any patients with drains and high-output intestinal fistulae.

More and more patients survive the initial acute phase of disease: they are particularly fragile and exposed to cumulated progressive complications including alterations of micronutrient status. Patients enter a state called chronic critical illness: it is a recent phenomenon which has changed the ICU world and increases in incidence [2].

10.1.1 Trace Elements

The essential trace elements were defined in the 1960s [1] as inorganic substances, mainly metals and metalloids, constituting <0.01 % of body mass, that are present in constant concentrations <50 μg/g tissue or fluid. Their absence causes reproducible biochemical, structural and functional deficiencies, while these alterations can be prevented/corrected by the intake of the single element. Among the 11 essential trace elements listed in Table 10.1, copper, iron, selenium and zinc are of special interest during critical illness and will be discussed hereafter.

10.1.1.1 Copper

This element was rarely considered a problem in the ICU, being confined to neurological pathologies such as insufficient (Menkes disease) or excess copper (Wilson's disease) [7]. Recent changes in the ICU population have emphasised the importance of this element. But Cu deficiency remains a differential diagnosis which is rarely mentioned. Its potent redox activity makes copper a key modulator of cell signal transduction pathways. Copper deficiency can result in impaired energy production, abnormal glucose and cholesterol metabolism, increased oxidative damage, delayed wound healing (altered due to insufficient elastin and collagen synthesis), structure and function of circulating blood and immune cells, abnormal neuropeptide synthesis and processing, aberrant cardiac electrophysiology, impaired myocardial contractility and persistent effects on the neurobehavioral and the immune system [8].

Severe copper deficiencies appear several months after bariatric surgery, particularly in patients having undergone malabsorptive procedures: this is a growing patient population resulting from the obesity epidemic. As copper is absorbed in the stomach and duodenum, deficiencies develop progressively [9]. In presence of cardiac and infectious complications, copper and ceruloplasmin concentrations should be determined, and copper prescribed by the intravenous route to be efficient as the gut is unable to absorb it.

Continuous renal replacement therapy is frequently required in chronic critical illness. The effluent losses contain several micronutrients, including copper [10]: the losses generally exceed one daily dose for standard PN. In patients undergoing prolonged renal replacement, blood copper should be monitored along with selenium to prevent development of extreme hypocupremia [11].

Major burns in patients have long been known to develop severe copper deficiencies caused by large losses from their burn wound exudates [12]. Death by cardiac arrest has been associated with extreme copper deficiency [13]. Early repletion of this element contributes to the restoration of immunity and of wound healing after major burns [14].

10.1.1.2 Iron

This element plays a central role in oxygen transport, being the core of haemoglobin, but also in electron transfer, nitrogen fixation or DNA synthesis and all essential reactions for living organisms. Iron deficiency is the main cause of anaemia worldwide, as well as a cause of fatigue and decreased effort capacity [15]. Anaemia is very frequent in the ICU, affecting nearly 70 % of patients. But systematic data on iron status in critically ill patients are few as the status is difficult to determine, the main indicators being affected by the omnipresent inflammatory response. A Belgian prospective study including 95 patients showed that the iron status measured by a combination of blood count, iron, ferritin, transferrin and transferrin receptor concentrations and transferrin saturation was rapidly altered in the majority of patients and remained so for many days [16]. True iron deficiency should be suspected as it is frequent in the general population [17], and therefore many patients start with iron deficiency or even anaemia. Critical illness worsens the status; hemorrhagic conditions and blood sampling contribute to depletion. It should also be considered when ferritin is in the lower range of normal, as this protein increases with inflammation. The clinical availability of the best marker of iron status in critical illness, hepcidin [15], is still to come.

10.1.1.3 Selenium

Selenium is essential for maintenance of overall health, especially for the thyroid, immunity and homeostasis. It is also important for reproduction [18]. It has a very important role in virology. Among the micronutrients with an antioxidant function, selenium is the one which has attracted most attention, followed by zinc. Indeed it constitutes the core of the glutathione peroxidase family of enzymes, which constitute the most important antioxidant defence system in the organism [19].

Critical illness and particularly those involving septic pathologies are characterised by inflammation and oxidative stress. Selenium concentrations are generally low, and the decrease of blood concentrations compared to reference ranges reflects the severity of disease [20].

A recent study combining in vitro and in vivo investigations confirmed that plasma concentrations of interleukin-6, other biomarkers of inflammation and markers of oxidative damage to proteins and lipids were elevated, particularly in patients with sepsis, and were inversely related to plasma selenium and zinc concentrations [5].

10.1.1.4 Zinc

Zinc is the structural and regulatory element in more than 300 enzymes, essential in all metabolic pathways, for genomic stability, DNA function and reparation, cell proliferation and apoptosis. It is also essential for the function of numerous hormones such as growth hormone, gustine, thyroid hormones, thymuline and insulin. It plays key roles in antioxidant and immune defences. The multiple functions of zinc require a dedicated review [21, 22].

In critical care research has focused on the antioxidant and immune functions mainly in sepsis, as well as on tissue repair.

10.1.1.5 Vanadium

This element is a new comer on the list, although no clear clinical deficiency state has yet been identified. The essential role of vanadium as an inorganic enzyme cofactor in maintaining haemostasis has long been known [23], although the mechanisms of action of vanadium salts remain poorly understood. Vanadium complexes are cofactors for several enzymes and also exhibit insulin-mimetic properties, making vanadium of interest to diabetes specialists [24]. The best accepted model of vanadium compounds' mechanism of action is to consider that they behave as phosphate analogues: vanadium would activate the protein tyrosine phosphorylation (PTP) of solubilised insulin receptor and autophosphorylation of this receptor in a mechanism analogous to insulin. Vanadium compounds increase glucose uptake and transport from the intracellular compartment to the cell surface through the insulin-dependent glucose transporter GLUT4 in the mechanism regulated by phosphoinositide 3-kinase and protein kinase B [25].

The average diet provides 10–160 μg of vanadium per day, mainly from mushrooms, seafood, black pepper, parsley, fennel seeds, grains and spinach. After entering the bloodstream, vanadium compounds are converted into vanadyl cations, which form complexes with transferrin and ferritin and, less frequently, with albumin, haemoglobin or low molecular components of plasma (citrate, lactate and phosphate) [23]. There are still no recommendations regarding this TE in artificial nutrition, as the toxicity limits are not yet well defined: hence actual multi-micronutrient preparations do not contain any vanadium.

10.1.2 Vitamins

They are by contrast with trace elements, organic substances that are required in minute amounts, which cannot be synthesised by the body in sufficient quantities to match the requirements to prevent deficiencies. While all those listed in Table 10.2 are essential, some seem to be of special interest during critical illness and are discussed below.

10.1.2.1 Vitamin B

Among the vitamin B family, thiamine is on the frontline in critically ill patients. This vitamin exists under various forms, the most important being thiamine pyrophosphate (TPP), which is the coenzyme for mitochondrial oxidative decarboxylation. It is hence essential for the metabolism of carbohydrates and branched amino acids. Thiamine influences reactions that protect against oxidative tissue damage by maintaining reduced NADP+, and thiamine deficiency decreases GPx activity [26].

Different studies have shown a high incidence of thiamine deficiency, varying between 28 and 71 % on admission to the emergency department or ICU [27]. It is particularly frequent in populations at risk of alcohol abuse. Further, depletion after admission has also been shown to occur within a few days [6]. Thiamine insufficiency should be kept in mind in different clinical scenarios such as severe sepsis, major burns, unexplained heart failure or lactic acidosis and neurological disorder in patients with a history of alcoholism, starvation, chronic malnutrition, long-term parenteral feeding, hyperemesis gravidarum or bariatric surgery [6]: it should also be suspected in patients who have been in hospital for a few days and submitted to investigations, which frequently result in acute starving sufficient to prompt a refeeding syndrome.

But the association of thiamine status with outcome is complex. While depletion of thiamine during the refeeding syndrome is rapidly lethal and may precipitate lactic acidosis and Wernicke–Korsakoff encephalopathy, a Brazilian study including 108 patients in septic shock showed that thiamine deficiency on admission despite being present in 71 % of patients was not associated with oxidative stress or mortality [28].

10.1.2.2 Vitamin C

Ascorbic acid is a water-soluble antioxidant vitamin circulating in plasma. It is taken up by the intestine via the sodium-dependent vitamin C transporter. Vitamin C scavenges reactive oxygen species such as superoxide and peroxynitrite in plasma and cells (preventing damage to proteins, lipids and DNA): it prevents occludin dephosphorylation and loosening of the tight junctions [29]. Ascorbate improves microcirculatory flow impairment by inhibiting tumour necrosis factor-induced intracellular adhesion molecule expression, which triggers leukocyte stickiness and slugging [30]. Severe vitamin C deficiency, or scurvy, is a clinical syndrome with lethargy, perifollicular petechiae, erythema, gingivitis, bleeding, impaired wound healing and depressed immunity, conditions rarely observed in ICU. But very low plasma concentrations have repeatedly been measured during critical illness and considered to reflect acute deficiency [31]. The low plasma concentrations are associated with inflammation, severity of organ failure and mortality [32]. It is of high potential interest in critically ill patients with a strong inflammatory response.

10.1.2.3 Vitamin D

This vitamin has recently become a major centre of interest. It was long confined to bone disease and to the maintenance adequate calcium levels for bone mineralisation and optimal skeletal muscle function [33]. It has been shown in the last decade to have pleiotropic effects, including on the immune system. In critically ill patients, the multiple effects of vitamin D including its role in immune function are of great interest, as deficiency defined by low to very low blood concentrations seems to be rather common [34]. On the basis of optimal bone health, vitamin D deficiency is defined as a serum 25(OH)D below 20 ng/ml (50 nmol/l), vitamin D insufficiency as a 25(OH)D of 20–30 ng/ml (50–75 nmol/l) and a normal vitamin D status as 25(OH)D above 30 ng/ml (75 nmol/l) [35]. These values have been directly applied to critically ill patients despite the fact that many factors differing from the general population may alter the blood concentrations such as fluid resuscitation and inflammatory state.

Two recent papers suggest that vitamin D deficiency is associated with adverse health outcomes including increased risk of cardiovascular disease, morbidity and mortality both in the general population and in critical illness [35, 36]. In a Brazilian study including 135 patients, the vitamin D level was an independent predictor of mortality [36]. Today it is not clear though whether vitamin D deficiency is a surrogate marker for increased morbidity or a therapeutic target.

10.1.2.4 Carnitine

It was isolated initially from a meat extract some 100 years ago. It was long not considered to be essential in mammals, having been discovered as an insect growth factor. It was later shown about 50 years ago to have important roles in metabolism as facilitator of β-oxidation and of transport of carboxylic acids (acyl group) across membranes, including that of coenzyme A [37]. It thereby performs a critical role in cellular energy metabolism. Carnitine is not required for transport of medium chain fatty acids, while facilitating their β-oxidation in skeletal muscles. It works as a key regulator of lipid metabolism in long chain fatty acid esterification and transport through the mitochondrial membrane [38]. It becomes conditionally essential in some clinical situations encountered in critical care.

Recent research has highlighted the importance of mitochondrial dysfunction in the metabolic and neuroendocrine changes observed in patients presenting with chronic critical illness [11]. Deficiency may develop as there is nearly no carnitine content in commercially available feeds nor in supplements. This small moiety may be lost in large amount through the effluents of patients on continuous renal replacement therapy causing acute and chronic deficiency states manifested as a generalised mitochondrial dysfunction and multiorgan failure including the liver, with clinical consequences such as muscle weakness, rhabdomyolysis, cardiomyopathy, arrhythmia or sudden death [11]. Upon diagnosis of deficiency based on blood samples, repletion may be carried out by the enteral or intravenous routes in the doses of 1–2 g/day. Normal requirements are 2–5 mg/kg/day. Carnitine is absorbed in the small intestine by a few transporters which vary according to the dose being supplemented.

Parenteral nutrition solutions do yet not contain carnitine. Nevertheless based on actual knowledge, at least in neonatology, carnitine should be routinely added to parenteral nutrition formulations [39].

10.1.2.5 Choline

Choline is not a vitamin as it is synthesised endogenously from methionine or absorbed from the portal circulation [40], but it is recognised as essential since the 1990s. It is ubiquitous in the diet. Nevertheless deficiency has been described in a series of animals, who develop cirrhosis. In humans it has been investigated in association with intestinal failure-associated liver disease and chronic cholestasis in the entity called parenteral nutrition-associated liver disease (PNALD). Its deficiency activates cellular apoptosis and is involved in lipid transport and transmembrane signalling [40].

In patients on parenteral nutrition, plasma-free choline has been found to be below normal in the majority of patients, with a significant inverse relationship between this concentration and ALT and AST levels. In 2012 the ASPEN published recommendations for changes in the composition of parenteral nutrition solutions: the working group conclude that choline should also be routinely added to adult and paediatric PN formulations. However, such commercially available parenteral product is still to be developed [39].

10.2 Which Micronutrients Should Be Considered Eligible for Intervention?

A major issue to consider when organising a micronutrient prescription is the fact that they do not intervene in metabolism independently from others, as single standalone entities. They should be administered in combination. In case of PN, which as available from industry by definition contains macronutrients but no micronutrients, the additional daily administration of trace elements and vitamins is required as stated in the ESPEN guidelines [41]. The products available in Europe are designed for home total PN, or for stable patients only, and most of these products are adequate but do not address the specific requirements and high metabolic needs of critically ill patients.

Some micronutrients have an easily identifiable therapeutic objective and indication, such as the plasma GPX3 activity in case of selenium deficiency, but a well defined therapeutic objective is generally unavailable in clinical settings. In patients presenting acute biological fluid losses, whatever their cause, replacement of the losses is warranted: it should nevertheless be kept in mind that one micronutrient loss rarely occurs alone. Trace elements are more affected than vitamins according to published literature. Several studies have confirmed the clinical benefice of the multi-micronutrient concept in pathologies characterised by biological fluid losses such as major trauma [42, 43] and major burns [14, 44]: significant reductions of infectious complications, of length of stay and of mortality have been observed.

10.2.1 Selenium

Several randomised trials have tested moderate to very high-dose selenium supplements aiming at attenuation of oxidative stress and inflammatory response. As many of the trials include small cohorts, meta-analysis has been conducted including various numbers of randomised controlled trials. Doses of selenium have been variable between 300 mcg and 4000 mcg/day, and selenium has frequently been used in combination with other antioxidant micronutrients. In patients with sepsis, selenium supplementation at doses higher than daily requirement may reduce mortality [45]. Trials delivering >500 mcg/day of selenium showed a trend towards a lower mortality whereas trials using doses lower than 500 mcg had no effect on mortality [46].

10.2.2 Zinc

High-output intestinal fistulae are a unique condition in which zinc is lost preferentially to any other micronutrient: 20–30 mg of zinc by the intravenous route may be required per day to compensate the losses [47].

Major burns is another condition requiring such high doses of zinc by the intravenous route, for 2–4 weeks, but the needs are not focused on zinc only but on a combination of trace elements, particularly copper and selenium, in association with thiamine and ascorbic acid.

10.2.3 Copper

As stated above, isolated copper deficiency is rare, but found in pathologies at risk. It is a component of multitrace element solutions, but in quantities insufficient to compensate for an acute deficiency. Copper sulphate is the usually available form, prepared by the hospital pharmacies. Our Lausanne university pharmacy prepares copper gluconate. Doses required for treatment of severe deficiency states vary between 2 and 6 mg/day administered as continuous intravenous infusion. Daily monitoring of liver tests AST and ALT is mandatory. In our own experience, no side effects are observed up to 8 mg/day in major burns [11].

10.2.4 Iron

It was long believed that iron supplementation would increase the risk of infections [48], and was therefore withhold in ICU patients, but this threat has not been confirmed, while the complications of iron deficiency and anaemia are obvious. A randomised placebo-controlled study in 200 anaemic cardiac surgery patients tested the enteral administration of ferrous sulphate 325 mg three times daily versus placebo and showed that the intervention was of limited efficiency, except for a reduced number of transfusions ($p=0.03$), but at least did not increase infectious complications [49]. Indeed in critically ill patients, the enteral route is uncertain. The most recent intravenous iron formulations, available since the 1990s, seem to replenish iron stores safely and effectively [17]: in case of deficiency with low ferritine levels, only intravenous administraiton is efficient.

10.2.5 Thiamine: Vitamin B

The European Society for Clinical Nutrition and Metabolism (ESPEN) guidelines for parenteral nutrition in intensive care, published in 2009 [41], recommend empirical thiamine supplementation (100–300 mg/day) during the first 3 days in the ICU for all patients at risk of thiamine deficiency. Thiamine supplementation should be prescribed liberally in ICU patients [6], without any blood determination being required prior to empirical administration: such a sampling should though be done in case of searching for a specific diagnosis such as cardiac beriberi.

10.2.6 Vitamin C

The doses required to achieve normalisation of blood concentrations during critical illness are much higher than the daily 100 mg recommended for healthy subjects. Up to 3 g daily for 2–6 days are needed to restore normal plasma concentrations in ICU patients [31].

Clinical trials in sepsis, trauma and major burns testing high-dose vitamin C have shown clinical benefits. Phase I studies in sepsis seem to confirm safety of very high doses (200 mg/kg/24 h) delivered for a short period of time [50] and potentially a clinical benefit reflected by faster and significant reductions of the sequential organ failure assessment (SOFA) scores in patients receiving high-dose treatment in a double-blind placebo-controlled setting. In major burns megadose vitamin supplements (66 mg/kg/h) delivered intravenously during the first 24 h reduce fluid requirements during resuscitation, resulting in lesser weight gain and improved blood oxygenation [51]. It is still too early to introduce this strategy in clinical practice: further large-scale studies are required to confirm the safety of such high doses.

10.2.7 Vitamin D

A large randomised Austrian trial including 475 critically ill patients with vitamin D deficiency [52] showed that the administration of high-dose vitamin D3 (540,000 IU) compared with placebo did not reduce hospital length of stay, hospital mortality or 6-month mortality. Nevertheless in the severe vitamin D deficiency subgroup, lower hospital mortality was observed: this finding should be considered hypothesis generating until further studies confirm these findings. Recently a study (VITD) including 25 ICU patients with vitamin D deficiency an oral ultra-high dose (540,000 IU corresponding to 13.5 mg) corrected the deficient blood concentrations within 2 days without any side effect (no hypercalcaemia or hypercalciuria) [53].

In major burns, vitamin D deficiency develops over time [54]. Focus has been in paediatric patients. The mechanism causing this deficiency is mainly limited exposure to sun after burn injury and decreased skin synthesis [55], which contribute to osteoporosis observed after burns. It was recently shown in a Belgian cohort of 24 adult patients on standard vitamin D intakes (400–600 ui/day) that 22/24 were vitamin D deficient or insufficient very early after injury and remained below references [56]. In another cohort of 29 burn patients, an oral dose of 100,000 IU D3 succeeded in increasing circulating levels by a median of 33 % [57].

Vitamin D has been investigated in paediatrics as deficiency threatens child growth. A meta-analysis of paediatric trials shows that rapid normalisation of vitamin D levels is best achieved by using loading therapy that considers disease status, baseline 25(OH)D and age (or weight). Nevertheless this meta-analysis concludes that loading doses of 300 000 IU should be avoided until trials are conducted that better evaluate risk and benefit [58].

Based on actual data, low vitamin D levels at ICU admission may serve as an indicator for vitamin D replacement. Available parenteral multivitamin preparations contain about 200 IU of vitamin D2 or D3, in addition to other fat-soluble vitamins: no intravenous vitamin D mono-preparation is available [52]. Oral preparations exist with doses up to 800 UI: considering the variable intestinal absorption existing in critical care patients, this route is the only actually available.

10.3 How Should Micronutrients Be Prescribed and Delivered?

The mode of administration during PN is highly variable depending on each institution's practice in the absence of strong guidelines. While TE are stable, but risk to cause separation of the lipid emulsions, vitamins are not: many studies have shown that the various vitamins but particularly vitamins A, E and C are very rapidly degraded, being extremely sensitive to light. This latter reason is probably the best argument in favour of an administration separate from the PN solution delivered separately over 6–12 h in light-protected bags as for vitamins [59].

Another argument is associated with the limited retention in the case of rapid administration: a very complete balance study was conducted in 1977 [60] with the intravenous micronutrient solutions available in the 1970s (Addam®, precursor of Addamel and Lipovit® solutions). It showed that some micronutrients were retained such as Fe, while others appeared not to be. Other elements retained were Ag, Co, Cr, Cu, Sb, Sc and W, while Br and Rb were lost by the patients. Negative balances were also found for As, Au, Cd, Cs, Mo, Se and Zn. Serum concentrations of thirteen TE (Ag, Br, Co, Cs, Cu, Fe, Hg, Mo, Rb, Sc, Se, W and Zn) were found to decrease during the period of total PN. The doses available in these preparations were not much different from those on the market in the twentieth century. Therefore these results remain pertinent and call for monitoring of trace elements.

Many preparations available on the market were developed more than 30 years ago. In 2012 the American Society for Parenteral and Enteral Nutrition (ASPEN) called for a revision of their composition in a very well-documented position paper [39]. Single trace element solutions are not easily available on the market: iron solutions have been developed, as well as selenium preparations. The situation seems a little better with vitamins which have been upgraded in the recent decade. Nevertheless the actual commercial vitamin solutions are also due for revision [61]. In patients on long-term PN and chronic critically ill patients, monitoring of blood levels is therefore required for both TE and vitamins.

Whatever the dose considered, the micronutrients should not be delivered as bolus in clinical settings. Micronutrients should be infused over as long a period as possible [59]. However, the problem is the potential interactions in the bag. Trace elements are entirely stable, but some of the water-soluble vitamins are not. Especially ascorbic acid is extremely labile and interacts with copper, resulting in ascorbic acid destruction.

10.4 Conclusion

In critically ill patients with inflammatory conditions, recent research shows that micronutrient prescription is not confined to parenteral nutrition. The solutions available in clinical practice are probably insufficient to cover the basal requirements in the vast majority of critically ill patients: therefore in conditions at risk as described in the above text including patients on long-term artificial nutrition, blood sampling remains the only tool available to detect deficiencies and should be considered in patients requiring critical care for more than a week as well as in those with important losses of biological fluids.

References

1. Cotzias GC (1967) Importance of trace element substances in experimental health, as exemplified by manganese. Proc First Conf Trace Subst Environ Health 1967:5–19
2. Cox CE (2012) Persistent systemic inflammation in chronic critical illness. Respir Care 57:859–864; discussion 64–66
3. Hotchkiss RS, Karl IE (2003) The pathophysiology and treatment of sepsis. New Engl J Med 348:138–150
4. Ghashut RA, McMillan DC, Kinsella J, Vasilaki AT, Talwar D, Duncan A (2015) The effect of the systemic inflammatory response on plasma zinc and selenium adjusted for albumin. Clin Nutr 2015 Feb 26; e-pub doi: 10.1016/j.clnu.2015.02.010
5. Mertens K, Lowes DA, Webster NR et al (2015) Low zinc and selenium concentrations in sepsis are associated with oxidative damage and inflammation. Brit J Anaesth 114:990–999
6. Manzanares W, Hardy G (2011) Thiamine supplementation in the critically ill. Curr Opin Clin Nutr Metab Care 14:610–617
7. Bandmann O, Weiss KH, Kaler SG (2015) Wilson's disease and other neurological copper disorders. Lancet Neurol 14:103–113
8. Hordyjewska A, Popiolek L, Kocot J (2014) The many "faces" of copper in medicine and treatment. Biometals 27:611–621
9. Wilson HO, Datta DB (2014) Complications from micronutrient deficiency following bariatric surgery. Ann Clin Biochem 51:705–709
10. Berger MM, Shenkin A, Revelly JP et al (2004) Copper, selenium, zinc and thiamine balances during continuous venovenous hemodiafiltration in critically ill patients. Am J Clin Nutr 80:410–416
11. Bonafé L, Berger MM, Que YA, Mechanick JI (2014) Carnitine deficiency in chronic critical illness. Curr Opin Clin Nutr Metab Care 17:200–209
12. Berger MM, Shenkin A (1998) Trace elements in trauma and burns. Curr Opin Clin Nutr Metab Care 1:513–517
13. Gosling P, Rothe HM, Sheehan TM, Hubbard LD (1995) Serum copper and zinc concentrations in patients with burns in relation to burn surface area. J Burn Care Rehab 16:481–486
14. Berger MM, Baines M, Raffoul W et al (2007) Trace element supplements after major burns modulate antioxidant status and clinical course by way of increased tissue trace element concentration. Am J Clin Nutr 85:1293–1300
15. Heming N, Montravers P, Lasocki S (2011) Iron deficiency in critically ill patients: highlighting the role of hepcidin. Crit Care 15:210
16. Piagnerelli M, Cotton F, Herpain A et al (2013) Time course of iron metabolism in critically ill patients. Acta Clin Belg 68:22–27
17. Lopez A, Cacoub P, Macdougall IC, Peyrin-Biroulet L (2015) Iron deficiency anaemia. Lancet 2015 Aug 24 epub: doi: 10.1016/S0140-6736(15)60865-0
18. Duntas LH, Benvenga S (2015) Selenium: an element for life. Endocrine 48:756–775
19. Brigelius-Flohe R, Maiorino M (1830) Glutathione peroxidases. Biochim Biophys Acta 2013:3289–3303
20. Forceville X, Vitoux D, Gauzit R, Combes A, Lahilaire P, Chappuis P (1998) Selenium, systemic immune response syndrome, sepsis, and outcome in critically ill patients. Crit Care Med 26:1536–1544

21. Prasad AS (2013) Discovery of human zinc deficiency: its impact on human health and disease. Adv Nutr 4:176–190
22. Sandstead HH (2013) Human zinc deficiency: discovery to initial translation. Adv Nutr 4:76–81
23. Gruzewska K, Michno A, Pawelczyk T, Bielarczyk H (2014) Essentiality and toxicity of vanadium supplements in health and pathology. J Physiol Pharmacol 65:603–611
24. Ozturk N, Olgar Y, Ozdemir S (2013) Trace elements in diabetic cardiomyopathy: an electrophysiological overview. World J Diabetes 4:92–100
25. Wu Y, Huang M, Zhao P, Yang X (2013) Vanadyl acetylacetonate upregulates PPAR gamma and adiponectin expression in differentiated rat adipocytes. J Biol Inorg Chem JBIC 18:623–631
26. Gioda CR, de Oliveira Barreto T, Primola-Gomes TN et al (2010) Cardiac oxidative stress is involved in heart failure induced by thiamine deprivation in rats. Am J Physiol Heart Circ Physiol 298:H2039–H2045
27. Lima LF, Leite HP, Taddei JA (2011) Low blood thiamine concentrations in children upon admission to the intensive care unit: risk factors and prognostic significance. Am J Clin Nutr 93:57–61
28. Costa NA, Gut AL, de Souza Dorna M et al (2014) Serum thiamine concentration and oxidative stress as predictors of mortality in patients with septic shock. J Crit Care 29:249–252
29. Berger MM, Oudemans-van Straaten HM (2015) Vitamin C supplementation in the critically ill patient. Curr Opin Clin Nutr Metab Care 18:193–201
30. Oudemans-van Straaten HM, Man A, de Waard MC (2014) Vitamin C revisited. Crit Care 18:460
31. Long CL, Maull KI, Krishnan RS et al (2003) Ascorbic acid dynamics in the seriously ill and injured. J Surg Res 109:144–148
32. de Grooth HM, Spoelstra-de Man AME, Oudemans-van Straaten HM (2014) Early plasma vitamin C concentration, organ dysfunction and ICU mortality. Abstract. Intens Care Med 40
33. Rizzoli R (2014) Nutritional aspects of bone health. Best Pract Res Clin Endocrinol Metab 28:795–808
34. Zajic P, Amrein K (2014) Vitamin D deficiency in the ICU: a systematic review. Minerva Endocrinol 39:275–287
35. Amrein K, Venkatesh B (2012) Vitamin D and the critically ill patient. Curr Opin Clin Nutr Metab Care 15:188–193
36. Moraes RB, Friedman G, Wawrzeniak IC et al (2015) Vitamin D deficiency is independently associated with mortality among critically ill patients. Clinics (Sao Paolo) 70:326–332
37. Borum PR (2009) Carnitine in parenteral nutrition. Gastroenterology 137:S129–S134
38. Hatamkhani S, Karimzadeh I, Elyasi S, Farsaie S, Khalili H (2013) Carnitine and sepsis: a review of an old clinical dilemma. J Pharm Pharm Sci 16:414–423
39. Vanek VW, Borum P, Buchman A et al (2012) A.S.P.E.N. Position paper: recommendations for changes in commercially available parenteral multivitamin and multi–trace element products. Nutr Clin Pract Off Publ Am Soc Parenter Enteral Nutr 27:440–491
40. Buchman AL (2009) The addition of choline to parenteral nutrition. Gastroenterology 137:S119–S128
41. Singer P, Berger MM, Van den Berghe G et al (2009) ESPEN guidelines on parenteral nutrition: intensive care. Clin Nutr 28:387–400
42. Collier BR, Giladi A, Dossett LA, Dyer L, Fleming SB, Cotton BA (2008) Impact of high-dose antioxidants on outcomes in acutely injured patients. JPEN J Parenter Enteral Nutr 32: 384–388
43. Berger MM, Soguel L, Shenkin A et al (2008) Influence of early antioxidant supplements on clinical evolution and organ function in critically ill cardiac surgery, major trauma and subarachnoid hemorrhage patients. Crit Care 12:R101
44. Barbosa E, Faintuch J, Machado Moreira EA et al (2009) Supplementation of vitamin E, vitamin C, and zinc attenuates oxidative stress in burned children: a randomized, double-blind, placebo-controlled pilot study. J Burn Care Res 30:859–866

45. Alhazzani W, Jacobi J, Sindi A et al (2013) The effect of selenium therapy on mortality in patients with sepsis syndrome: a systematic review and meta-analysis of randomized controlled trials. Crit Care Med 41:1555–1564
46. Manzanares W, Dhaliwal R, Jiang X, Murch L, Heyland DK (2012) Antioxidant micronutrients in the critically ill: a systematic review and meta-analysis. Crit Care 16:R66
47. Jeejeebhoy KN (2007) Human zinc deficiency. Nutr Clin Pract 22:65–67
48. Scrimshaw NS, SanGiovanni JP (1997) Synergism of nutrition, infection, and immunity – an overview. Am J Clin Nutr 66:464S–477S
49. Pieracci FM, Henderson P, Rodney JR et al (2009) Randomized, double-blind, placebo-controlled trial of effects of enteral iron supplementation on anemia and risk of infection during surgical critical illness. Surg Infect (Larchmt) 10:9–19
50. Fowler AA 3rd, Syed AA, Knowlson S et al (2014) Phase I safety trial of intravenous ascorbic acid in patients with severe sepsis. J Transl Med 12:32
51. Tanaka H, Matsuda T, Miyagantani Y, Yukioka T, Matsuda H, Shimazaki S (2000) Reduction of resuscitation fluid volumes in severely burned patients using ascorbic acid administration. Arch Surg 135:326–331
52. Amrein K, Schnedl C, Holl A et al (2014) Effect of high-dose vitamin D3 on hospital length of stay in critically ill patients with vitamin D deficiency: the VITdAL-ICU randomized clinical trial. JAMA 312:1520–1530
53. Amrein K, Sourij H, Wagner G et al (2011) Short-term effects of high-dose oral vitamin D3 in critically ill vitamin D deficient patients: a randomized, double-blind, placebo-controlled pilot study. Crit Care 15:R104
54. Gottschlich MM, Mayes T, Khoury J, Warden GD (2004) Hypovitaminosis D in acutely injured pediatric burn patients. J Am Diet Assoc 104:931–941; quiz 1031
55. Klein GL, Holick MF, Langman CB, Celis MM, Herndon DN (2004) Synthesis of vitamin D in skin after burns. Lancet 363:291–292
56. Rousseau AF, Damas P, Ledoux D, Cavalier E (2014) Effect of cholecalciferol recommended daily allowances on vitamin D status and fibroblast growth factor-23: an observational study in acute burn patients. Burns 40:865–870
57. Rousseau AF, Damas P, Ledoux D et al (2015) Vitamin D status after a high dose of cholecalciferol in healthy and burn subjects. Burns 41:1028–1034
58. McNally JD, Iliriani K, Pojsupap S et al (2015) Rapid normalization of vitamin D levels: a meta-analysis. Pediatrics 135:e152–e166
59. Berger MM, Shenkin A (2006) Vitamins and trace elements: practical aspects of supplementation. Nutrition 22:952–955
60. Jacobson S, Wester PO (1977) Balance study of twenty trace elements during total parenteral nutrition in man. Br J Nutr 37:107–126
61. Buchman AL, Howard LJ, Guenter P, Nishikawa RA, Compher CW, Tappenden KA (2009) Micronutrients in parenteral nutrition: too little or too much? The past, present, and recommendations for the future. Gastroenterology 137:S1–S6
62. Shenkin A (2008) Basics in clinical nutrition: trace elements and vitamins in parenteral and enteral nutrition. e-SPEN e293–7
63. Bailay LB, Baumgartner TG, Borum PR et al (1997) Clinical guide to parenteral micronutrition, 3rd edn, pp. 271–395, and 403–620

Part II
Hormonal Regulation

Chapter 11
Thyroidal Changes During Critical Illness

Lies Langouche and Greet Van den Berghe

Abstract Patients suffering from a variety of critical illnesses present with uniform alterations within the thyroid axis with low plasma triiodothyronine (T3), but increased plasma reverse T3 (rT3). As these changes occur in the presence of low-normal thyroid stimulating hormone (TSH), this constellation is also referred to as Nonthyroidal Illness Syndrome (NTI). Both central and peripheral components of the thyroidal axis play a role in the development of NTI. Furthermore, nutritional intake can affect the extent and composition of NTI. The severity of NTI is associated with a poor prognosis, but it is still unclear whether this indicates a causal relationship, or in contrast, an adaptation to more severe illness.

11.1 The Thyroid Axis During Health

Thyroid hormones (TH) are essential for differentiation and growth, from fetal development throughout adult live [1]. They are important regulators of thermoregulation and energy metabolism and are involved in lipid and glucose metabolism [2]. The circulating concentrations of TH are tightly regulated by a classical hypothalamic-pituitary-thyroid feedback system. The hypothalamus releases thyrotropin-releasing hormone (TRH), which stimulates the anterior pituitary to synthesize and release thyroid-stimulating hormone (TSH). TSH sequentially stimulates the thyroid gland to produce and release thyroxine (T4) [3]. The thyroid gland mainly generates T4, but the biological activity of TH is predominantly regulated by triiodothyronine (T3) [1]. Both T4 and T3 have inhibitory feedback control on both TRH and TSH secretion [4, 5].

L. Langouche, MSc, PhD • G. Van den Berghe, MD, PhD (✉)
Department of Cellular and Molecular Medicine, Clinical Division and Laboratory of Intensive Care Medicine, KU Leuven, Herestraat 49, Leuven B-3000, Belgium
e-mail: greet.vandenberghe@med.kuleuven.be

J.-C. Preiser (ed.), *The Stress Response of Critical Illness: Metabolic and Hormonal Aspects*, DOI 10.1007/978-3-319-27687-8_11

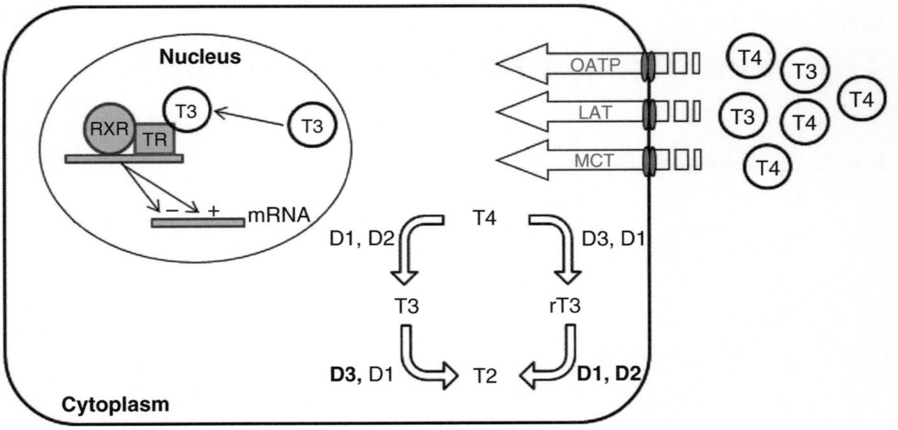

Fig. 11.1 Schematic outline of cellular uptake and metabolism of thyroid hormones

TH are transported in the blood by thyroxine-binding globulin (TBG), transthyretin, and albumin [6]. TBG is the dominant binding protein with the highest binding affinity for T4, around 50-fold higher than that of transthyretin and 7000-fold higher than that of albumin. Several transporters mediate the uptake of TH across the plasma membrane. The organic anion-transporting polypeptide-1C1, the monocarboxylate transporter (MCT) 8 and MCT10, and the L-type amino acid transporter (LAT) 1 and LAT2, and more recently LAT3 and LAT4 have been identified as relatively specific TH transporters [7, 8] (Fig. 11.1). The intracellular action of TH is further regulated by several subtypes of iodothyronine deiodinases. These enzymes are responsible for the deiodination of T4 to the active T3 or to the biologically inactive reverse T3 (rT3) [9, 10]. T3 mainly exerts its actions through interaction with its specific nuclear receptors TRα and TRβ to regulate gene transcription but can also induce nongenomic effects [11].

11.2 Alterations in the Thyroid Axis in Acute and Prolonged Critical Illness

Patients suffering from a variety of critical illnesses present with uniform alterations within the thyroid axis (Fig. 11.2). During acute and severe physical stress, caused by illness, surgery, or trauma, T3 plasma concentrations decline rapidly, whereas circulating rT3 concentrations increase. The concentration of T4 is only shortly elevated and subsequently returns to the normal physiological range, although in more severely ill patients, T4 concentration can also decrease [12]. In contrast with primary hypothyroidism, low plasma T3 concentration perseveres in the presence of normal TSH. This constellation, with low plasma T3 but normal TSH in the context of illness, has been described as “euthyroid sick syndrome,” “low T3 syndrome,” or “nonthyroidal illness (NTI).” The reduction in circulating T3 during the first hours after ICU admission reflects the severity of illness and correlates with outcome [13, 14].

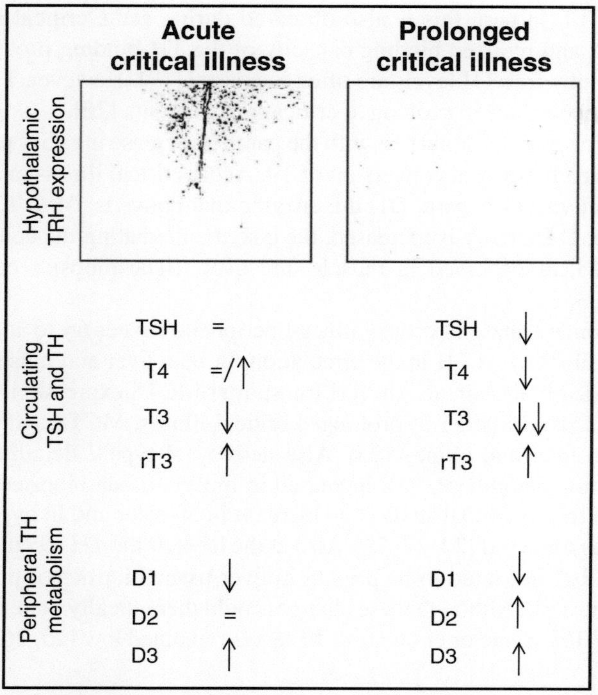

Fig. 11.2 Changes in the thyroid axis during acute and chronic critical illness. The upper panel displays reduced TRH gene expression in the hypothalamus of prolonged critically ill rabbits (Adapted from [28]). The middle panel illustrates schematically the observed adaptations in circulating TSH and TH of acute and prolonged critically ill patients. The bottom panel summarizes the findings in deiodinase tissue activity of acute and prolonged critically ill patients

The TSH profile is already affected in this acute phase of critical illness; while single-sample TSH levels are normal, the typical nocturnal TSH surge is no longer present [15]. When patients do not immediately recover and require prolonged intensive care, the pulsatile TSH release becomes substantially suppressed in addition to the absent nocturnal TSH surge [16]. Circulating T4 declines, with as a result much less elevated rT3, and circulating T3 can decrease even further. In this later phase of illness, reduced TSH, lowered T4 and T3, and elevated rT3 levels are associated with worse outcome [17].

11.3 Underlying Pathology of the Low T3 Syndrome

11.3.1 Binding Proteins and Peripheral Metabolism of Thyroid Hormones

In normal conditions, total plasma TH concentration is kept proportional to the concentration of TH-binding proteins, in order to maintain free hormone levels in equilibrium [18]. In part, this is also observed during acute critical illnesses with reduced levels and reduced binding capacity of the TH-binding proteins TBG and albumin, whereby free TH levels are often increased [19]. However, TBG returns to normal reference values in prolonged critically ill patients [20].

The acute lowering of (total) T3 with the parallel increase in rT3 is predominantly due to an altered peripheral conversion of T4. Acute critical illness or inflammation reduces the activity of hepatic D1, the enzyme that converts T4 to T3 [21, 22]. At the same time, D3 activity is increased, the enzyme mediating the conversion of T4 to inactive rT3, as observed in muscle and liver tissue biopsies of critically ill patients [21, 23, 24].

In the prolonged phase of critical illness, peripheral tissues try to adapt to the sustained low availability of TH in the circulation. In both liver and muscle biopsies of prolonged critically ill patients, the TH transporter MCT8 expression was increased [25]. Also in a rabbit model of prolonged critical illness, MCT8 and MCT10 were upregulated in liver and kidney [25]. Also activity of type 2 deiodinase (D2), the second activating deiodinase, was increased in muscle tissue biopsies of prolonged ICU patients [26]. In animal studies, an increase in alveolar and in hypothalamic D2 expression was observed [22, 27–29]. Also at the level of the TH receptor, an upregulated TRα1/TRα2 appeared to be present in liver tissue biopsies of prolonged critically ill patients [30]. Although these changes could theoretically increase local tissue availability of TH, tissue or circulating T3 levels remained low [25, 26, 28].

11.3.2 The Impact of the Nutritional Status of the Patient

Loss of appetite and poor oral/enteral nutritional intake are very common in critical illness [31]. Of interest, the thyroidal alterations during the first days of critical illness are comparable to those observed for otherwise healthy subjects in the fasting state [32–34]. The contribution of restricted nutrition during human critical illnesses to the NTI has been documented in a few small clinical studies that indeed indicated that decreased caloric intake during critical illness is associated with more pronounced NTI changes [35–37]. More recently, the large randomized controlled EPaNIC trial compared two nutritional regimens in adult ICU patients [38]. This study demonstrated that tolerating a nutritional deficit during the first week of critical illness as compared with the early administration of supplemental parenteral nutrition resulted in fewer complications and accelerated recovery [38]. Furthermore, a subanalysis of this EPaNIC trial demonstrated that while not feeding early reduced complications and accelerated recovery of patients with NTI, it aggravated the decrease in circulating levels of TSH, total T4 and T3, and the T3 to rT3 ratio. The opposite was observed with early feeding that appeared to "improve" the NTI [39]. Similar findings were reported from an animal study which compared the effect of fasting versus feeding over 7 days of critical illness [40]. This study furthermore demonstrated that while early feeding diminished the lowering of T3, it also normalized peripheral D1 and D3 activity [40].

The instant drop in circulating T3 during nutrient restriction in otherwise healthy subjects has been explained as an attempt of the human body to avert protein breakdown by reducing energy expenditure [34]. Also in critically ill patients, tolerating a fasting response induced a more significant inactivation of T4 with lower T3 and higher rT3, which explained part of the outcome benefit of not feeding early [39]. Also targeting fasting blood glucose levels with insulin therapy in critically ill children, which mimics the blood glucose levels of a fasting response, resulted in improved outcome while further accentuating the NTI [41]. Together these findings indicate that at least a part of the immediate decrease in circulating T3 is induced by the reduced nutritional intake in critically ill patients rather than by the underlying illness and that this might be an adaptive response.

11.3.3 Central Regulation

The observation that despite the low circulating T3 and low-normal T4 single-sample TSH levels are low normal in the prolonged phase of critical illness, suggests a centrally suppressed thyroid axis [16]. This is further corroborated by the observed reduced hypothalamic TRH gene expression in brain sections of patients dying after chronic critical illness and in prolonged critically ill rabbits [28, 42]. In contrast, in the pituitaries of these prolonged critically ill rabbits, TSH gene and protein expression remained normal [43]. The substantial increase in TSH secretion and in peripheral TH concentrations, which is observed after TRH administration in prolonged critically ill patients and animals, supports this interpretation [44, 45]. Also the observation that the onset of recovery is preceded by a rise in TSH suggests that a suppressed hypothalamic stimulation of the pituitary plays a role in the prolonged phase of critical illness [46].

This central suppression of TRH could be the consequence of a changed set point for TH-induced feedback inhibition, due to a local upregulation of TH concentration. As stated above, in animal studies, an increase in hypothalamic D2 expression was observed after LPS injection [22, 29]. Also a rabbit study of prolonged critical illness demonstrated increased D2 levels as well as TH transporters in the hypothalamus [28]. However, as local hypothalamic T4 and T3 content were low normal in these rabbits, these findings could also suggest a compensatory response to a relative hypothyroid hypothalamic state rather than an altered set point. This attempt to compensate for sustained low thyroid levels also suggests that the hypothalamic suppression of the thyroid axis could be a deleterious consequence of prolonged or more severe critical illness. This was also suggested by the EPaNIC subanalysis, where the further lowering of T4 in nutrient-restricted patients was associated with worse outcome [39]. Also consistent with this interpretation is the observation that especially the more severely ill patients present a decline in circulating T4 levels, whereas all other critically ill patients reveal low T3 and high rT3 levels already from admission to the ICU [17]. Furthermore, ICU patients who received an infusion of TRH combined with a GH secretagogue displayed normalized TH levels coinciding with lowered markers of hypercatabolism [44].

11.3.4 Contributing Factors

Cytokines can mimic the acute changes of the thyroid axis and are assumed be involved in the pathogenesis of NTI [47, 48]. Especially TNF was clearly associated with the alterations in TH metabolism in human clinical samples [49, 50]. However, administration of cytokine antagonists did not restore normal thyroid function after endotoxemic challenge [51, 52].

Administered as well as endogenous dopamine or corticosteroids could also play a role as these can trigger or aggravate hypothyroidism in critical illness [53, 54]. The low selenium concentrations observed already from admission to the ICU is another potential interfering factor [55]. Indeed, deiodinases require selenium for their catalytic activity and defects in the synthesis of selenoproteins or nutritional selenium deficiency can lead to reduced deiodinase activity [2]. Furthermore, selenium supplementation in trauma patients was associated with modest changes in thyroid hormones, with an earlier normalization of T4, T3, and reverse T3 [56]. In patients with acute myocardial infarction, the administration of N-acetyl-cysteine, an antioxidant that can stimulate activity of the deiodinases by restoring intracellular cysteine and/or glutathione levels, prevented the T3 increase and lowered rT3 compared to placebo-treated patients [57].

11.4 TH Actions During Critical Illness

During the acute phase of critical illness, the peripheral alteration in deiodinase activity causes a reduction in circulating levels of the biologically active T3. As explained above, this acute part of the thyroidal response appears to be, at least in part, adaptive. Besides the overall downregulation of metabolism in the organism in order to save energy, also a direct effect of increased D3 could be beneficial, such as in granulocytes, where it could optimize bacterial killing capacity [58, 59].

In patients who require prolonged intensive care, the origin and impact of the thyroidal changes appear to differ. Several clinical symptoms observed during prolonged critical illness, such as muscle and skin atrophy and hair loss and also hypothermia, impaired consciousness, and hampered myocardial function, resemble those observed in hypothyroidism. Furthermore, during the prolonged phase of critical illness, peripheral tissues seem to adapt to the sustained low circulating TH levels with tissue-specific changes in TH transporters, deiodinases, and receptors. For example, endotoxin increased D2 expression in macrophages, which was shown to be essential for cytokine production and phagocytosis [60]. Also alveolar D2 upregulation during sepsis appeared to be adaptive during acute lung injury and sepsis [27].

11.5 Substitution Treatment?

Whether or not critically ill patients would benefit from TH treatment is yet unclear. The biphasic nature of the origin and consequences of low T3 during critical illness indicates that certainly in the early phase of critical illness, such benefit can be questioned. As the reduced nutritional intake that goes along with the acute response to illness is to a large extent responsible for the observed thyroidal alterations, these responses are likely selected by evolution and do not warrant interference. On the other hand, prolonged critically ill patients, who are fully fed, still suffer from sustained low T3 and T4 and display signs or symptoms of hypothyroidism and might benefit from a treatment that aims at normalizing thyroid hormones.

Unfortunately, only very limited clinical studies testing this hypothesis are available, often underpowered, with a high variability in patient selection (age, disease type, and timing) or treatment choice. Administration of T4 failed to demonstrate a clinical benefit, although this could be partly because of a compromised conversion of T4 to T3 [61]. Treatment with T3 substitution doses to children after cardiopulmonary bypass surgery was associated with improved postoperative cardiac function; however, the children received dopamine which induces iatrogenic hypothyroidism [62]. One also has to bear in mind that circulating TH levels do not necessarily reflect normalized tissue levels [24]. A continuous infusion of TRH combined with a growth hormone secretagogue not only normalized TH to physiological levels, but markers of hypercatabolism were also lowered [44]. Sufficiently powered randomized controlled trials in a well-selected patient population are required to test a potential beneficial effect on outcome.

11.6 Primary Thyroid Disorders in ICU Patients

Patients, who suffer from long-term primary hypothyroidism, depend physiologically on exogenous thyroid replacement, usually administered as oral levothyroxine. However, at admission to the ICU, the primary focus of care is the acute medical problem of the patient and not the prescription and continuation of chronic therapy. A retrospective chart review study in a tertiary referral university hospital demonstrated that thyroid replacement therapy was discontinued in up to 40 % of the patients for at least 7 days during their ICU stay. This was either due to lack of prescription or because the patient was intolerant to oral feeding and no parenteral preparation was prescribed [63]. Inadequate replacement or omission of therapy will lead to hypothyroidism in these patients, which can lead to adverse outcome including loss of consciousness and bradycardia [63].

The high prevalence of NTI and the extent of the thyroid axis changes in ICU patients can make it difficult to distinguish NTI from untreated primary hypothyroidism. For the diagnosis of untreated primary hypothyroidism in ICU patients, the most useful parameter is elevated plasma TSH in the presence of low TH. In patients clinically suspected to have severe hypothyroidism and with demonstrated low plasma TH, a normal plasma TSH virtually excludes primary hypothyroidism. However, one should bear in mind that in hypothyroid patients, high serum TSH concentration may decrease during critical illness especially if the patient receives dopamine or high doses of glucocorticoids [53, 54]. On the other hand, although high plasma TSH in combination with low plasma T4 is indicative of hypothyroidism, this constellation can also be found in patients recovering from NTI [46]. A more clear distinction between primary hypothyroidism and NTI would be presence of a high plasma T3/T4 ratio in combination with low plasma rT3, as these changes are opposite to those of NTI, but these measurements only have limited diagnostic accuracy.

A very dangerous complication of untreated hypothyroidism is the development of myxedema coma. A secondary insult such as hypothermia, vascular accidents, or infection may trigger this life-threatening condition [64]. Diagnosis is based on elevated plasma TSH with low or undetectable T4 and T3 and the presence of clinical features such as changes in mental status (lethargy, stupor, delirium, or coma) and hypothermia. Again, the presence of NTI may reduce the degree of TSH elevation. Myxedema coma is potentially fatal (mortality up to 50 %), thus immediate treatment is required and depends on the recognition of the clinical features. Treatment should aim at TH replacement therapy, combined with ventilatory and hemodynamic support. In addition, stress dose glucocorticoids are advised as concomitant autoimmune primary adrenal insufficiency may be present, especially in patients with hypoglycemia [65].

Patients suffering from thyrotoxicosis, or hyperthyroidism, may present with high free T4 in combination with low serum TSH. The combination of suppressed TSH, high FT4, and normal T3 may point to the combination of thyrotoxicosis and NTI. Clinical features (thyroid enlargement, proptosis) and the presence of thyroid antibodies (anti-TPO, TBII) can give further confirmation.

Decompensated hyperthyroidism (or thyroid storm) is characterized by the acute onset of enhanced symptoms of hyperthyroidism. It is important to recognize that this condition is a clinical diagnosis; laboratory measurements cannot distinguish severe thyrotoxicosis from thyroid storm. The classic clinical features include fever, supraventricular tachycardia, gastrointestinal symptoms, and confusion, delirium, or sometimes coma [64]. Of note, altered mentation was the only clinical feature which was significantly different between patients with thyroid storm and patients with compensated thyrotoxicosis [66]. Precipitating factors include surgery, parturition, infection, iodinated contrast materials, stroke, diabetic ketoacidosis, and withdrawal or discontinuation of antithyroid medications. Treatment includes ICU monitoring and aims at restoring thyroid gland function while diminishing TH effects on peripheral tissues using a combination of beta-blockers, glucocorticoids, antithyroid drugs, and eventually high dose of iodide compounds [67].

11.7 Conclusion

Critically ill patients display low plasma T3 with increased plasma rT3, in the presence of low or normal TSH and low or normal T4. This constellation is referred to as nonthyroidal illness or NTI. Although the severity of illness strongly correlates with the severity of the changes in thyroidal hormone concentrations, the causality of this association is not fully elucidated. In the acute phase of illness, NTI is predominantly induced by the reduced nutritional intake and seems to be a beneficial adaptation in times of high metabolic demand. On the other hand, in prolonged critically ill patients also a central hypothalamic suppression seems to occur which appears to be related to worse outcome.

Sufficiently powered randomized controlled trials in a well-selected patient population, targeting especially prolonged critically ill patients, are required to test a potential beneficial effect on outcome. Treatment with hypothalamic-releasing factors might be the optimal choice to normalize circulating T4 and T3 levels in these patients.

Acknowledgments *Supported* by the Methusalem Program of the Flemish Government (METH/14/06) to GVdB via the KU Leuven, by an ERC Advanced Grant (AdvG-2012-321670) to GVdB from the Ideas Program of the European Union seventh framework program.

Conflicts of Interest The authors have no conflicts of interest to disclose.

References

1. Yen PM (2001) Physiological and molecular basis of thyroid hormone action. Physiol Rev 81(3):1097–1142
2. Mullur R, Liu YY, Brent GA (2014) Thyroid hormone regulation of metabolism. Physiol Rev 94(2):355–382
3. Goldsmith RE, Stanbury JB, Brownell GL (1951) The effect of thyrotropin on the release of hormone from the human thyroid. J Clin Endocrinol Metab 11(10):1079–1094
4. Weintraub BD, Wondisford FE, Farr EA et al (1989) Pre-translational and post-translational regulation of TSH synthesis in normal and neoplastic thyrotrophs. Horm Res 32(1–3):22–24
5. Bodenner DL, Mroczynski MA, Weintraub BD, Radovick S, Wondisford FE (1991) A detailed functional and structural analysis of a major thyroid hormone inhibitory element in the human thyrotropin beta-subunit gene. J Biol Chem 266(32):21666–21673
6. Oppenheimer JH (1968) Role of plasma proteins in the binding, distribution and metabolism of the thyroid hormones. N Engl J Med 278(21):1153–1162
7. Visser WE, Friesema EC, Jansen J, Visser TJ (2008) Thyroid hormone transport in and out of cells. Trends Endocrinol Metab 19(2):50–56
8. Zevenbergen C, Meima ME, Lima de Souza EC et al (2015) transport of iodothyronines by human l-type amino acid transporters. Endocrinology 156(11):4345–4355. doi:10.1210/en2015-1140
9. Bianco AC, Salvatore D, Gereben B, Berry MJ, Larsen PR (2002) Biochemistry, cellular and molecular biology, and physiological roles of the iodothyronine selenodeiodinases. Endocr Rev 23(1):38–89

10. Friesema EC, Jansen J, Visser TJ (2005) Thyroid hormone transporters. Biochem Soc Trans 33(Pt 1):228–232
11. Cheng SY, Leonard JL, Davis PJ (2010) Molecular aspects of thyroid hormone actions. Endocr Rev 31(2):139–170
12. Van den Berghe G (2000) Novel insights into the neuroendocrinology of critical illness. Eur J Endocrinol 143(1):1–13
13. Rothwell PM, Lawler PG (1995) Prediction of outcome in intensive care patients using endocrine parameters. Crit Care Med 23(1):78–83
14. Rothwell PM, Udwadia ZF, Lawler PG (1993) Thyrotropin concentration predicts outcome in critical illness. Anaesthesia 48(5):373–376
15. Romijn JA, Wiersinga WM (1990) Decreased nocturnal surge of thyrotropin in nonthyroidal illness. J Clin Endocrinol Metab 70(1):35–42
16. Van den Berghe G, de Zegher F, Veldhuis JD et al (1997) Thyrotropin and prolactin release in prolonged critical illness: dynamics of spontaneous secretion and effects of growth hormone-secretagogues. Clin Endocrinol (Oxf) 47(5):599–612
17. Peeters RP, Wouters PJ, van Toor H, Kaptein E, Visser TJ, Van den Berghe G (2005) Serum rT3 and T3/rT3 are prognostic markers in critically ill patients and are associated with post-mortem tissue deiodinase activities. J Clin Endocrinol Metab 90(8):4559–4565
18. Refetoff S, Robin NI, Fang VS (1970) Parameters of thyroid function in serum of 16 selected vertebrate species: a study of PBI, serum T4, free T4, and the pattern of T4 and T3 binding to serum proteins. Endocrinology 86(4):793–805
19. Docter R, van Toor H, Krenning EP, de Jong M, Hennemann G (1993) Free thyroxine assessed with three assays in sera of patients with nonthyroidal illness and of subjects with abnormal concentrations of thyroxine-binding proteins. Clin Chem 39(8):1668–1674
20. Van den Berghe G, de Zegher F, Vlasselaers D et al (1996) Thyrotropin-releasing hormone in critical illness: from a dopamine-dependent test to a strategy for increasing low serum triiodothyronine, prolactin, and growth hormone concentrations. Crit Care Med 24(4):590–595
21. Peeters RP, Wouters PJ, Kaptein E, van Toor H, Visser TJ, Van den Berghe G (2003) Reduced activation and increased inactivation of thyroid hormone in tissues of critically ill patients. J Clin Endocrinol Metab 88(7):3202–3211
22. Boelen A, Kwakkel J, Thijssen-Timmer DC, Alkemade A, Fliers E, Wiersinga WM (2004) Simultaneous changes in central and peripheral components of the hypothalamus-pituitary-thyroid axis in lipopolysaccharide-induced acute illness in mice. J Endocrinol 182(2):315–323
23. Rodriguez-Perez A, Palos-Paz F, Kaptein E et al (2008) Identification of molecular mechanisms related to nonthyroidal illness syndrome in skeletal muscle and adipose tissue from patients with septic shock. Clin Endocrinol (Oxf) 68(5):821–827
24. Peeters RP, Geyten S, Wouters PJ et al (2005) Tissue thyroid hormone levels in critical illness. J Clin Endocrinol Metab 90(12):6498–6507
25. Mebis L, Paletta D, Debaveye Y et al (2009) Expression of thyroid hormone transporters during critical illness. Eur J Endocrinol 161(2):243–250
26. Mebis L, Langouche L, Visser TJ, Van den Berghe G (2007) The type II iodothyronine deiodinase is up-regulated in skeletal muscle during prolonged critical illness. J Clin Endocrinol Metab 92(8):3330–3333
27. Ma SF, Xie L, Pino-Yanes M et al (2011) Type 2 deiodinase and host responses of sepsis and acute lung injury. Am J Respir Cell Mol Biol 45(6):1203–1211
28. Mebis L, Debaveye Y, Ellger B et al (2009) Changes in the central component of the hypothalamus-pituitary-thyroid axis in a rabbit model of prolonged critical illness. Crit Care 13(5):R147
29. Fekete C, Gereben B, Doleschall M et al (2004) Lipopolysaccharide induces type 2 iodothyronine deiodinase in the mediobasal hypothalamus: implications for the nonthyroidal illness syndrome. Endocrinology 145(4):1649–1655
30. Thijssen-Timmer DC, Peeters RP, Wouters P et al (2007) Thyroid hormone receptor isoform expression in livers of critically ill patients. Thyroid 17(2):105–112

31. Schutz P, Bally M, Stanga Z, Keller U (2014) Loss of appetite in acutely ill medical inpatients: physiological response or therapeutic target? Swiss Med Wkly 144:w13957
32. Everts ME, Jong M, Lim CF et al (1996) Different regulation of thyroid hormone transport in liver and pituitary: its possible role in the maintenance of low T3 production during nonthyroidal illness and fasting in man. Thyroid 6(4):359–368
33. Boelen A, Wiersinga WM, Fliers E (2008) Fasting-induced changes in the hypothalamus-pituitary-thyroid axis. Thyroid 18(2):123–129
34. Gardner DF, Kaplan MM, Stanley CA, Utiger RD (1979) Effect of tri-iodothyronine replacement on the metabolic and pituitary responses to starvation. N Engl J Med 300(11): 579–584
35. Chourdakis M, Kraus MM, Tzellos T et al (2012) Effect of early compared with delayed enteral nutrition on endocrine function in patients with traumatic brain injury: an open-labeled randomized trial. JPEN J Parenter Enteral Nutr 36(1):108–116
36. Richmand DA, Molitch ME, O'Donnell TF (1980) Altered thyroid hormone levels in bacterial sepsis: the role of nutritional adequacy. Metabolism 29(10):936–942
37. Ouchi K, Matsubara S, Matsuno S (1991) Effects of supplementary parenteral nutrition on thyroid hormone patterns in surgical patients with liver cirrhosis. Nutrition 7(3):189–192
38. Casaer MP, Mesotten D, Hermans G et al (2011) Early versus late parenteral nutrition in critically ill adults. N Engl J Med 365(6):506–517
39. Langouche L, Vander PS, Marques M et al (2013) Impact of early nutrient restriction during critical illness on the nonthyroidal illness syndrome and its relation with outcome: a randomized, controlled clinical study. J Clin Endocrinol Metab 98(3):1006–1013
40. Mebis L, Eerdekens A, Guiza F et al (2012) Contribution of nutritional deficit to the pathogenesis of the nonthyroidal illness syndrome in critical illness: a rabbit model study. Endocrinology 153(2):973–984
41. Gielen M, Mesotten D, Wouters PJ et al (2012) Effect of tight glucose control with insulin on the thyroid axis of critically ill children and its relation with outcome. J Clin Endocrinol Metab 97(10):3569–3576
42. Fliers E, Guldenaar SE, Wiersinga WM, Swaab DF (1997) Decreased hypothalamic thyrotropin-releasing hormone gene expression in patients with nonthyroidal illness. J Clin Endocrinol Metab 82(12):4032–4036
43. Langouche L, Princen L, Gunst J, Guiza F, Derde S, Van den Berghe G (2013) Anterior pituitary morphology and hormone production during sustained critical illness in a rabbit model. Horm Metab Res 45(4):277–282
44. Van den Berghe G, de Zegher F, Baxter RC et al (1998) Neuroendocrinology of prolonged critical illness: effects of exogenous thyrotropin-releasing hormone and its combination with growth hormone secretagogues. J Clin Endocrinol Metab 83(2):309–319
45. Van den Berghe G, Wouters P, Weekers F et al (1999) Reactivation of pituitary hormone release and metabolic improvement by infusion of growth hormone-releasing peptide and thyrotropin-releasing hormone in patients with protracted critical illness. J Clin Endocrinol Metab 84(4):1311–1323
46. Bacci V, Schussler GC, Kaplan TB (1982) The relationship between serum triiodothyronine and thyrotropin during systemic illness. J Clin Endocrinol Metab 54(6):1229–1235
47. Boelen A, Platvoet-ter Schiphorst MC, Bakker O, Wiersinga WM (1995) The role of cytokines in the lipopolysaccharide-induced sick euthyroid syndrome in mice. J Endocrinol 146(3):475–483
48. Van der Poll T, Romijn JA, Wiersinga WM, Sauerwein HP (1990) Tumor necrosis factor: a putative mediator of the sick euthyroid syndrome in man. J Clin Endocrinol Metab 71(6):1567–1572
49. Mooradian AD, Reed RL, Osterweil D, Schiffman R, Scuderi P (1990) Decreased serum triiodothyronine is associated with increased concentrations of tumor necrosis factor. J Clin Endocrinol Metab 71(5):1239–1242
50. Chopra IJ, Sakane S, Teco GN (1991) A study of the serum concentration of tumor necrosis factor-alpha in thyroidal and nonthyroidal illnesses. J Clin Endocrinol Metab 72(5):1113–1116

51. Van der Poll T, Van Zee KJ, Endert E et al (1995) Interleukin-1 receptor blockade does not affect endotoxin-induced changes in plasma thyroid hormone and thyrotropin concentrations in man. J Clin Endocrinol Metab 80(4):1341–1346
52. Van der Poll T, Endert E, Coyle SM, Agosti JM, Lowry SF (1999) Neutralization of TNF does not influence endotoxin induced changes in thyroid hormone metabolism in humans. Am J Physiol 276(2 Pt 2):R357–R362
53. Van den Berghe G, de Zegher F, Lauwers P (1994) Dopamine and the sick euthyroid syndrome in critical illness. Clin Endocrinol (Oxf) 41(6):731–737
54. Faglia G, Ferrari C, Beck-Peccoz P, Spada A, Travaglini P, Ambrosi B (1973) Reduced plasma thyrotropin response to thyrotropin releasing hormone after dexamethasone administration in normal subjects. Horm Metab Res 5(4):289–292
55. Forceville X, Vitoux D, Gauzit R, Combes A, Lahilaire P, Chappuis P (1998) Selenium, systemic immune response syndrome, sepsis, and outcome in critically ill patients. Crit Care Med 26(9):1536–1544
56. Berger MM, Reymond MJ, Shenkin A et al (2001) Influence of selenium supplements on the post-traumatic alterations of the thyroid axis: a placebo-controlled trial. Intensive Care Med 27(1):91–100
57. Vidart J, Wajner SM, Leite RS et al (2014) N-acetylcysteine administration prevents nonthyroidal illness syndrome in patients with acute myocardial infarction: a randomized clinical trial. J Clin Endocrinol Metab 99(12):4537–4545
58. Boelen A, Kwakkel J, Fliers E (2011) Beyond low plasma T3: local thyroid hormone metabolism during inflammation and infection. Endocr Rev 32(5):670–693
59. Boelen A, Boorsma J, Kwakkel J et al (2008) Type 3 deiodinase is highly expressed in infiltrating neutrophilic granulocytes in response to acute bacterial infection. Thyroid 18(10):1095–1103
60. Kwakkel J, Surovtseva OV, de Vries EM, Stap J, Fliers E, Boelen A (2014) A novel role for the thyroid hormone-activating enzyme type 2 deiodinase in the inflammatory response of macrophages. Endocrinology 155(7):2725–2734
61. Brent GA, Hershman JM (1986) Thyroxine therapy in patients with severe nonthyroidal illnesses and low serum thyroxine concentration. J Clin Endocrinol Metab 63(1):1–8
62. Bettendorf M, Schmidt KG, Grulich-Henn J, Ulmer HE, Heinrich UE (2000) Tri-iodothyronine treatment in children after cardiac surgery: a double-blind, randomised, placebo-controlled study. Lancet 356(9229):529–534
63. Barrett NA, Jones A, Whiteley C, Yassin S, McKenzie CA (2012) Management of long-term hypothyroidism: a potential marker of quality of medicines reconciliation in the intensive care unit. Int J Pharm Pract 20(5):303–306
64. Ringel MD (2001) Management of hypothyroidism and hyperthyroidism in the intensive care unit. Crit Care Clin 17(1):59–74
65. Fliers E, Wiersinga WM (2003) Myxedema coma. Rev Endocr Metab Disord 4(2):137–141
66. Angell TE, Lechner MG, Nguyen CT, Salvato VL, Nicoloff JT, LoPresti JS (2015) Clinical features and hospital outcomes in thyroid storm: a retrospective cohort study. J Clin Endocrinol Metab 100(2):451–459
67. Papi G, Corsello SM, Pontecorvi A (2014) Clinical concepts on thyroid emergencies. Front Endocrinol (Lausanne) 5:102

Chapter 12
Stress Response: Adrenal Function

Paul E. Marik

Abstract Exposure of the host to diverse noxious stimuli results in a stereotypic and coordinated stress response which serves to restore homeostasis and enhance survival. The stress response is mediated primarily by the hypothalamic-pituitary-adrenal (HPA) axis with the release of ACTH and cortisol and the sympatho-adrenal system with the release of catecholamines. Classically the stress response is short lived with cortisol and catecholamine levels returning to baseline once the stress has dissipated. Critically ill and injured patients, however, have a prolonged stress response which may last for weeks, with the chronic stress response differing both qualitatively and quantitatively from the acute stress response. Furthermore, critical illness is frequently associated with multiple derangements of the HPA axis including decreased production of ACTH and cortisol, decreased expression and dysfunction of the glucocorticoid receptor as well as decreased cortisol metabolism. This chapter provides an overview of the complex and dynamic changes of the HPA axis in the critically ill patient.

Exposure of the host to diverse noxious stimuli results in a stereotypic and coordinated response, referred to by Hans Selye as the "*general adaption syndrome*" (or stress response) which serves to restore homeostasis and enhance survival [1]. The stress response is mediated primarily by the hypothalamic-pituitary-adrenal (HPA) axis as well as the sympathoadrenal system (SAS). Activation of the HPA axis results in increased secretion from the paraventricular nucleus of the hypothalamus of corticotrophin-releasing hormone (CRH) and arginine vasopressin (AVP) (see Fig. 12.1) [2]. CRH plays a major role in orchestrating and coordinating the stress response. CRH stimulates the production of ACTH by the anterior pituitary, causing the zona fasciculata of the adrenal cortex to produce more glucocorticoids (cortisol in humans)

P.E. Marik, MD, FCCP, FCCM
Division of Pulmonary and Critical Care Medicine, Department of Medicine,
Eastern Virginia Medical School, 825 Fairfax Av, Suite 410, Norfolk, VA 23507, USA
e-mail: marikpe@evms.edu

J.-C. Preiser (ed.), *The Stress Response of Critical Illness: Metabolic and Hormonal Aspects*, DOI 10.1007/978-3-319-27687-8_12

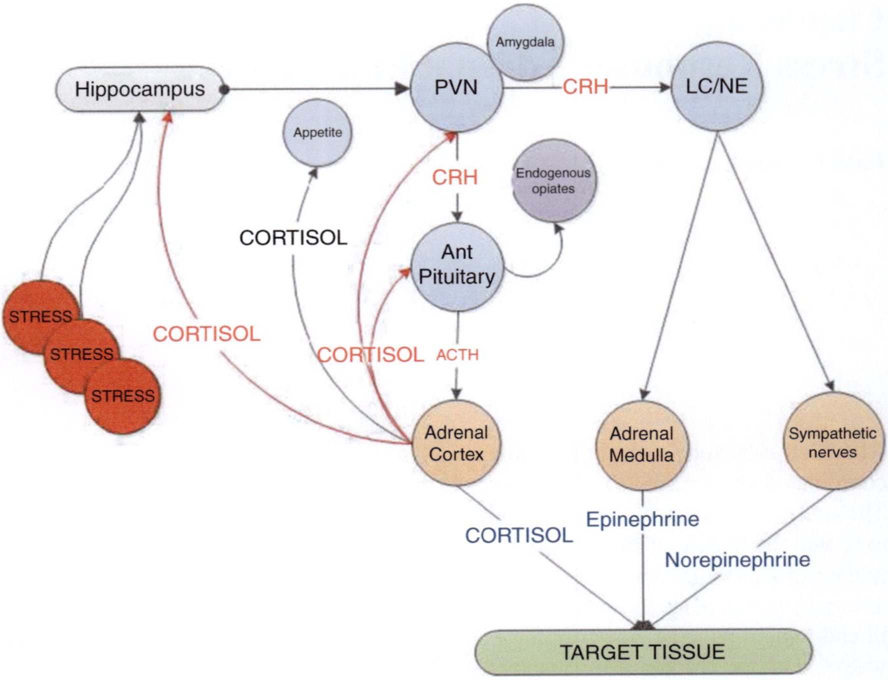

Fig. 12.1 Activation of the stress response. *CRH* corticotrophin-releasing hormone, *PVN* paraventricular nucleus, *LC/NE* locus coeruleus norepinephrine system, *ACTH* adrenocorticotrophic hormone, *CRH* corticotrophin

[3]. ACTH stimulates steroidogenesis by binding to the melanocortin-2 receptor on adrenocortical cells. ACTH upregulates expression of this receptor and mediates cholesterol release from lipid droplets. In addition, ACTH activates the expression of genes encoding cholesterol uptake and synthesis as well as key enzymes responsible for cortisol synthesis [4]. In healthy individuals, the release of ACTH and cortisol occurs predominantly in discreet pulses superimposed upon nonpulsatile release, with a characteristic diurnal pattern with low levels during sleep and maximal levels around waking. Activation of the SAS results in the secretion of epinephrine and norepinephrine from the adrenal medulla and sympathetic nerves and to an increased production of inflammatory cytokines such as interleukin-6 (IL-6) [2]. In general, there is a graded response to the degree of stress. Cortisol and catecholamine levels correlate with the intensity of the stressor, the type of surgery, the severity of injury, and the APACHE score [3]. With acute severe stress, adrenal cortisol output increases approximately tenfold (~300 mg hydrocortisone/day) [3]. In patients with shock, plasma concentrations of epinephrine increase 50-fold, and norepinephrine levels increase tenfold [5]. The adrenal medulla is the major source of these released catecholamines [5]. An intact HPA axis is required to protect the host against diverse stressors (fight and flight response) and to ensure survival. Adrenalectomized animals succumb rapidly to hemorrhagic and septic shock with steroid replacement

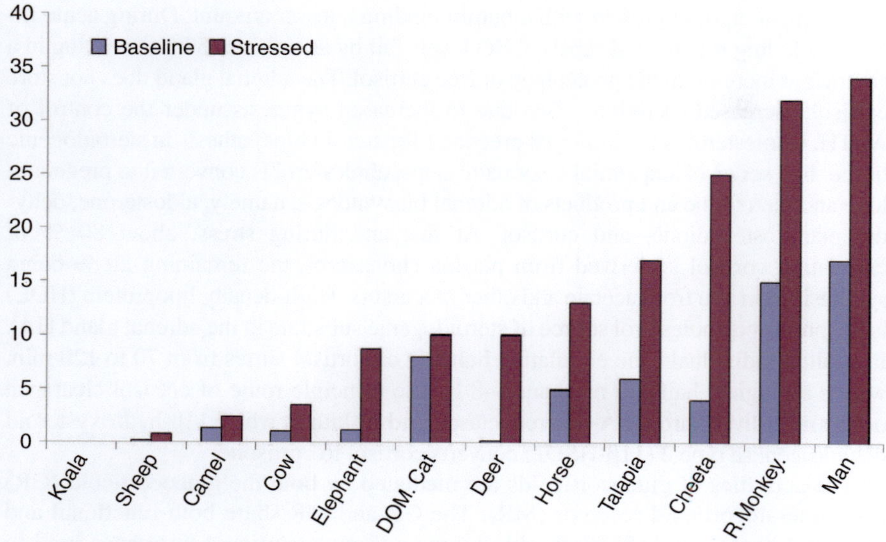

Fig. 12.2 Baseline and stress cortisol level among various species (Reproduced with permission from Springer Publications. From Marik and Levitov [13])

being protective against these challenges [6, 7]. Likewise adrenalectomy increases the lethality of lipopolysaccharide, tumor necrosis factor-α (TNF-α), and interleukin-1(IL-1) [8]. In critically ill patients, suppression of cortisol synthesis (with etomidate used for sedation) dramatically increases mortality [9].

The stress response acts via multiple genomic and nongenomic mechanisms to enhance cardiovascular reserve and provide a ready source of fuel (glucose and lactate) for the brain, and heart, allowing the organism to take appropriate action (flight or fight) while preventing excessive activation of the immune system [2, 10, 11]. The increase in serum cortisol during stress protects the organism against developing post-traumatic stress disorder (PTSD) [12]. The fight and flight response is essential for survival and is present in the most primitive of species. Furthermore, within species the degree of activation of the HPA axis has evolved to match the degree of stress to which the organism is exposed (see Fig. 12.2) [13]. In humans, a number of factors modulate the degree of activation of the stress response including (i) alcohol and medications, (ii) genetic factors including glucocorticoid receptor (GR) and CRH receptor polymorphisms, (iii) sex hormone levels, (iv) previous exposure to stress, (v) maternal stress and fetal programming, (vi) obesity, and (vii) educational level.

12.1 Cortisol Physiology

Cortisol (hydrocortisone) is the major endogenous glucocorticoid secreted by the adrenal cortex. Over 90 % of circulating cortisol is bound to corticosteroid-binding globulin (CBG) with less than 10 % in the free, biologically active form. CBG is the predominant binding protein with albumin binding a lesser amount. During acute illness, including trauma and sepsis, CBG levels fall by as much as 50 %, resulting in a significant increase in the percentage of free cortisol. The adrenal gland does not store cortisol; increased secretion arises due to increased synthesis under the control of ACTH. Cholesterol is the principal precursor for steroid biosynthesis in steroidogenic tissue. In a series of sequential enzymatic steps, cholesterol is converted to pregnenolone and then to the end products of adrenal biosynthesis, namely, aldosterone, dehydroepiandrostenedione, and cortisol. At rest and during stress, about 80 % of circulating cortisol is derived from plasma cholesterol, the remaining 20 % being synthesized in situ from acetate and other precursors. High-density lipoprotein (HDL) is the preferred cholesterol source of steroidogenic substrate in the adrenal gland [14]. In healthy individuals, the circulating half-life of cortisol varies from 70 to 120 min, with a biological half-life of about 6–8 h. The principle route of cortisol clearance occurs in the liver (through A-ring reductases) and the kidney where 11β-hydroxysteroid dehydrogenase type 2 (11β-HSD2) converts cortisol to cortisone.

The activities of glucocorticoids are mediated by both the glucocorticoid (GR) and mineralocorticoid receptor (MR). The GR and MR share both functional and structural homology [15]. Both aldosterone and glucocorticoid hormones bind to both the GR and MR. At low basal levels, cortisol binds to the high-affinity, low-capacity mineralocorticoid receptor (MR). However, with increased cortisol secretion, the MR are saturated, and cortisol then binds to the low-affinity, high-capacity GR. In addition, the 11β-hydroxysteroid dehydrogenase (11β-HSD) enzymes play an important role in preventing glucocorticoid access to cells that express the MR [16, 17]. This enzyme has two isoforms, a NAD+-dependent form (11β-HSD-2) and a NADP+-dependent form (11β-HSD-1). 11β-HSD-2 is found in tissues with high levels of MR activity such as the kidney, sweat and salivary glands, placenta, and colon. 11β-HSD-2 converts cortisol to cortisone, its inactive reduced metabolite which is unable to bind to the GR and MR. 11β-HSD-1, which is found in glucocorticoid target tissues, catalyzes the conversion of cortisone to the active glucocorticoid cortisol. Pro-inflammatory cytokines modulate the activity of the 11β-HSD enzymes, with interleukin-1β (IL-1β) and tumor necrosis factor-α (TNF-α) increasing the activity of 11β-HSD-1 while decreasing that of 11β-HSD-2 [18, 19].

Cortisol diffuses rapidly across cell membranes binding to the GR. Two isoforms of the GR have been isolated, namely, GR-α and GR-β. The GR-β isoform fails to bind cortisol and activate gene expression and thus functions as a negative inhibitor of GR-α [20]. Seven isoforms of GR-α have been reported; these isoforms may be selectively expressed by different tissues with each isoform eliciting a distinct response [21, 22]. Through the association and disassociation of chaperone molecules, the glucocorticoid-GR-α complex moves into the nucleus where it binds as a homodimer to DNA sequences called glucocorticoid-responsive elements (GREs) located in the promoter regions of target genes which then activate or repress transcription of the associated genes. In addition, the cortisol-GR complex may affect cellular function indirectly by binding to and modulating the transcriptional activity of other nuclear transcription factors such as nuclear factor-κB (NF-κB) and activator protein-1 (AP-1). Overall, glucocorticoids affect the transcription of thousands of genes in every cell of the body. It has been estimated that glucocorticoids affect 20 % of the genome of mononuclear blood cells [23]. Cortisol has several important physiologic actions on metabolism, cardiovascular function, and the immune system. Cortisol increases the synthesis of catecholamines and catecholamine receptors which is partially responsible for its positive inotropic effects. In addition, cortisol has potent anti-inflammatory actions including the reduction in number and function of various immune cells, such as T and B lymphocytes, monocytes, neutrophils, and eosinophils at sites of inflammation. Cortisol is the most important inhibitor of the transcription of pro-inflammatory mediators (inhibits NF-kB and AP-1 by multiple mechanisms) [3].

12.2 The Stress Response in Critical Illness

Classically the stress response is short lived (lasting less than 60 min, e.g., physical fight, being chased by a predator, parachuting) allowing the host to successfully deal with the acute threat, following which the stress response rapidly dissipates with cortisol and catecholamine levels returning to baseline. Critically ill and injured patients, however, have a prolonged stress response which may last for weeks, with the chronic stress response differing both qualitatively and quantitatively from the acute stress response. In addition, it is likely that the type of acute illness, for example, sepsis, non-septic critical illness, trauma, or burns, will have a moderating effect on the stress response. While a number of studies have characterized the stress response and the HPA axis early in the course of the disease (i.e., on ICU admission), very few studies have investigated the temporal trends of CRH, ACTH, and cortisol over time. These studies have demonstrated that the pattern of the HPA activation during critical illness differs quite considerably from the acute stress response [24]. Most strikingly there appears to be a dissociation between the serum cortisol and ACTH levels, known as the "cortisol-ACTH dissociation" [25]. In addition, there is a marked hourly variability in plasma cortisol levels with loss of the circadian rhythm [26]. Annane and colleagues performed a cosyntropin stimulation and metyrapone test within 24 h of ICU admission in critically ill patients with sepsis, critically ill patients without sepsis, and healthy volunteers [27]. In this study the mean basal cortisol was 17.8 ug/dl, 27.8 ug/dl, and 12.6 ug/dl, respectively, while the simultaneous ACTH levels were 8 pg/ml, 6 pg/ml, and 33 pg/ml respectively. This study demonstrates that while the basal cortisol was elevated in the majority of critically ill patients, the ACTH levels were subnormal. In addition, it should be noted that the basal cortisol levels were lower in the critically ill septic as compared to non-septic patients. Only a few studies have evaluated the course of serum cortisol and ACTH levels over time. Vermes et al measured the cortisol and ACTH levels daily for 8 days in 30 critically ill patients and 15 matched hospitalized controls [28]. The plasma cortisol levels were elevated in the critically ill patients and remained high during the whole observation period. In contrast, plasma ACTH levels decreased between days 3 and 5, reaching significantly lower levels on day 5 compared to those in the control group. Vassiliadi et al measured cortisol, ACTH, and stimulated cortisol levels every 3–4 days until day 30, recovery, or death in 51 critically ill patients with sepsis [29]. In this study basal cortisol was elevated (all above 10 ug/dl) and remained elevated throughout the duration of the study. The

ACTH levels, however, were low on presentation and normalized after day 10. In the most comprehensive study to date, Boonen et al evaluated the time course of the HPA axis and cortisol metabolism over 7 days in 158 ICU patients [24]. Similar to the study of Vassiliadi et al, plasma cortisol levels were elevated on presentation (all above 10 ug/dl) and remained elevated over the 7 days of the study; however, ACTH levels were reduced on presentation (lower than controls) and tended to increase over the next 6 days. Furthermore, although the ACTH levels were subnormal, cortisol production was increased by 83 % while plasma clearance was reduced by 53 %. Patients with a cortisol response to corticotrophin less than 21 ug/dl had substantially reduced plasma clearance of cortisol than patients with a normal response to corticotrophin. The calculated plasma clearance after the administration of 100 mg of hydrocortisone was 60 % lower in patients than in controls. These authors noted that the levels of 11β-HSD2 and A-ring reductases were markedly reduced in patients as compared to controls. These studies suggest that pituitary-independent mechanisms, most notably impaired cortisol clearance contribute to the increased cortisol levels found in critically ill patients. It is further postulated that the increased cortisol levels via negative feedback inhibit ACTH release accounting for the low ACTH levels [24, 30, 31]. Increased cortisol levels do not appear to be due to increased adrenocortical sensitivity to ACTH [25]. Boonen et al demonstrated that pulsatile ACTH secretion was 31 % lower in ICU patients than controls, largely due to decreased ACTH burst mass [25]. In experimental sepsis models, levels of ACTH expression are rapidly suppressed, possibly due to nitric oxide or due to decreased orexin signaling [32–34]. It is has been suggested that increased levels of pro-inflammatory cytokines, particularly interleukin-6 (IL-6), may act synergistically with ACTH to increase cortisol synthesis [24, 29].

As ACTH levels are subnormal during critical illness and as ACTH plays an important role in steroidogenesis and has tropic effects on the adrenal cortex, it has been postulated that the low ACTH levels would lead to atrophy of the adrenal gland and decreased ACTH responsiveness. Boonen and colleagues harvested the adrenal glands from long-stay ICU patients, short-stay ICU patients, and controls within 24 h of their death [35]. These authors demonstrated 78 % less cholesterol ester and at least 58 % less mRNA expression of ACTH-regulated steroidogenic enzymes in the long-stay ICU patients as compared to the controls and short-stay patients. This finding may contribute to the "relative adrenal insufficiency" noted in chronic ICU patients.

12.3 Alternative Explanations for Altered HPA Function During Critical Illness

The finding that critically ill patients have reduced cortisol metabolism resulting in increased cortisol levels with low concomitant low ACTH levels has recently gained much attention [24, 30, 31]. However, it is likely that other derangements of the HPA axis as well as abnormal glucocorticoid signaling may occur in the critically ill. It is therefore probable that a variety of phenotypic patterns exist and that these patterns may change over time. Festti et al evaluated the HPA axis in 34 patients within the first 24 h of the onset of septic shock [36]. In this study 32 % of patients had adrenal insufficiency (Δ cortisol <9 mg/dl) with the baseline ACTH being significantly higher in the nonresponders compared to the responders (55.5 pg/mL vs. 18.3 pg/mL, $p=0.01$). The high ACTH in the nonresponders may be a consequence of abnormalities in steroidogenesis. While the baseline cortisol levels were increased in the studies by Boonen et al and Vassiliadi et al, other studies have demonstrated low cortisol levels (<10 ug/dl) in approximately 20 % of patients [27, 37]. In the study by Annane et al. 18 % of the septic patients had a basal cortisol <10 ug/dl [27]. Kwon et al. evaluated the HPA axis in 82 critically ill patients [37]. In this study 16 (20 %) patients had a basal cortisol < 10 ug/dl, while an additional 20 (24 %) patients had a delta cortisol of <9 ug/dl after a cosyntropin stimulation test. The ACTH profile of the patients with a low cortisol has not been compared to those with an elevated cortisol, and the mechanism leading to a low cortisol in these patients has not been well studied. In addition to these studies, a strong body of evidence suggest that substrate deficiency (HDL) may lead to inadequate cortisol synthesis during acute illness.

High-density lipoprotein (HDL) is an important lipoprotein present in human plasma and plays a major role in reverse cholesterol transport [38]. The major apoprotein present in HDL is apolipoprotein A1 (Apo-A1), which provides structural stability to the spherical molecule. Free cholesterol is esterified by lecithin-cholesterol acyltransferase (LCAT) which then combines with the disk-shaped pre-HDL complex forming a spherical structure, HDL_3 (see Fig. 12.3) [39]. HDL_3 molecules continue to engulf additional lipid molecules and apoproteins, thereby forming mature HDL_2. HDL_2 is removed from the circulation by the liver where it binds to the scavenger receptor class B type I (or the human homolog Cla-1) and Apo-A1 receptors. HDL has been shown to be substantially reduced in patients with many acute illnesses, including sepsis and burns, following myocardial infarction and in patients undergoing surgical interventions [40, 41]. Pro-inflammatory cytokines, particularly IL-6, appear to decrease the synthesis of

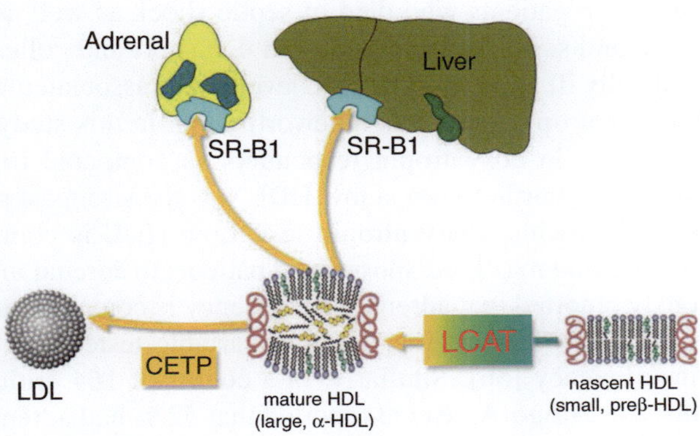

Fig. 12.3 HDL metabolism. *LCAT* lecithin-cholesterol acyltransferase, *CETP* cholesterol ester transfer protein, *SR-B1* scavenger receptor class B type I (Cla-1 in humans)

Apo-1 [42, 43]. In addition, during the acute phase response, Apo-A1 is replaced by serum amyloid A (SAA) in the HDL particle [38]. Ly et al demonstrated that plasma LCAT activity and hepatic LCAT mRNA levels are decreased by lipopolysaccharide and TNF-α treatment [44]. Similarly, Ettinger et al demonstrated that TNF-α, IL-1, and IL-6 decreased synthesis of LCAT in cultured Hep G2 cells [45]. It is likely that LCAT levels are reduced in critically ill and injured patients leading to reduced HDL_2 levels.

Low HDL levels have been demonstrated to have important prognostic implications. Mesotton et al demonstrated that ICU patients with a HDL level less than 15 mg/dl had a substantially higher mortality than patients with a HDL level above this value [46]. In a series of 2989 surgical patients Delgado-Rodriquez and colleagues demonstrated that a HDL level <37 mg/dl was highly predictive of nosocomial infection, length of stay, and hospital death [47]. Barlage et al. reported that Apo-AI levels were an independent predictor of 30-day mortality in patients with sepsis [48]. HDL is believed to modulate the inflammatory process by a number of mechanisms including binding and neutralization of bacterial toxins, inhibition of adhesion molecule expression, and stimulation of endothelial nitric oxide synthase (eNOS) production [38]. However, HDL may have a major role in modulating the inflammatory response in its role as the major precursor of cortisol.

Experimental studies suggest that HDL is the preferred cholesterol source of steroidogenic substrate in the adrenal gland [14]. Mouse SR-B1 (scavenger receptor, class B, type 1) and its human homolog (Cla-1) have been identified as the high-affinity HDL receptor mediating selective cholesterol uptake [49–53]. These receptors are expressed at high levels in the parenchymal cells of the liver and the steroidogenic cells of the adrenal glands, ovary, and testis [52]. Cai et al. demonstrated that SR-BI knockout mice had marked glucocorticoid insufficiency and higher mortality in LPS shock compared with control mice [53]. In this study SR-BI-null mice showed a lack of inducible glucocorticoid synthesis in response to LPS, bacterial infection, stress, or ACTH. Decreased production of cortisol during acute illness may therefore occur due to substrate deficiency (HDL). Polito et al demonstrated diffuse lipid depletion in the zona fasciculata of the adrenal glands in patients who died of septic shock as well as in experimental endotoxemia and sepsis models [54]. Van der Voort and colleagues demonstrated that in critically ill patients, low HDL levels were associated with an attenuated response to cosyntropin [55]. It is noteworthy that in this study, the mean HDL level was 27 mg/dl in cosyntropin responders as compared to 12.7 mg/dl in the nonresponders. Furthermore, a low HDL was the strongest predictor of nonresponsiveness following a cosyntropin test. Low HDL is common in patients with liver disease and may predispose these patients to adrenal insufficiency. We have previously reported that adrenal insufficiency is common in patients with liver disease, with a low HDL being the only variable tested that was predictive of adrenal insufficiency [56]. Similarly, in a cohort of 164 critically ill patients with liver disease, Atogo-Asse et al reported that 52 % had adrenal insufficiency (Δ cortisol <9 mg/dl) with the increment in the cortisol following a cosyntropin test being inversely related to the HDL level [57].

12.4 Tissue Glucocorticoid Resistance

Tissue corticosteroid resistance is a well-known manifestation of chronic inflammatory diseases such as chronic obstructive pulmonary disease (COPD), severe asthma, systemic lupus erythematosus (SLE), ulcerative colitis, and rheumatoid arthritis. Defective GR nuclear translocation and altered histone acetylation have been described in corticosteroid-resistant asthmatics [58, 59]. Increased expression of the beta-isoform of the GR has been reported in patients with glucocorticoid-insensitive asthma and patients with idiopathic pulmonary fibrosis [60, 61]. It is likely that patients with acute inflammatory diseases such as sepsis, acute lung injury (ALI), pancreatitis, traumatic injuries, and burns may develop tissue resistance to glucocorticoids during the course of their disease. In a mouse fibroblast cell line model, Pariante and colleagues demonstrated that IL-1 reduced GR translocation and function [62]. In cell culture as well as in ex vivo human lymphocytes, Webster et al demonstrated that TNF-α disproportionately increased the levels of the GR-β over the GR-α isoform and that this was associated with the development of glucocorticoid resistance [63]. Guerrero et al demonstrated increased expression of the GR-β isoform in mononuclear cells from septic patients [64]. In a murine *Staphylococcus aureus* sepsis model, Bergquist et al demonstrated markedly decreased GR expression and decreased nuclear translocation of the GR complex into the nucleus [65]. In this study it is noteworthy that GR expression decreased with time which paralleled the time-dependent decreased efficacy of glucocorticoids in preventing weight loss in the animals. Similarly, in an LPS model, these authors demonstrated decreased GR nuclear translocation compared to control animals [66]. In this study, glucocorticoid treatment improved survival only when started early (2 h) after LPS administration. Van den Akker et al demonstrated that neutrophils from pediatric patients with sepsis had decreased expression of GR mRNA, with the GR levels being inversely related to the level of IL-6 [67]. Similarly, Indyk et al demonstrated lower total and cytoplasmic GR levels in critically ill children [68]. In an ex vivo model, Meduri and colleagues compared the cytoplasmic to nuclear density of the GR complex in patients with ARDS who were improvers with those of non-improvers [69]. These authors demonstrated a markedly reduced nuclear density of the GR complex in non-improvers, while the cytoplasmic density was similar between improvers and non-improvers. This experiment provides further evidence that the nuclear GC-GR activity may be impaired in critically ill patients despite adequate cytoplasmic (serum) levels of cortisol.

12.5 Critical Illness-Related Corticosteroid Insufficiency (CIRCI)

Critical illness is associated with multiple derangements of the HPA axis including decreased production of CRH, ACTH, and cortisol, decreased expression and dysfunction of the GR as well as decreased cortisol metabolism. These abnormalities may coexist and change dynamically over time. As there is currently no test or measure of cellular glucocorticoid activity, the net result of these interacting factors may be almost impossible to determine at the bedside. Standard methods of assessing adrenal activity based on measuring plasma cortisol concentration have been shown to suffer numerous problems, including lack of reproducibility, large interassay variation, lack of agreement on diagnostic criteria, excessive variation, and poor correlation with outcome [26, 70–73]. As a result, it has proven difficult to reliably identify patients who have suppressed adrenal activity and who may benefit from administration of exogenous corticosteroids.

A few patients may develop "absolute adrenal insufficiency" due to acute destruction of the adrenal gland (i.e., due to hemorrhage); however, these patients are uncommon. The concept of "relative adrenal insufficiency (RAI)" has been proposed to resolve this conundrum; however, the pathophysiology and diagnosis of this condition remain elusive [73, 74]. One approach to resolving the question of whether too little glucocorticoid signal ultimately "gets through" is to examine target genes and cellular pathways whose function is primarily regulated by glucocorticoids. Ultimately activation of primary GR target genes will allow quantification of glucocorticoid activity at the tissue and cellular level [75]. However, this approach is currently not widely available. In critically ill patients, particularly those with sepsis, the inhibitory effects of glucocorticoids on NF-κβ signaling pathways may be used as a surrogate marker of activation of GR target genes. Through their inhibitory effects on NF-κβ signaling pathways, glucocorticoids are the most potent anti-inflammatory hormones in the body and thereby serve to suppress the production and activity of pro-inflammatory cytokines during exposure to stress. Inadequate glucocorticoid-mediated feedback inhibition of the immune response will result in excess circulating levels of pro-inflammatory mediators. This has led to the concept of "critical illness-related corticosteroid insufficiency (CIRCI)" [3, 76]. CIRCI is defined as inadequate cellular corticosteroid activity for the severity of the patients' illness; i.e., CIRCI may be due to inadequate levels of circulating cortisol, systemic or local abnormities in cortisol metabolism, corticosteroid tissue resistance, or a combination of these factors. CIRCI manifests with insufficient corticosteroid-mediated downregulation of inflammatory transcription factors. Inadequate glucocorticoid-mediated feedback inhibition of the immune response will result in excess levels of pro-inflammatory mediators. Patients with severe sepsis, septic shock, and acute lung injury as well as those with severe traumatic injuries and burns have immune dysregulation with an exaggerated pro-inflammatory response. These patients by definition have CIRCI.

The paradigm proposed by Roger Bone suggested that patients with an exaggerated pro-inflammatory response (systemic inflammatory response syndrome) transition after a period of time into a state of immuno-paresis which he termed the compensatory anti-inflammatory response syndrome (CARS) [77]. However, examination of previous studies provides evidence that both pro-inflammatory and an opposing anti-inflammatory response occur concomitantly in sepsis and following traumatic injuries [78, 79]. Osuchowski et al were first to report that production of anti- and pro-inflammatory cytokines occurs simultaneously in a polymicrobial sepsis model [80]. Xiao et al. demonstrated that following severe trauma, burn injuries, and administration of endotoxin in humans, the early leukocyte genomic response is characterized by simultaneously increased expression of genes involved in the systemic inflammatory, innate immune, and compensatory anti-inflammatory responses [81]. Furthermore, patients with a complicated clinical course had an increased magnitude and duration of these genomic changes. Almansa et al. compared the gene expression profiles of surgical patients with sepsis as compared to surgical patients without sepsis [82]. These authors demonstrated the simultaneous coexistence of increased innate and depressed adaptive immunity. Tang and colleagues performed a systematic review examining gene profiles in sepsis [83]. These authors concluded that "the arbitrary distinction of separating sepsis into pro-inflammatory and anti-inflammatory phases is not supported by gene-expression data." It is likely that the excessive pro-inflammatory response characteristic of CIRCI may potentiate the simultaneous anti-inflammatory response. It is therefore proposed that early treatment with exogenous corticosteroids which would dampen the excessive pro-inflammatory response in patients with sepsis, trauma, and burns may "paradoxically" limit the simultaneous anti-inflammatory response thereby restoring homeostases without a prolonged pro- or anti-inflammatory response. This postulate is supported by the landmark study of Keh and colleagues who in a randomized crossover study evaluated the clinical and immunological response of "low"-dose corticosteroids in patients with septic shock [84]. In this study hydrocortisone simultaneously decreased circulating levels of both pro- and anti-inflammatory cytokines while at the same time preserving competence of adaptive immunity. Importantly, in vitro granulocyte function (respiratory burst and phagocytosis) remained intact, indicating that low-dose hydrocortisone did not suppress innate defense mechanisms. Furthermore, interleukin-12 (IL-12), a central regulatory cytokine directing Th1 development and monocyte activation, increased during hydrocortisone treatment. The results of the study by Keh and colleagues are supported by the HYPOLYTE study where 150 patients with severe trauma were randomly assigned to a continuous intravenous infusion of either hydrocortisone (200 mg/d for 5 days) or placebo [85]. By intention to treat analysis, 35.6 % of hydrocortisone patients developed hospital-acquired pneumonia (the primary endpoint) as compared to 51.3 % of placebo patients (hazard ratio, 0.51; 95 % confidence interval 0.30–0.83; $P = .007$). Macrophage dysfunction plays an important role in mediating the immunosuppression which characterizes critical illness [86]. It should be noted that glucocorticoids cause a phenotypic switch of macrophages (M1 to M2) with the differentiation of a specific anti-inflammatory phenotype which is actively involved in resolution of inflammation [87]. M2 cells show efficient phagocytic activity and high expression of scavenger receptors and have different chemokine expression profiles compared with M1 macrophages [88, 89].

12.6 Conclusions

The alterations of the HPA axis and GR function following critical illness are complex, dynamic, and difficult to quantitate at the bedside. Nevertheless, critical illness-related corticosteroid insufficiency (CIRCI) is exceedingly common, and treatment with "low-dose" glucocorticoids appears to downregulate both the pro- and anti-inflammatory response while preserving Th1 lymphocyte responsiveness and thereby restoring homeostasis and likely improving patient outcomes.

References

1. Selye H (1936) A syndrome produced by diverse nocuous agents. Nature 136:32
2. Chrousos GP, Gold PW (1992) The concepts of stress and stress system disorders. Overview of physical and behavioral homeostasis. JAMA 267:1244–1252
3. Marik PE (2009) Critical illness related corticosteroid insufficiency. Chest 135:181–193
4. Lehoux JG, Fleury A, Ducharme L (1998) The acute and chronic effects of adrenocorticotropin on the levels of messenger ribonucleic acid and protein of steroidogenic enzymes in rat adrenal in vivo. Endocrinology 139:3913–3922
5. Chernow B, Rainey TR, Lake CR (1982) Endogenous and exogenous catecholamines in critical care medicine. Crit Care Med 10:409–416
6. Hinshaw LB, Beller BK, Chang AC et al (1985) Corticosteroid/antibiotic treatment of adrenalectomized dogs challenged with lethal E. coli. Circ Shock 16:265–277
7. Darlington DN, Chew G, Ha T et al (1990) Corticosterone, but not glucose, treatment enables fasted adrenalectomized rats to survive moderate hemorrhage. Endocrinology 127:766–772
8. Bertini R, Bianchi M, Ghezzi P (1988) Adrenalectomy sensitizes mice to the lethal effects of interleukin 1 and tumor necrosis factor. J Exp Med 167:1708–1712
9. Ledingham IM, Watt I (1983) Influence of sedation on mortality in critically ill multiple trauma patients [letter]. Lancet 1:1270
10. Garcia-Alvarez M, Marik PE, Bellomo R (2013) Stress hyperlactemia; present understanding and controversy. Lancet Endo Diabetes 2:339–347
11. Marik PE, Bellomo R (2013) Stress hyperglycemia: an essential survival response! Crit Care 17:305
12. Cohen H, Zohar J, Gidron Y et al (2006) Blunted HPA axis response to stress influences susceptibility to posttraumatic stress response in rats. Biol Psychiatry 59:1208–1218
13. Marik PE, Levitov A (2010) The "koala stress syndrome" and adrenal responsiveness in the critically ill. Intensive Care Med 36:1805–1806
14. Yaguchi H, Tsutsumi K, Shimono K et al (1998) Involvement of high density lipoprotein as substrate cholesterol for steroidogenesis by bovine adrenal fasciculo-reticularis cells. Life Sci 62:1387–1395
15. Rogerson FM, Fuller PJ (2003) Interdomain interactions in the mineralocorticoid receptor. Mol Cell Endocrinol 200:45–55
16. Edwards CR, Stewart PM, Burt D et al (1988) Localisation of 11 beta-hydroxysteroid dehydrogenase--tissue specific protector of the mineralocorticoid receptor. Lancet 2:986–989
17. Funder JW, Pearce PT, Smith R et al (1988) Mineralocorticoid action: target tissue specificity is enzyme, not receptor, mediated. Science 242:583–585
18. Tomlinson JW, Moore J, Cooper MS et al (2001) Regulation of expression of 11beta-hydroxysteroid dehydrogenase type 1 in adipose tissue: tissue-specific induction by cytokines. Endocrinology 142:1982–1989

19. Cai TQ, Wong B, Mundt SS et al (2001) Induction of 11beta-hydroxysteroid dehydrogenase type 1 but not -2 in human aortic smooth muscle cells by inflammatory stimuli. J Steroid Biochem Mol Biol 77:117–122
20. Oakley RH, Jewell CM, Yudt MR et al (1999) The dominant negative activity of the human glucocorticoid receptor beta isoform. Specificity and mechanisms of action. J Biol Chem 274:27857–27866
21. Lu NZ, Collins JB, Grissom SF et al (2007) Selective regulation of bone cell apoptosis by translational isoforms of the glucocorticoid receptor. Mol Cell Biol 27:7143–7160
22. Duma D, Jewell CM, Cidlowski JA (2006) Multiple glucocorticoid receptor isoforms and mechanisms of post-translational modification. J Steroid Biochem Mol Biol 102:11–21
23. Galon J, Franchimont D, Hiroi N et al (2002) Gene profiling reveals unknown enhancing and suppressive actions of glucocorticoids on immune cells. FASEB J 16:61–71
24. Boonen E, Vervenne H, Meersseman P et al (2013) Reduced cortisol metabolism during critical illness. N Engl J Med 368:1477–1488
25. Boonen E, Meersseman P, Vervenne H et al (2014) Reduced nocturnal ACTH-driven cortisol secretion during critical illness. Am J Physiol Endocrinol Metab 306:E883–E892
26. Venkatesh B, Mortimer RH, Couchman B et al (2005) Evaluation of random plasma cortisol and the low dose corticotropin test as indicators of adrenal secretory capacity in critically ill patients: a prospective study. Anaesth Intensive Care 33:201–209
27. Annane D, Maxime V, Ibrahim F et al (2006) Diagnosis of adrenal insufficiency in severe sepsis and septic shock. Am J Respir Crit Care Med 174:1319–1326
28. Vermes I, Beishuizen A, Hampsink RM et al (1995) Dissociation of plasma adrenocorticotropin and cortisol levels in critically ill patients: possible role of endothelin and atrial natriuretic hormone. J Clin Endocrinol Metab 80:1238–1242
29. Vassiliadi DA, Dimopoulou I, Tzanela M et al (2014) Longitudinal assessment of adrenal function in the early and prolonged phases of critical illness in septic patients: relations to cytokine levels and outcomes. J Clin Endocrinol Metab 99:4471–4480
30. Boonen E, van den Berghe G (2015) Understanding the HPA response to critical illness: novel insights with clinical implications. Intensive Care Med 41:131–133
31. Boonen E, van den Berghe G (2014) Cortisol metabolism in critical illness: implications for clinical care. Curr Opin Endocrinol Diabetes Obes 21:185–192
32. Gibbison B, Angelini GD, Lightman SL (2013) Dynamic output and control of the hypothalamic-pituitary-adrenal axis in critical illness and major surgery. Br J Anaesth 111:347–360
33. Polito A, Sonneville R, Guidoux C et al (2011) Changes in CRH and ACTH synthesis during experimental and human septic shock. PLoS One 6:e25905
34. Deutschman CS, Raj NR, McGuire EO et al (2013) Orexinergic activity modulates altered vital signs and pituitary hormone secretion in experimental sepsis. Crit Care Med 41:e368–e375
35. Boonen E, Langouche L, Janssens T et al (2014) Impact of duration of critical illness on the adrenal glands of human intensive care patients. J Clin Endocrinol Metab 99:4212–4222
36. Festti J, Grion CM, Festti L et al (2014) Adrenocorticotropic hormone but not high-density lipoprotein cholesterol or salivary cortisol was a predictor of adrenal insufficiency in patients with septic shock. Shock 42:16–21
37. Kwon YS, Suh GY, Jeon K et al (2010) Cytokine levels and dysfunction in the hypothalamus-pituitary-adrenal axis in critically-ill patients. Intensive Care Med 36:1845–1851
38. Murch O, Collin M, Hinds CJ et al (2007) Lipoproteins in inflammation and sepsis. I. Basic science. Intensive Care Med 33:13–24
39. Rye KA, Clay MA, Barter PJ (1999) Remodelling of high density lipoproteins by plasma factors. Atherosclerosis 145:227–238
40. Chien JY, Jerng JS, Yu CJ et al (2005) Low serum level of high-density lipoprotein cholesterol is a poor prognostic factor for severe sepsis. Crit Care Med 33:1688–1693
41. van Leeuwen HJ, Heezius EC, Dallinga GM et al (2003) Lipoprotein metabolism in patients with severe sepsis. Crit Care Med 31:1359–1366

42. Gordon BR, Parker TS, Levine DM et al (2001) Relationship of hypolipidemia to cytokine concentrations and outcomes in critically ill surgical patients. Crit Care Med 29:1563–1568
43. Bonville DA, Parker TS, Levine DM et al (2004) The relationships of hypocholesterolemia to cytokine concentrations and mortality in critically ill patients with systemic inflammatory response syndrome. Surg Infect (Larchmt) 5:39–49
44. Ly H, Francone OL, Fielding CJ et al (1995) Endotoxin and TNF lead to reduced plasma LCAT activity and decreased hepatic LCAT mRNA levels in Syrian hamsters. J Lipid Res 36:1254–1263
45. Ettinger WH, Varma VK, Sorci-Thomas M et al (1994) Cytokines decrease apolipoprotein accumulation in medium from Hep G2 cells. Arterioscler Thromb 14:8–13
46. Mesotten D, Swinnen JV, Vanderhoydonc F et al (2004) Contribution of circulating lipids to the improved outcome of critical illness by glycemic control with intensive insulin therapy. J Clin Endocrinol Metab 89:219–226
47. Delgado-Rodriguez M, Medina-Cuadros M, Gomez-Ortega A et al (2002) Cholesterol and serum albumin levels as predictors of cross infection, death, and length of hospital stay. Arch Surg 137:805–812
48. Barlage S, Gnewuch C, Liebisch G et al (2009) Changes in HDL-associated apolipoproteins relate to mortality in human sepsis and correlate to monocyte and platelet activation. Intensive Care Med 35:1877–1885
49. Acton S, Rigotti A, Landschultz KT et al (1996) Identification of scavenger receptor SR-BI as a high density lipoprotein receptor. Science 271:518–520
50. Calco D, Gomez-Coronado D, Lasuncion MA et al (1997) CLA-I is an 85-kD plasma membrane glycoprotein that acts as a high affinity receptor for both native (HDL, LDL, and VLDL) and modified (OxLDL and AcLDL) lipoproteins. Arterioscler Thromb Vasc Biol 17:2341–2349
51. de la Llera-Moya M, Connelly MA, Drazul D et al (2001) Scavenger receptor class B type 1 affects cholestrol homeostasis by magnifying cholestrol flux between cells and HDL. J Lipid Res 42:1969–1978
52. Liu J, Heikkila P, Meng QH et al (2000) Expression of low and high density lipoprotein receptor genes in human adrenals. Eur J Endocrinol 142:677–682
53. Cai L, Ji A, de Beer FC et al (2008) SR-B1 protects against endotoxemia in mice through its roles in glucocorticoid production and hepatic clearance. J Clin Invest 118:364–375
54. Polito A, de la Grandmaison GL, Mansart A et al (2010) Human and experimental septic shock are characterized by depletion of lipid droplets in the adrenals. Intensive Care Med 36:1852–1858
55. van der Voort PH, Gerritsen RT, Bakker AJ et al (2003) HDL-cholestrol level and cortisol response to synacthen in critically ill patients. Intensive Care Med 29:2199–2203
56. Marik PE, Gayowski T, Starzl TE et al (2005) The hepatoadrenal syndrome: a common yet unrecognized clinical condition. Crit Care Med 33:1254–1259
57. Etogo-Asse FE, Vincent RP, Hughes SA et al (2012) High density lipoprotein in patients with liver failure; relation to sepsis, adrenal function and outcome of illness. Liver Int 32:128–136
58. Matthews JG, Ito K, Barnes PJ et al (2004) Defective glucocorticoid receptor nuclear translocation and altered histone acetylation patterns in glucocorticoid-resistant patients. J Allergy Clin Immunol 113:1100–1108
59. Hew M, Bhavsar P, Torrego A et al (2006) Relative corticosteroid insensitivity of peripheral blood mononuclear cells in severe asthma. Am J Respir Crit Care Med 174:134–141
60. Goleva E, LI LB, Eves PT et al (2006) Increased glucocorticoid receptor Beta alters steroid response in glucocorticoid-insensitive asthma. Am J Respir Crit Care Med 173:607–616
61. Wikstrom AC (2003) Glucocorticoid action and novel mechanisms of steroid resistance: role of glucocorticoid receptor-interacting proteins for glucocorticoid responsiveness. J Endocrinol 178:331–337
62. Pariante CM, Pearce BD, Pisell TL et al (1999) The proinflammatory cytokine, interleukin-1alpha, reduces glucocorticoid receptor translocation and function. Endocrinology 140:4359–4366

63. Webster JC, Oakley RH, Jewell CM et al (2001) Proinflammatory cytokines regulate human glucocorticoid receptor gene expression and lead to the accumulation of the dominant negative beta isoform: a mechanism for the generation of glucocorticoid resistance. Proc Natl Acad Sci U S A 98:6865–6870
64. Guerrero J, Gatica HA, Rodriguez M et al (2013) Septic serum induces glucocorticoid resistance and modifies the expression of glucocorticoid isoform receptors: a prospective cohort study and in vitro experimental assay. Crit Care 17:R107
65. Bergquist M, Nurkkala M, Rylander C et al (2013) Expression of the glucocorticoid receptor is decreased in experimental Staphylococcus aureus sepsis. J Infect 67:574–583
66. Bergquist M, Jirholt P, Nurkkala M et al (2015) Glucocorticoid receptor function is decreased in neutrophils during endotoxic shock. J Infect 69:113–122
67. van den Akker EL, Koper JW, Joosten K et al (2013) Glucocorticoid receptor mRNA levels are selectively decreased in neutrophils of children with sepsis. Intensive Care Med 35:1247–1254
68. Indyk JA, Candido-Vitto C, Wolf M et al (2013) Reduced glucocorticoid receptor protein expression in children with critical illness. Horm Res Paediatr 79:169–178
69. Meduri GU, Muthiah MP, Carratu P et al (2005) Nuclear factor-kappaB- and glucocorticoid receptor alpha- mediated mechanisms in the regulation of systemic and pulmonary inflammation during sepsis and acute respiratory distress syndrome. Evidence for inflammation-induced target tissue resistance to glucocorticoids. Neuroimmunomodulation 12:321–338
70. Cohen J, Venkatesh B (2009) Assessment of tissue cortisol activity. Crit Care Resusc 11:287–289
71. Cohen J, Ward G, Prins J et al (2006) Variability of cortisol assays can confound the diagnosis of adrenal insufficiency in the critically ill population. Intensive Care Med 32:1901–1905
72. Cohen J, Smith ML, Deans RV et al (2012) Serial changes in plasma total cortisol, plasma free cortisol and tissue cortisol activity in patients with septic shock: an observational study. Shock 37:28–33
73. Cooper MS, Stewart PM (2003) Corticosteroid insufficiency in acutely ill patients. N Engl J Med 348:727–734
74. Venkatesh B, Cohen J, Cooper M (2015) Ten false beliefs about cortisol in critically ill patients. Intensive Care Med 41(10):1817–1819
75. Wang JC, Derynck MK, Nonaka D et al (2004) Chromatin immunoprecipitation (ChIP) scanning identifies primary glucocorticoid receptor target genes. Proc Natl Acad Sci U S A 101:15603–15608
76. Marik PE, Pastores SM, Annane D et al (2008) Recommendations for the diagnosis and management of corticosteroid insufficiency in critically ill adult patients: consensus statements from an international task force by the American College of Critical Care Medicine. Crit Care Med 36:1937–1949
77. Bone RC (1996) Sir Isaac Newton, sepsis, SIRS and CARS. Crit Care Med 24:1125–1128
78. Hotchkiss RS, Monneret G, Payen D (2013) Immunosuppression in sepsis: a novel understanding of the disorder and a new therapeutic approach. Lancet Infect Dis 13:260–268
79. Vanzant EL, Lopez CM, Ozrazgat-Baslanti T et al (2014) Persistent inflammation, immunosuppression, and catabolism syndrome after severe blunt trauma. J Trauma Acute Care Surg 76:21–30
80. Osuchowski MF, Welch K, Siddiqui J et al (2006) Circulating cytokine/inhibitor profiles reshape the understanding of the SIRS/CARS continuum in sepsis and predict mortality. J Immunol 177:1967–1974
81. Xiao W, Mindrinos MN, Seok J et al (2011) A genomic storm in critically injured humans. J Exp Med 208:2581–2590
82. Almansa R, Heredia-Rodriguez M, Gomez-Sanchez E et al (2015) Transcriptomic correlates of organ failure extent in sepsis. J Infect 70:445–456
83. Tang BM, Huang SJ, McLean AS (2010) Genome-wide transcription profiling of human sepsis: a systematic review. Crit Care 14:R237

84. Keh D, Boehnke T, Weber-Cartens S et al (2003) Immunologic and hemodynamic effects of "low-dose" hydrocortisone in septic shock: a double-blind, randomized, placebo-controlled, crossover study. Am J Respir Crit Care Med 167:512–520
85. Roquilly A, Mahe PJ, Seguin P et al (2011) Hydrocortisone therapy for corticosteroid insufficiency related to trauma. The HYPOLYT study. JAMA 305:1201–1209
86. Munoz C (1991) Dysregulation of in vitro cytokine production by monocytes during sepsis. J Clin Invest 88:1747–1754
87. Ehrchen J, Steinmuller L, Barczyk K et al (2007) Glucocorticoids induce differentiation of a specifically activated, anti-inflammatory subtype of human monocytes. Blood 109:1265–1274
88. Bystrom J, Evans I, Newson J et al (2008) Resolution-phase macrophages possess a unique inflammatory phenotype that is controlled by cAMP. Blood 112:4117–4127
89. Sica A, Mantovani A (2012) Macrophage plasticity and polarization: in vivo veritas. J Clin Invest 122:787–795

Chapter 13
Enterohormones and the Response to Critical Illness

Mark P. Plummer, Annika Reintam Blaser, and Adam M. Deane

Abstract The secretion of a number of enterohormones is disordered in the critically ill which may mediate abnormalities in motility and glycaemia. However, these mediators can also potentially serve a protective role, dampening inflammation and modulating the enteral immune response. There are over 30 recognised enterohormones, and therapeutic manipulation of specific enterohormones or their receptors is a burgeoning area of critical care research with promising preclinical data and an increasing number of small clinical trials. Further characterisation of the effect of critical illness on the endocrine gut and how it can be manipulated to improve outcomes in critical illness warrants evaluation.

13.1 Introduction

The enteroendocrine cells constitute less than 1 % of the total epithelial cell population of the gastrointestinal tract yet together form the largest endocrine system in the body [1]. These cells are responsible for the production of over 30 peptides which in health modulate gastrointestinal motility, secretory, absorptive and immune functions and mucosal growth and repair [2]. The physiological stress of critical illness and the

M.P. Plummer, MMBS (✉)
Discipline of Acute Care Medicine, University of Adelaide, Adelaide, Australia
e-mail: mark.philip.plummer@gmail.com

A.R. Blaser, PhD
Department of Anaesthesiology and Intensive Care, University of Tartu, Tartu, Estonia

A.M. Deane, PhD
Discipline of Acute Care Medicine, University of Adelaide, Adelaide, Australia

Department of Critical Care Services, Royal Adelaide Hospital, Adelaide, Australia
e-mail: adam.m.deane@gmail.com

J.-C. Preiser (ed.), *The Stress Response of Critical Illness: Metabolic and Hormonal Aspects*, DOI 10.1007/978-3-319-27687-8_13

Table 13.1 Function of enterohormones and impact of critical illness

Enterohormone	Site of secretion	Dominant effects	Effect of critical illness
Ghrelin	Parietal cells	↑ Growth hormone	↑ Total concentration ? ↓ Active concentration
	Gastric fundus	↑ Appetite	
		↑ Gastric emptying	
		Energy homeostasis	
Motilin	M cells	↑ Fasting intestinal motility	Unknown
	Proximal duodenum	↑ Gastric emptying (supraphysiological)	
CCK	I cells	↑ Gallbladder contraction	↑ Concentration
	Duodenum and jejunum	↓ Gastric emptying	
		↑ Pancreatic enzyme secretion	
		↓ Appetite	
GLP-1	L cells	↑ Insulin (glucose dependent)	↑ Concentration
	Distal ileum and colon	↓ Glucagon (glucose dependent)	
		↓ Gastric emptying	
		↓ Appetite	
GIP	K cells	↑ Insulin (glucose dependent)	No effect
	Duodenum and jejunum	↑ Glucagon (glucose dependent)	
GLP-2	L cells	↑ Intestinal mucosal growth	Unknown
	Distal ileum and colon	↑ Intestinal absorptive capacity	
		↓ Intestinal permeability	
		↑ Intestinal mucosal blood flow	
Peptide YY	L cells	↓ Gastric emptying	↑ Concentration
	Distal ileum, colon and rectum	↓ Gallbladder contraction	
		↓ Gastric acid secretion	
		↓ Pancreatic exocrine secretion	

treatments administered are associated with substantially disordered gastrointestinal and metabolic functions [3], many of which have been shown to be associated with adverse outcomes [4]. While it is not a clinical practice to measure plasma enterohormone levels, which may contribute to the current paucity of data, it is increasingly evident that a number of enterohormones mediate, or have the potential to mediate, many of the functional gastrointestinal and metabolic abnormalities that occur during critical illness. This chapter will review the enterohormones most likely to be of clinical significance: ghrelin, motilin, cholecystokinin (CCK), glucagon-like peptide 1 (GLP-1), glucose-dependent insulinotropic polypeptide (GIP), glucagon-like peptide 2 (GLP-2) and polypeptide YY (PYY). A summary for each hormone is provided with a focus on location of the secretory cell and receptor for hormone function, stimulus for secretion, and if there are sufficient data, the effect of critical illness on plasma concentrations and action is outlined (Table 13.1). In addition, studies relating to enterohormone receptor pharmacological agonism or antagonism and therapeutic potential in critical illness are presented where relevant.

13.2 Ghrelin

13.2.1 Ghrelin in Health

Ghrelin is primarily secreted during fasting from parietal cells of the gastric fundus in the inactive (nonacylated) form [5]. Its secretion is suppressed in the postprandial phase as a result of the interaction of nutrient with the small intestine [5]. Ghrelin is a prohormone and requires posttranslational acylation for the majority of its biological activity [6]. Acylated ghrelin is the endogenous ligand for the growth hormone secretagogue receptor (GHS-R1a) on the anterior pituitary, and therefore it is a natural secretagogue for growth hormone [7]. The GHS-R1a is expressed widely beyond the anterior pituitary including on pancreatic islets, B and T lymphocytes, neutrophils, myocardium, thyroid tissue and at multiple sites throughout the central nervous system, which explains the diverse physiological actions of this hormone [8]. As well as regulating growth hormone secretion, ghrelin plays important roles in stimulating appetite and modulating glucose homeostasis, decreasing insulin secretion and increasing insulin sensitivity [8]. It also modulates stress, anxiety and sleep, protects against muscle atrophy, modulates taste sensation and has vasodilatory effects [8]. Studies using exogenous ghrelin at supraphysiological concentrations indicate that ghrelin accelerates gastric emptying in humans and in animal models of sepsis-induced gastroparesis [9, 10]. In ambulant patients with diabetic gastroparesis, a ghrelin agonist has been shown to stimulate gastrokinesis [11].

13.2.2 Ghrelin in Critical Illness

In the largest study to date of endogenous ghrelin concentrations in critical illness, Koch et al. analysed plasma ghrelin in 170 critically ill patients and 60 healthy persons as a control group [12]. While they demonstrated that total ghrelin concentrations are increased during critical illness, they did not differentiate between the active (acylated) and inactive form [12]. This is important as the majority of circulating ghrelin is in the inactive form and is renally cleared, unlike the active form which undergoes organ-independent enzyme metabolism with a short half-life of 10 min [13]. Inactive ghrelin accumulates in renal failure [11], and Koch et al. demonstrated an inverse association between renal function and ghrelin concentration in non-septic critically ill patients [12]. In the only study to date to measure both active and inactive ghrelin in critical illness, Crona and MacLaren demonstrated that compared to patients tolerating enteral nutrition, patients with feed intolerance had higher concentrations of total ghrelin but lower concentrations of active ghrelin [6]. These data suggest that while total ghrelin concentrations may be elevated during critical illness, active ghrelin levels may be decreased and contribute to slow gastric emptying. Studies into the effect of exogenous ghrelin, or its agonists, to manage feed intolerance in this population are warranted.

As well as influencing gut motility, there is mechanistic plausibility that ghrelin may be protective in sepsis; in multiple animal models, exogenous ghrelin has been found to downregulate proinflammatory cytokines [14], protect against endotoxaemia-induced acute kidney injury [15], ameliorate gut mucosal barrier function [16], attenuate sepsis-induced acute lung injury [17] and improve tissue perfusion [18]. Exogenous ghrelin has not been evaluated as a therapy in the critically ill but has been shown to reduce cachexia, increase appetite and improve exercise tolerance in patients with cancer, heart failure, end-stage renal disease and chronic obstructive pulmonary disease [19]. This is likely due to both anabolic growth hormone dependent and independent effects, for example, improved appetite [4].

While growth hormone is suppressed in critical illness, trials with suprapharmacological doses of growth hormone have reported adverse outcomes [20]. Despite this adverse effect of growth hormone administration, careful evaluation of ghrelin therapy in the critically ill appears warranted to establish the effects on gastric emptying, appetite and anabolism.

13.3 Motilin

13.3.1 Motilin in Health

Motilin is synthesised by M cells in the proximal duodenum and regulates the fasting pattern of motility of the gut by binding to the motilin-specific G-protein-coupled receptor [21]. Motilin is predominantly secreted in the interdigestive state, and the peak plasma motilin concentration coincides with the onset of the antegrade contractions during the fasting phase III-migrating motor complex [22]. Pharmacological concentrations of exogenously administered motilin accelerate gastric emptying in healthy individuals and in patients with gastroparesis [23]. The macrolide antibiotic erythromycin is a motilin receptor agonist and potently stimulates gastric emptying which has led to its additional use as a gastric prokinetic agent for the treatment of gastroparesis of multiple aetiologies [24].

13.3.2 Motilin in Critical Illness

Erythromycin potently stimulates gastric emptying in critically ill patients with feed intolerance and large gastric residual volumes [25–27]. Tachyphylaxis to stimulation of the motilin receptor develops quickly with erythromycin, and the effects are diminished in 60 % of critically ill patients within 1 week of regular administration [25]. While a more effective gastrokinetic drug than metoclopramide, observational data indicate that erythromycin is administered less frequently [28], perhaps because of concerns regarding adverse effects, such as the potential to exacerbate bacterial resistance, interaction with other medications metabolised by the cytochrome P450 3A4 system and prolongation of the QT interval [29]. For these reasons there is increasing effort to identify a selective motilin receptor agonist without macrolide antibiotic properties for clinical use. There are preliminary data from a small phase 2 study that a non-macrolide selective motilin receptor agonist accelerates gastric emptying in the critically ill compared to placebo, and larger randomised controlled trials are keenly awaited [30].

13.4 Cholecystokinin

13.4.1 Cholecystokinin in Health

Cholecystokinin (CCK) is a peptide hormone secreted by I cells in the mucosa of the duodenum and jejunum in response to dietary fat, protein and, to a lesser extent, carbohydrates [31]. It binds to its specific G-protein-coupled receptor on the gastric, gallbladder and small intestinal mucosa, vagal afferents and centrally in the hypothalamus and hindbrain where it acts as a neuropeptide [32]. Endogenous CCK is the principal regulator of gallbladder contraction and has been shown to slow gastric emptying, relax the sphincter of Oddi and stimulate pancreatic enzyme secretion [33, 34]. Interaction of CCK with central satiation receptors in the hypothalamus reduces hunger and energy intake [35].

13.4.2 Cholecystokinin in Critical Illness

Our group has previously demonstrated elevated fasting and nutrient-stimulated plasma CCK levels in critical illness compared to healthy subjects [36]. Furthermore, fasting plasma CCK concentrations were higher in critically ill patients with delayed gastric emptying compared to those with normal emptying, suggesting a role for CCK in the pathogenesis of delayed gastric emptying [37]. However, our experience from studies performed in healthy participants with normal rates of gastric emptying is that the magnitude of acceleration that occurs when antagonising endogenous hormones is much less than during administration of pharmacological concentrations [38, 39]. Given that gastric emptying is slow in many patients and can be due to many causes, our opinion is that CCK antagonists would have only a modest effect on gastric emptying and feed intolerance in the critically ill.

There are preclinical data to suggest that endogenous cholecystokinin mediates the beneficial immune and antiinflammatory effects attributable to enteral nutrition in critical illness [40, 41]. In a rat model of haemorrhagic shock, CCK released in response to an enteral lipid load activates immunomodulatory receptors via vagal pathways, dampening the systemic inflammatory response and attenuating gastric epithelial permeability and bacterial translocation [40, 41]. Further studies are required to characterise the effect of critical illness on plasma CCK, the associations between plasma CCK and gastric emptying and the potential immunomodulatory role of CCK.

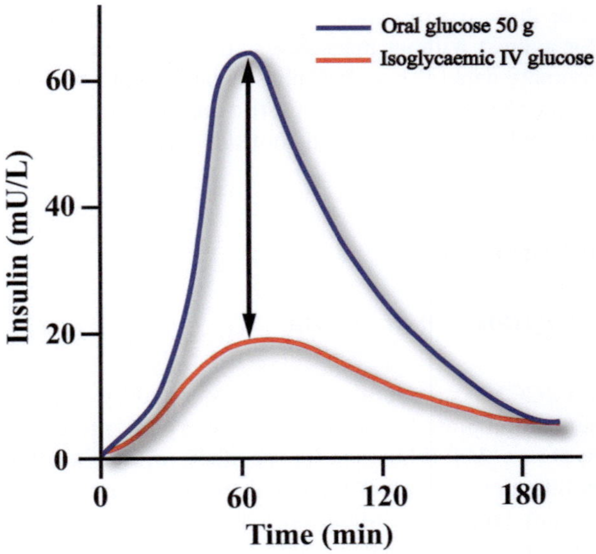

Fig. 13.1 The incretin effect (Adapted from Nauck et al. [45]). There is a substantially greater release of insulin in response to oral glucose as compared to an isoglycaemic intravenous infusion of glucose. The difference between the plasma insulin, as demonstrated by the *arrow*, is the incretin effect and is mediated by the enterohormones glucagon-like peptide 1(GLP-1) and glucose-dependent insulinotropic polypeptide (GIP)

13.5 Glucagon-Like Peptide 1 (GLP-1)

13.5.1 GLP-1 in Health and Diabetes

GLP-1 is an incretin hormone stored in enteric L cells located predominantly in the distal small intestine and colon and is secreted in response to luminal fat, carbohydrate, protein and bile acids [42, 43]. Incretins are gut hormones that potentiate insulin secretion after a meal in a glucose-dependent manner [44]. Together with glucose-dependent insulinotropic polypeptide (GIP), GLP-1 accounts for the two to threefold greater insulinotropic response to an oral glucose load compared to the equivalent intravenous glucose load (Fig. 13.1) [46]. The primary physiological role of endogenous GLP-1 is to lower blood glucose [47] via direct effects on pancreatic islet cell G-protein-coupled receptors to propagate secondary messenger signals that stimulate insulin and suppress glucagon release and indirect effects on the gut to slow gastric emptying and small intestinal motility [38, 47, 48]. The insulinotropic and glucagonostatic effect on the pancreatic α and β cells are strictly glucose dependent such that below a blood glucose of ~6 mmol/L, even pharmacological doses of GLP-1 (and its agonists) have little or no impact on blood glucose [49]. In contrast, the ability of exogenously administered GLP-1 to slow gastric emptying persists during hypoglycaemia [39]. GLP-1 receptors are expressed widely beyond the pancreas and gut including in the lung, kidney, skin, heart and brain [50]. A detailed review of the extrapancreatic effects of endogenous GLP-1 is beyond the scope of this chapter; however, GLP-1 is thought to play a role in regulating appetite, learning and memory, preventing cardiac cell apoptosis, increasing bone formation and decreasing dermal cytokine expression [51].

The glucose-dependent insulinotropic effect of GLP-1 is preserved in patients with type 2 diabetes [52], making the GLP-1 receptor an attractive therapeutic target in this group [53]. Native GLP-1 is rapidly metabolised by dipeptidyl peptidase-4 (DPP-4) predominantly on capillary endothelia, imparting the enterohormone with a short half-life of 1–2 min [54, 55] which makes therapeutic delivery of native GLP-1 impractical. This has led to the development of subcutaneously administered GLP-1 receptor agonists that are resistant to DPP-4 degradation such as exenatide and lixisenatide, as well as oral DPP-4 inhibitors such as sitagliptin, linagliptin and vildagliptin that have now been incorporated into standard algorithms for the management of type 2 diabetes [56].

13.5.2 GLP-1 in Critical Illness

In the critically ill, endogenous GLP-1 concentrations are increased [57–59] when compared to nutrient-stimulated physiological levels in healthy persons [60]. There appear to be associations between plasma concentration and biomarkers of inflammation, illness severity [58] and feed intolerance [59]. Murine studies have demonstrated inducible GLP-1 secretion by a range of inflammatory stimuli including endotoxin, IL-1 and IL-6 [58, 61]. Interestingly, when systemic inflammation is induced in healthy volunteers by a TNF-α infusion, there is no demonstrable change in the incretin effect [62].

13.5.3 Therapeutic Potential of GLP-1-Based Therapy in the Critically Ill

The rapid, organ-independent metabolism of a therapy that causes controlled, glucose-dependent glucagon suppression and insulin release makes GLP-1 a promising agent for the management of stress hyperglycaemia [43, 63]. To date, the use of GLP-1 in the critically ill is limited to small studies to establish proof of principle, albeit with promising results [64]. With pharmacological concentrations of intravenous GLP-1, marked glucose lowering has been observed in patients with type 2 diabetes postcardiac surgery [65, 66]. In a heterogeneous cohort of mechanically ventilated patients, exogenous GLP-1 has been observed to reduce the glycaemic response to small intestinal nutrient delivery in patients with type 2 diabetes [67] and to intragastric and intestinal nutrient delivery in patients without pre-existing diabetes [68, 69]. In a small ($n=18$) randomised, double-blind, placebo-controlled crossover study in critically ill surgical patients, GLP-1 in combination with intensive insulin therapy was also shown to reduce glycaemic variability when compared to intensive insulin therapy alone [70].

Administration of the commercially available GLP-1 agonist exenatide is also being explored. In an open-label, nonrandomised pilot study, Abuannadi and colleagues administered intravenous exenatide to 40 patients following major cardiac surgery [71]. Intravenous exenatide was associated with significantly reduced glycaemic variability compared to conventional intravenous insulin therapy and achieved equipotent blood glucose lowering with no episodes of severe hypoglycaemia [71]. Exenatide has also been administered subcutaneously in an open-label study in paediatric burn patients where it was shown to reduce exogenous insulin requirements [72].

While GLP-1 and its agonists have an inherently low risk of hypoglycaemia, there is a dose-dependent relationship between GLP-1 and the slowing of gastric emptying, and this has raised concerns that pharmacologically induced slower emptying may predispose to aspiration in mechanically ventilated critically ill patients [63]. Somewhat reassuringly, in a population of nondiabetic critically ill patients, our group has demonstrated that acute infusion of GLP-1 at pharmacological concentration slows gastric emptying when gastromotor function is normal at baseline but has no effect when gastric emptying is already delayed [68].

There have been no human studies into the therapeutic potential of DPP-4 inhibitors in the critically ill which may be due to their oral route of administration and resultant variable pharmacokinetics.

Whether GLP-1, its agonists or the DPP-4 inhibitors could be used as standalone therapy or in combination with insulin for the management of stress hyperglycaemia warrants further investigation.

13.6 Glucose-Dependent Insulinotropic Polypeptide (GIP)

13.6.1 GIP in Health and Type 2 Diabetes

Glucose-dependent insulinotropic polypeptide, previously known as gastric inhibitory polypeptide, is secreted from duodenal and jejunal K cells in response to luminal fat and carbohydrate [44]. GIP exerts its incretin effect through distinct G-protein-coupled receptors that are highly expressed in islet β-cells, and like GLP-1, the insulinotropic action of GIP is strictly glucose dependent [44]. GIP also has glucose-dependent effects on the α-cell, dose dependently stimulating glucagon secretion during hypo- and euglycaemia with no effect during hyperglycaemia [73]. GIP has no direct enterogastrone effect on either gastric acid secretion or gastric emptying but may slightly accelerate gastric emptying via indirect mechanisms through lowering systemic glycaemia [32]. GIP receptors are expressed widely and have been identified in the fat, bone, brain and cardiac tissue with in vitro and murine studies, suggesting potential roles for GIP in triglyceride metabolism, bone formation and neuroprotection [44]. GIP is also metabolised by DPP-4 with a resultantly short half-life of ~4 min [74].

Unlike GLP-1, the insulinotropic effect of GIP is profoundly reduced in patients with type 2 diabetes and long-standing chronic hyperglycaemia [45]. This is likely due, at least in part, to the direct toxic effects of chronic hyperglycaemia downregulating GIP receptor expression on the β-cell [75], an effect which may be reversible with Hϕjberg et al. reporting that the insulinotropic property of GIP increased severalfold following 4 weeks of near-normal glycaemia in patients with type 2 diabetes [76].

13.6.2 GIP in Critical Illness

It does not appear that critical illness alters fasting or nutrient-stimulated GIP levels [57, 77]. There is a persuasive rationale for a potential therapeutic role for exogenous GIP in the management of stress hyperglycaemia, specifically its inherent safety profile; it stimulates glucagon release during hypoglycaemia and insulin release during hyperglycaemia and does not slow gastric emptying [78, 79].

In the only studies in the critically ill to date, our group has investigated GIP both as a solo agent and in combination with GLP-1 for the management of stress hyperglycaemia [78, 80]. Consistent with the lack of effect in patients with type 2 diabetes, we have shown that GIP has a negligible effect on glycaemia, gastric emptying, glucose absorption, insulin or glucagon secretion during critical illness [80] and provides no additional glucose lowering or insulinotropic effect when administered in conjunction with GLP-1 [78]. Together, these data suggest that future studies should focus on GLP-1 or its agonists, rather than GIP for the management of stress hyperglycaemia.

13.7 Glucagon-Like Peptide-2

13.7.1 GLP-2 in Health

GLP-2 is co-secreted with GLP-1 in response to luminal nutrient from L cells that are located primarily in the distal ileum and colon [81]. GLP-2 is a pleiotropic hormone influencing multiple facets of intestinal physiology, the foremost of which is stimulation of intestinal mucosal growth in the small and, to a lesser extent, the large bowel [82]. GLP-2 acts through G-protein-coupled receptors primarily located in the small intestine [82]. While the receptor has been demonstrated on gastrointestinal endocrine cells, enteric neurons and myofibroblasts, its absence on both crypt epithelial cells and enterocytes suggests an indirect mechanism of its primary intestinotrophic action [81]. Like GLP-1 and GIP, GLP-2 is rapidly inactivated by the ubiquitous enzyme DPP-4, conferring a short half-life of ~7 min [83].

The majority of the gastrointestinal effects of GLP-2 have been elucidated following exogenous administration of GLP-2 or degradation-resistant GLP-2 analogues such as teduglutide. The intestinotrophic effects of GLP-2 are mediated via an increase in intestinal crypt cell proliferation, a reduction in villous cell apoptosis and improved mesenteric blood flow, collectively increasing mucosal mass and surface area with an accompanied increase in intestinal digestive and absorptive capacity [81, 83]. GLP-2 administration also decreases gastric acid secretion and is glucagonotropic, but unlike GLP-1 has no effect on insulin secretion, gastric emptying or postprandial glycaemia [4].

13.7.2 Therapeutic Role of GLP-2 in Gastrointestinal Disease

Exogenously administered GLP-2 and GLP-2 analogues significantly improve morbidity and increase gastrointestinal absorptive capacity in a diverse range of preclinical intestinal injury models, including small bowel resection [84], enteritis [85], necrotizing pancreatitis [86] and ischaemic-reperfusion injury [87]. Furthermore, GLP-2 enhances epithelial barrier capacity, decreasing transcellular and paracellular permeability and reducing bacterial translocation [81, 86, 88]. These promising preclinical results encouraged human trials of the GLP-2 analogue, teduglutide, which has since gained FDA approval for the management of short bowel syndrome after demonstrating increased gastrointestinal absorptive capacity and a reduction in faecal weight, energy expenditure and total parenteral nutrition (TPN) requirement [89].

13.7.3 Therapeutic Potential of GLP-2 in Critical Illness Implicate

Critically ill patients fasted for >4 days, demonstrating significant duodenal mucosal atrophy and increased gut permeability [90], and bacterial translocation has been implicated to play a role in the development of sepsis and multi-organ failure [91]. The physiological concentrations and potential effects of pharmacological concentrations of GLP-2 are yet to be studied in the critically ill. It is plausible that during critical illness the administration of GLP-2 may attenuate mucosal atrophy, improve nutrient absorption and reduce secondary infections.

13.8 Peptide YY

13.8.1 Peptide YY in Health

Peptide YY (PYY) also known as peptide tyrosine-tyrosine is secreted by L cells located throughout the gastrointestinal tract but with the highest density in the colon [92]. PYY is released in response to enteral nutrient with fat being the most potent stimulus [93]. As PYY levels increase within 15 min of meal ingestion, an indirect mechanism mediated via CCK-dependent pathways has been proposed to initiate the initial secretory response which is later maintained via direct enteral stimulation of the lower gastrointestinal tract [93]. PYY exerts predominantly inhibitory functions in health, slowing gastric and gallbladder emptying and inhibiting gastric acid and pancreatic exocrine secretion [32]. PYY receptors are also located centrally, and exogenous PYY has been shown to be anorectic, inhibiting appetite and energy intake in overweight humans [94].

13.8.2 PYY in Critical Illness

Fasting and nutrient-stimulated PYY concentrations are elevated two to threefold in critical illness which progressively normalise as critical illness resolves [95]. The PYY response is substantially greater in those critically ill patients with feed intolerance, suggesting a role for PYY in critical illness-induced delayed gastric emptying [96]. This highlights a potential role for PYY receptor antagonists in the management of feed intolerance in the critically ill; however, at present there are no PYY antagonists available for clinical use.

13.9 Conclusion

The secretion of a number of enterohormones is disordered in the critically ill which may mediate abnormalities in motility and glycaemia while also potentially serving a protective role, dampening inflammation and modulating the enteral immune response. There are over 30 recognised enterohormones, and therapeutic manipulation of specific enterohormones or their receptors is a burgeoning area of critical care research with promising preclinical data and an increasing number of small clinical trials. Further characterisation of the effect of critical illness on the endocrine gut and how it can be manipulated to improve outcomes in critical illness warrants evaluation.

References

1. Rehfeld JF (2012) Beginnings: a reflection on the history of gastrointestinal endocrinology. Regul Pept 177(Suppl):S1–S5
2. Schmidt WE (1997) The intestine, an endocrine organ. Digestion 58(Suppl 1):56–58
3. Thompson JS (1995) The intestinal response to critical illness. Am J Gastroenterol 90(2): 190–200
4. Deane A, Chapman MJ, Fraser RJ, Horowitz M (2010) Bench-to-bedside review: the gut as an endocrine organ in the critically ill. Crit Care 14(5):228
5. Parker BA, Doran S, Wishart J, Horowitz M, Chapman IM (2005) Effects of small intestinal and gastric glucose administration on the suppression of plasma ghrelin concentrations in healthy older men and women. Clin Endocrinol 62(5):539–546
6. Crona D, MacLaren R (2012) Gastrointestinal hormone concentrations associated with gastric feeding in critically ill patients. JPEN J Parenter Enteral Nutr 36(2):189–196

7. Kojima M, Hosoda H, Date Y, Nakazato M, Matsuo H, Kangawa K (1999) Ghrelin is a growth-hormone-releasing acylated peptide from stomach. Nature 402(6762):656–660
8. Muller TD, Nogueiras R, Andermann ML, Andrews ZB, Anker SD, Argente J, Batterham RL, Benoit SC, Bowers CY, Broglio F et al (2015) Ghrelin. Mol Metab 4(6):437–460
9. Tack J, Depoortere I, Bisschops R, Delporte C, Coulie B, Meulemans A, Janssens J, Peeters T (2006) Influence of ghrelin on interdigestive gastrointestinal motility in humans. Gut 55(3):327–333
10. De Winter BY, De Man JG, Seerden TC, Depoortere I, Herman AG, Peeters TL, Pelckmans PA (2004) Effect of ghrelin and growth hormone-releasing peptide 6 on septic ileus in mice. J Neurogastroenterol Motil 16(4):439–446
11. Ejskjaer N, Vestergaard ET, Hellstrom PM, Gormsen LC, Madsbad S, Madsen JL, Jensen TA, Pezzullo JC, Christiansen JS, Shaughnessy L et al (2009) Ghrelin receptor agonist (TZP-101) accelerates gastric emptying in adults with diabetes and symptomatic gastroparesis. Aliment Pharmacol Ther 29(11):1179–1187
12. Koch A, Sanson E, Helm A, Voigt S, Trautwein C, Tacke F (2010) Regulation and prognostic relevance of serum ghrelin concentrations in critical illness and sepsis. Crit Care 14(3):R94
13. Cummings DE, Overduin J (2004) Circulating Ghrelin levels in pathophysiological conditions. In: Ghigo E (ed) Ghrelin. Springer Science+Business Media, Boston, pp 213–214
14. Wu R, Dong W, Cui X, Zhou M, Simms HH, Ravikumar TS, Wang P (2007) Ghrelin down-regulates proinflammatory cytokines in sepsis through activation of the vagus nerve. Ann Surg 245(3):480–486
15. Wang W, Bansal S, Falk S, Ljubanovic D, Schrier R (2009) Ghrelin protects mice against endotoxemia-induced acute kidney injury. Am J Physiol Renal Physiol 297(4):F1032–F1037
16. Wu R, Dong W, Qiang X, Wang H, Blau SA, Ravikumar TS, Wang P (2009) Orexigenic hormone ghrelin ameliorates gut barrier dysfunction in sepsis in rats. Crit Care Med 37(8):2421–2426
17. Wu R, Dong W, Zhou M, Zhang F, Marini CP, Ravikumar TS, Wang P (2007) Ghrelin attenuates sepsis-induced acute lung injury and mortality in rats. Am J Respir Crit Care Med 176(8):805–813
18. Wu R, Dong W, Zhou M, Cui X, Hank Simms H, Wang P (2005) Ghrelin improves tissue perfusion in severe sepsis via downregulation of endothelin-1. Cardiovasc Res 68(2):318–326
19. Garin MC, Burns CM, Kaul S, Cappola AR (2013) Clinical review: the human experience with ghrelin administration. J Clin Endocrinol Metab 98(5):1826–1837
20. Doig GS, Simpson F, Finfer S, Delaney A, Davies AR, Mitchell I, Dobb G (2008) Nutrition Guidelines Investigators of the ACTG: effect of evidence-based feeding guidelines on mortality of critically ill adults: a cluster randomized controlled trial. JAMA 300(23):2731–2741
21. Poitras P, Peeters TL (2008) Motilin. Curr Opin Endocrinol Diabetes Obes 15(1):54–57
22. Vantrappen G, Janssens J, Peeters TL, Bloom SR, Christofides ND, Hellemans J (1979) Motilin and the interdigestive migrating motor complex in man. Dig Dis Sci 24(7):497–500
23. Peeters TL, Muls E, Janssens J, Urbain JL, Bex M, Van Cutsem E, Depoortere I, De Roo M, Vantrappen G, Bouillon R (1992) Effect of motilin on gastric emptying in patients with diabetic gastroparesis. Gastroenterology 102(1):97–101
24. Janssens J, Peeters TL, Vantrappen G, Tack J, Urbain JL, De Roo M, Muls E, Bouillon R (1990) Improvement of gastric emptying in diabetic gastroparesis by erythromycin. Preliminary studies. N Engl J Med 322(15):1028–1031
25. Nguyen NQ, Chapman MJ, Fraser RJ, Bryant LK, Holloway RH (2007) Erythromycin is more effective than metoclopramide in the treatment of feed intolerance in critical illness. Crit Care Med 35(2):483–489
26. MacLaren R, Kiser TH, Fish DN, Wischmeyer PE (2008) Erythromycin vs metoclopramide for facilitating gastric emptying and tolerance to intragastric nutrition in critically ill patients. JPEN J Parenter Enteral Nutr 32(4):412–419
27. Dive A, Miesse C, Galanti L, Jamart J, Evrard P, Gonzalez M, Installe E (1995) Effect of erythromycin on gastric motility in mechanically ventilated critically ill patients: a double-blind, randomized, placebo-controlled study. Crit Care Med 23(8):1356–1362

28. Gungabissoon U, Hacquoil K, Bains C, Irizarry M, Dukes G, Williamson R, Deane AM, Heyland DK (2015) Prevalence, risk factors, clinical consequences, and treatment of enteral feed intolerance during critical illness. JPEN J Parenter Enteral Nutr 39(4):441–448
29. Sanger GJ, Wang Y, Hobson A, Broad J (2013) Motilin: towards a new understanding of the gastrointestinal neuropharmacology and therapeutic use of motilin receptor agonists. Br J Pharmacol 170(7):1323–1332
30. Chapman MJ, Fraser R, Nguyen NQ, Deane AM, O'Conner SN, Duncan R, Hacquoil K, Vasist L, Barton M, Dukes G (2011) The effect of GSK962040, a selective motilin agonist, on gastric emptying in critically ill patients with enteral feed intolerance (Mot112572). Crit Care Med 39(12):195
31. Pilichiewicz AN, Chaikomin R, Brennan IM, Wishart JM, Rayner CK, Jones KL, Smout AJ, Horowitz M, Feinle-Bisset C (2007) Load-dependent effects of duodenal glucose on glycemia, gastrointestinal hormones, antropyloroduodenal motility, and energy intake in healthy men. Am J Physiol Endocrinol Metab 293(3):E743–E753
32. Luttikhold J, de Ruijter FM, van Norren K, Diamant M, Witkamp RF, van Leeuwen PA, Vermeulen MA (2013) Review article: the role of gastrointestinal hormones in the treatment of delayed gastric emptying in critically ill patients. Aliment Pharmacol Ther 38(6):573–583
33. Wank SA (1995) Cholecystokinin receptors. Am J Physiol 269(5 Pt 1):G628–G646
34. Fried M, Erlacher U, Schwizer W, Lochner C, Koerfer J, Beglinger C, Jansen JB, Lamers CB, Harder F, Bischof-Delaloye A et al (1991) Role of cholecystokinin in the regulation of gastric emptying and pancreatic enzyme secretion in humans. Studies with the cholecystokinin-receptor antagonist loxiglumide. Gastroenterology 101(2):503–511
35. Rayner CK, Park HS, Doran SM, Chapman IM, Horowitz M (2000) Effects of cholecystokinin on appetite and pyloric motility during physiological hyperglycemia. Am J Physiol Gastrointest Liver Physiol 278(1):G98–G104
36. Nguyen NQ, Fraser RJ, Chapman MJ, Bryant LK, Holloway RH, Vozzo R, Wishart J, Feinle-Bisset C, Horowitz M (2007) Feed intolerance in critical illness is associated with increased basal and nutrient-stimulated plasma cholecystokinin concentrations. Crit Care Med 35(1): 82–88
37. Nguyen NQ, Fraser RJ, Chapman M, Bryant LK, Wishart J, Holloway RH, Horowitz M (2006) Fasting and nutrient-stimulated plasma peptide-YY levels are elevated in critical illness and associated with feed intolerance: an observational, controlled study. Crit Care 10(6):R175
38. Deane AM, Nguyen NQ, Stevens JE, Fraser RJ, Holloway RH, Besanko LK, Burgstad C, Jones KL, Chapman MJ, Rayner CK et al (2010) Endogenous glucagon-like peptide-1 slows gastric emptying in healthy subjects, attenuating postprandial glycemia. J Clin Endocrinol Metab 95(1):215–221
39. Plummer MP, Jones KL, Annink CE, Cousins CE, Meier JJ, Chapman MJ, Horowitz M, Deane AM (2014) Glucagon-like peptide 1 attenuates the acceleration of gastric emptying induced by hypoglycemia in healthy subjects. Diabetes Care 37(6):1509–1515
40. Luyer MD, Greve JW, Hadfoune M, Jacobs JA, Dejong CH, Buurman WA (2005) Nutritional stimulation of cholecystokinin receptors inhibits inflammation via the vagus nerve. J Exp Med 202(8):1023–1029
41. de Haan JJ, Lubbers T, Hadfoune M, Luyer MD, Dejong CH, Buurman WA, Greve JW (2008) Postshock intervention with high-lipid enteral nutrition reduces inflammation and tissue damage. Ann Surg 248(5):842–848
42. Schirra J, Katschinski M, Weidmann C, Schafer T, Wank U, Arnold R, Goke B (1996) Gastric emptying and release of incretin hormones after glucose ingestion in humans. J Clin Invest 97(1):92–103
43. Plummer MP, Chapman MJ, Horowitz M, Deane AM (2014) Incretins and the intensivist: what are they and what does an intensivist need to know about them? Crit Care 18(1):205
44. Campbell JE, Drucker DJ (2013) Pharmacology, physiology, and mechanisms of incretin hormone action. Cell Metab 17(6):819–837
45. Nauck M, Stockmann F, Ebert R, Creutzfeldt W (1986) Reduced incretin effect in type 2 (non-insulin-dependent) diabetes. Diabetologia 29(1):46–52

46. Perley MJ, Kipnis DM (1967) Plasma insulin responses to oral and intravenous glucose: studies in normal and diabetic subjects. J Clin Invest 46(12):1954–1962
47. Schirra J, Nicolaus M, Roggel R, Katschinski M, Storr M, Woerle HJ, Goke B (2006) Endogenous glucagon-like peptide 1 controls endocrine pancreatic secretion and antro-pyloro-duodenal motility in humans. Gut 55(2):243–251
48. Edwards CM, Todd JF, Mahmoudi M, Wang Z, Wang RM, Ghatei MA, Bloom SR (1999) Glucagon-like peptide 1 has a physiological role in the control of postprandial glucose in humans: studies with the antagonist exendin 9–39. Diabetes 48(1):86–93
49. Nauck MA, Heimesaat MM, Behle K, Holst JJ, Nauck MS, Ritzel R, Hufner M, Schmiegel WH (2002) Effects of glucagon-like peptide 1 on counterregulatory hormone responses, cognitive functions, and insulin secretion during hyperinsulinemic, stepped hypoglycemic clamp experiments in healthy volunteers. J Clin Endocrinol Metab 87(3):1239–1246
50. Pyke C, Heller RS, Kirk RK, Orskov C, Reedtz-Runge S, Kaastrup P, Hvelplund A, Bardram L, Calatayud D, Knudsen LB (2014) GLP-1 receptor localization in monkey and human tissue: novel distribution revealed with extensively validated monoclonal antibody. Endocrinology 155(4):1280–1290
51. Muscogiuri G, Cignarelli A, Giorgino F, Prodram F, Santi D, Tirabassi G, Balercia G, Modica R, Faggiano A, Colao A (2014) GLP-1: benefits beyond pancreas. J Endocrinol Invest 37:1143–53
52. Nauck MA, Heimesaat MM, Orskov C, Holst JJ, Ebert R, Creutzfeldt W (1993) Preserved incretin activity of glucagon-like peptide 1 [7–36 amide] but not of synthetic human gastric inhibitory polypeptide in patients with type-2 diabetes mellitus. J Clin Invest 91(1): 301–307
53. Nauck M (1996) Therapeutic potential of glucagon-like peptide 1 in type 2 diabetes. Diabet Med 13(9 Suppl 5):S39–S43
54. Nauck MA (2009) Unraveling the science of incretin biology. Am J Med 122(6 Suppl): S3–S10
55. Holst JJ (2007) The physiology of glucagon-like peptide 1. Physiol Rev 87(4):1409–1439
56. Inzucchi SE, Bergenstal RM, Buse JB, Diamant M, Ferrannini E, Nauck M, Peters AL, Tsapas A, Wender R, Matthews DR et al (2012) Management of hyperglycemia in type 2 diabetes: a patient-centered approach: position statement of the American Diabetes Association (ADA) and the European Association for the Study of Diabetes (EASD). Diabetes Care 35(6): 1364–1379
57. Deane AM, Rayner CK, Keeshan A, Cvijanovic N, Marino Z, Nguyen NQ, Chia B, Summers MJ, Sim JA, van Beek T et al (2014) The effects of critical illness on intestinal glucose sensing, transporters, and absorption. Crit Care Med 42:57–65
58. Kahles F, Meyer C, Mollmann J, Diebold S, Findeisen HM, Lebherz C, Trautwein C, Koch A, Tacke F, Marx N et al (2014) GLP-1 secretion is increased by inflammatory stimuli in an IL-6-dependent manner, leading to hyperinsulinemia and blood glucose lowering. Diabetes 63(10):3221–3229
59. Summers MJ, DI Bartolomeo AE, Zaknic AV, Chapman MJ, Nguyen NQ, Zacharakis B, Rayner CK, Horowitz M, Deane AM (2014) Endogenous amylin and glucagon-like peptide-1 concentrations are not associated with gastric emptying in critical illness. Acta Anaesthesiol Scand 58(2):235–242
60. Muscelli E, Mari A, Casolaro A, Camastra S, Seghieri G, Gastaldelli A, Holst JJ, Ferrannini E (2008) Separate impact of obesity and glucose tolerance on the incretin effect in normal subjects and type 2 diabetic patients. Diabetes 57(5):1340–1348
61. Nguyen AT, Mandard S, Dray C, Deckert V, Valet P, Besnard P, Drucker DJ, Lagrost L, Grober J (2014) Lipopolysaccharides-mediated increase in glucose-stimulated insulin secretion: involvement of the GLP-1 pathway. Diabetes 63(2):471–482
62. Nielsen ST, Lehrskov-Schmidt L, Krogh-Madsen R, Solomon TP, Lehrskov-Schmidt L, Holst JJ, Moller K (2013) Tumour necrosis factor-alpha infusion produced insulin resistance but no change in the incretin effect in healthy volunteers. Diabetes Metab Res Rev 29(8):655–663

63. Combes J, Borot S, Mougel F, Penfornis A (2011) The potential role of glucagon-like peptide-1 or its analogues in enhancing glycaemic control in critically ill adult patients. Diabetes Obes Metab 13(2):118–129
64. Pinelli NR, Jones MC, Monday LM, Smith Z, Rhoney DH (2012) Exogenous glucagon-like peptide-1 for hyperglycemia in critically ill patients. Ann Pharmacother 46(1):124–129
65. Meier JJ, Weyhe D, Michaely M, Senkal M, Zumtobel V, Nauck MA, Holst JJ, Schmidt WE, Gallwitz B (2004) Intravenous glucagon-like peptide 1 normalizes blood glucose after major surgery in patients with type 2 diabetes. Crit Care Med 32(3):848–851
66. Sokos GG, Bolukoglu H, German J, Hentosz T, Magovern GJ Jr, Maher TD, Dean DA, Bailey SH, Marrone G, Benckart DH et al (2007) Effect of glucagon-like peptide-1 (GLP-1) on glycemic control and left ventricular function in patients undergoing coronary artery bypass grafting. Am J Cardiol 100(5):824–829
67. Deane AM, Summers MJ, Zaknic AV, Chapman MJ, Fraser RJ, Di Bartolomeo AE, Wishart JM, Horowitz M (2011) Exogenous glucagon-like peptide-1 attenuates the glycaemic response to postpyloric nutrient infusion in critically ill patients with type-2 diabetes. Crit Care 15(1):R35
68. Deane AM, Chapman MJ, Fraser RJ, Summers MJ, Zaknic AV, Storey JP, Jones KL, Rayner CK, Horowitz M (2010) Effects of exogenous glucagon-like peptide-1 on gastric emptying and glucose absorption in the critically ill: relationship to glycemia. Crit Care Med 38(5):1261–1269
69. Deane AM, Chapman MJ, Fraser RJ, Burgstad CM, Besanko LK, Horowitz M (2009) The effect of exogenous glucagon-like peptide-1 on the glycaemic response to small intestinal nutrient in the critically ill: a randomised double-blind placebo-controlled cross over study. Crit Care 13(3):R67
70. Galiatsatos P, Gibson BR, Rabiee A, Carlson O, Egan JM, Shannon RP, Andersen DK, Elahi D (2014) The glucoregulatory benefits of glucagon-like peptide-1 (7–36) amide infusion during intensive insulin therapy in critically ill surgical patients: a pilot study. Crit Care Med 42(3):638–645
71. Abuannadi M, Kosiborod M, Riggs L, House JA, Hamburg MS, Kennedy KF, Marso SP (2013) Management of hyperglycemia with the administration of intravenous exenatide to patients in the cardiac intensive care unit. Endocr Pract 19(1):81–90
72. Mecott GA, Herndon DN, Kulp GA, Brooks NC, Al-Mousawi AM, Kraft R, Rivero HG, Williams FN, Branski LK, Jeschke MG (2010) The use of exenatide in severely burned pediatric patients. Crit Care 14(4):R153
73. Meier JJ, Gallwitz B, Siepmann N, Holst JJ, Deacon CF, Schmidt WE, Nauck MA (2003) Gastric inhibitory polypeptide (GIP) dose-dependently stimulates glucagon secretion in healthy human subjects at euglycaemia. Diabetologia 46(6):798–801
74. Deacon CF, Ahren B (2011) Physiology of incretins in health and disease. Rev Diabet Stud 8(3):293–306
75. Zhou J, Livak MF, Bernier M, Muller DC, Carlson OD, Elahi D, Maudsley S, Egan JM (2007) Ubiquitination is involved in glucose-mediated downregulation of GIP receptors in islets. Am J Physiol Endocrinol Metab 293(2):E538–E547
76. Hojberg PV, Vilsboll T, Rabol R, Knop FK, Bache M, Krarup T, Holst JJ, Madsbad S (2009) Four weeks of near-normalisation of blood glucose improves the insulin response to glucagon-like peptide-1 and glucose-dependent insulinotropic polypeptide in patients with type 2 diabetes. Diabetologia 52(2):199–207
77. Layon AJ, Florete OG Jr, Day AL, Kilroy RA, James PB, McGuigan JE (1991) The effect of duodenojejunal alimentation on gastric pH and hormones in intensive care unit patients. Chest 99(3):695–702
78. Lee MY, Fraser JD, Chapman MJ, Sundararajan K, Umapathysivam MM, Summers MJ, Zaknic AV, Rayner CK, Meier JJ, Horowitz M et al (2013) The effect of exogenous glucose-dependent insulinotropic polypeptide in combination with glucagon-like peptide-1 on glycemia in the critically ill. Diabetes Care 36(10):3333–3336

79. Kar P, Cousins CE, Annink CE, Jones KL, Chapman MJ, Meier JJ, Nauck MA, Horowitz M, Deane AM (2015) Effects of glucose-dependent insulinotropic polypeptide on gastric emptying, glycaemia and insulinaemia during critical illness: a prospective, double blind, randomised, crossover study. Crit Care 19(1):20
80. Kar P, Jones KL, Horowitz M, Chapman MJ, Deane AM (2015) Measurement of gastric emptying in the critically ill. Clin Nutr 34(4):557–564
81. Dube PE, Brubaker PL (2007) Frontiers in glucagon-like peptide-2: multiple actions, multiple mediators. Am J Physiol Endocrinol Metab 293(2):E460–E465
82. Wallis K, Walters JR, Forbes A (2007) Review article: glucagon-like peptide 2--current applications and future directions. Aliment Pharmacol Ther 25(4):365–372
83. Estall JL, Drucker DJ (2006) Glucagon-like Peptide-2. Annu Rev Nutr 26:391–411
84. Scott RB, Kirk D, MacNaughton WK, Meddings JB (1998) GLP-2 augments the adaptive response to massive intestinal resection in rat. Am J Physiol 275(5 Pt 1):G911–G921
85. Boushey RP, Yusta B, Drucker DJ (1999) Glucagon-like peptide 2 decreases mortality and reduces the severity of indomethacin-induced murine enteritis. Am J Physiol 277(5 Pt 1): E937–E947
86. Kouris GJ, Liu Q, Rossi H, Djuricin G, Gattuso P, Nathan C, Weinstein RA, Prinz RA (2001) The effect of glucagon-like peptide 2 on intestinal permeability and bacterial translocation in acute necrotizing pancreatitis. Am J Surg 181(6):571–575
87. Prasad R, Alavi K, Schwartz MZ (2000) Glucagonlike peptide-2 analogue enhances intestinal mucosal mass after ischemia and reperfusion. J Pediatr Surg 35(2):357–359
88. Cameron HL, Perdue MH (2005) Stress impairs murine intestinal barrier function: improvement by glucagon-like peptide-2. J Pharmacol Exp Ther 314(1):214–220
89. Wilhelm SM, Lipari M, Kulik JK, Kale-Pradhan PB (2014) Teduglutide for the treatment of short bowel syndrome. Ann Pharmacother 48(9):1209–1213
90. Hernandez G, Velasco N, Wainstein C, Castillo L, Bugedo G, Maiz A, Lopez F, Guzman S, Vargas C (1999) Gut mucosal atrophy after a short enteral fasting period in critically ill patients. J Crit Care 14(2):73–77
91. Deitch EA (1990) The role of intestinal barrier failure and bacterial translocation in the development of systemic infection and multiple organ failure. Arch Surg 125(3):403–404
92. Adrian TE, Ferri GL, Bacarese-Hamilton AJ, Fuessl HS, Polak JM, Bloom SR (1985) Human distribution and release of a putative new gut hormone, peptide YY. Gastroenterology 89(5):1070–1077
93. Lin HC, Chey WY, Zhao X (2000) Release of distal gut peptide YY (PYY) by fat in proximal gut depends on CCK. Peptides 21(10):1561–1563
94. Batterham RL, Cohen MA, Ellis SM, Le Roux CW, Withers DJ, Frost GS, Ghatei MA, Bloom SR (2003) Inhibition of food intake in obese subjects by peptide YY3-36. N Engl J Med 349(10):941–948
95. Nematy M, O'Flynn JE, Wandrag L, Brynes AE, Brett SJ, Patterson M, Ghatei MA, Bloom SR, Frost GS (2006) Changes in appetite related gut hormones in intensive care unit patients: a pilot cohort study. Crit Care 10(1):R10
96. Nguyen NQ, Fraser RJ, Bryant LK, Chapman MJ, Wishart J, Holloway RH, Butler R, Horowitz M (2007) The relationship between gastric emptying, plasma cholecystokinin, and peptide YY in critically ill patients. Crit Care 11(6):R132

Chapter 14
Adipokines in Critical Illness

Katherine Robinson, John Prins, and Bala Venkatesh

14.1 Adipose Tissue: Definition

Adipose tissue in human can be divided into two main categories, being white adipose tissue and brown adipose tissue. White adipose tissue (WAT) is located in the subcutis (subcutaneous) and in intra-abdominal locations in association with the viscera (visceral). WAT functions as a storage facility, sequestering energy in the form of triglyceride, which is found in the cytoplasmic, unilocular lipid droplet within mature adipocytes. Accumulation or mobilisation of these fat stores occurs in the face of varying energy requirements.

Brown adipose tissue (BAT) is responsible for 'non-shivering' thermogenesis, which is the production of heat from glucose and fat. In human infants, the interscapular, neck, axillae, mediastinal, para-aortic and perirenal regions are depots for BAT [1]. In adult humans, brown adipocytes are found in the cervical-supraclavicular region in the ventral neck and may also extend inferiorly along the thoracic and abdominal paraspinal region [2]. Sympathetic nerve stimulation of these adipocytes results in uncoupled oxidative phosphorylation within their abundant mitochondria to generate heat. In contrast to WAT, the triglyceride in these cells is stored in numerous small cytoplasmic droplets, enabling rapid mobilisation of fuel for heat production [3].

K. Robinson, MBBS • J. Prins, MD, PhD, FRACP • B. Venkatesh, MD, FCICM (✉)
Intensive Care Unit, Wesley Hospital,
University of Queensland, St Lucia, QLD, Australia
e-mail: katherine.robinson2@uqconnect.edu.au; john.prins@mater.uq.edu.au; bmvenkat@bigpond.net.au

J.-C. Preiser (ed.), *The Stress Response of Critical Illness: Metabolic and Hormonal Aspects*, DOI 10.1007/978-3-319-27687-8_14

14.2 White Adipose Tissue

Adipose tissue has functions more complex and far reaching than its role in fat storage. In addition to mature adipocytes, WAT contains stromal vascular cells. This stromal component consists of adipocyte precursors (preadipocytes), fibroblasts, endothelial cells and immune cells, including macrophages and lymphocytes. Both the adipocyte and stromal fractions of WAT have secretory functions.

Healthy adipose tissue, when unchallenged by excess nutrition and a positive energy balance, contains macrophages which are of M2 morphology, or ‘alternately activated’. These secrete interleukin-10 (IL-10), which is an insulin-sensitising cytokine.

The difference between subcutaneous and visceral deposits may extend beyond anatomical location. It is the visceral adiposity which correlates more strongly with obesity-associated disease [4]. Reduction of subcutaneous fat mass via liposuction does not improve the metabolic profile of patients; however, bariatric surgery that includes visceral fat reduction does produce improvements in glucose metabolism [4].

Thus, in addition to storage, the secretory function of WAT enables it to have significant impact on metabolism, circadian body clocks, energy homeostasis and inflammation. As the fat mass expands, the inflammatory consequences become significant.

The observation of the inflammatory changes that occur in the presence of excessive fat stores has helped define adipose tissue as a key regulator of immunity and inflammation and an endocrine organ in its own right.

14.3 Adipose Tissue: Chronic Inflammation

Adipose tissue is the connection between metabolism, energy regulation and inflammation. The visceral compartment of white adipose tissue is believed to be most related to alterations of metabolic health. Visceral adipose tissue contains significant numbers of resident leucocytes, including T and B lymphocytes, regulatory T cells (Tregs), natural killer T cells, eosinophils, mast cells and macrophages. Whether it be during times of starvation and illness, when mobilisation of fat stores is required to meet increased intrinsic energy needs or when chronic overfeeding resulting excessive fat storage, signalling between the resident leucocytes and adipocytes is a vital component of the metabolic and inflammatory processes which occur within adipose tissue [5].

Expansion of adipose tissue in the obese state results in WAT inflammation. This inflammation that develops in the growing fat stores is likely to be multifactorial in aetiology. Contributing factors are postulated to be lipotoxicity, endoplasmic reticulum stress, local tissue hypoxia and Toll-like receptor activation [5]. The ‘stressed’ and now insulin-resistant adipocytes secrete proinflammatory mediators such as TNF-α, monocyte chemoattractant protein (MCP) and fatty acids. These proinflammatory substances result in the activation of resident leucocytes, increased local inflammation and an increased macrophage population with an influx of ‘classically’

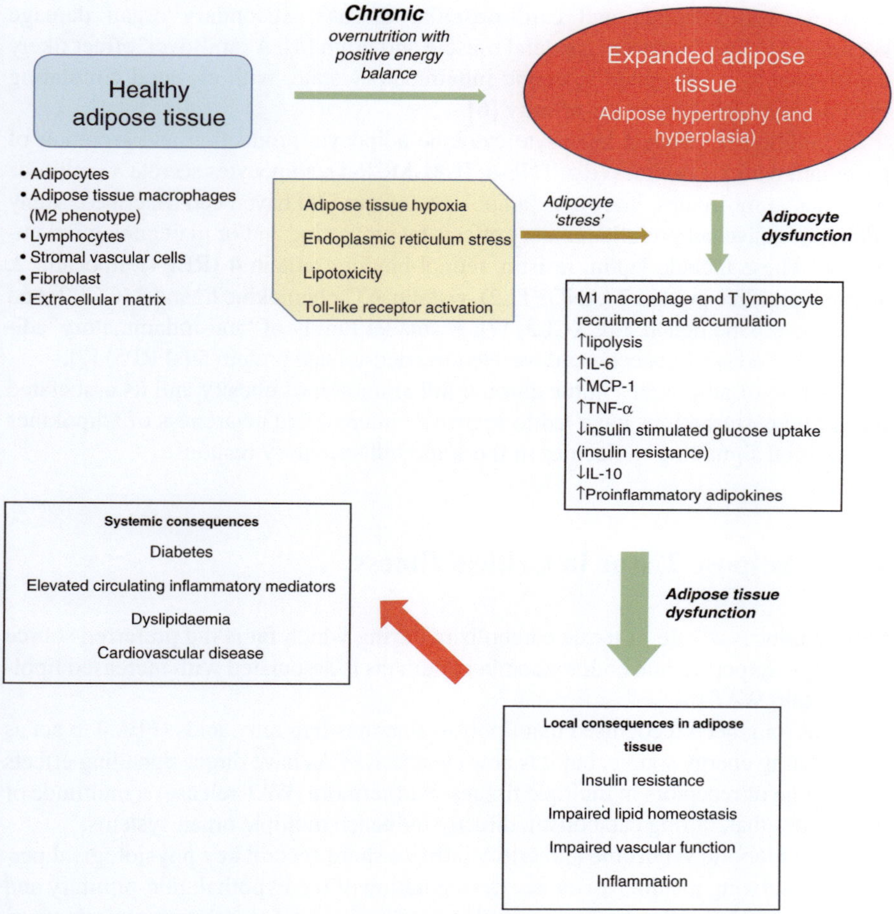

Fig. 14.1 The consequences of an expanding fat mass. As the result of a prolonged positive energy balance, there is an expansion of fat mass, with both adipocyte hypertrophy and hyperplasia. It is the increase in cell volume seen in adipocyte hypertrophy that is most strongly associated with adipocyte dysfunction. This hypertrophy places adipocytes under 'stress' and subsequent activation of signalling pathways, which results in the transformation and accumulation of inflammatory cells in adipose tissue and the subsequent release of proinflammatory cytokines and adipokines with local insulin resistance. Development of the 'metabolic syndrome' – a systemic manifestation of adipose tissue dysfunction – ensues, characterised by obesity, insulin resistance, dyslipidaemia and hypertension

activated or 'M1' macrophages into adipose tissue and transformation of resident M2 macrophages to the M1 phenotype. M1 macrophages produce proinflammatory cytokines TNF-α and IL-6. This then feeds back upon local adipocytes and a cycle of adipose tissue dysfunction and inflammation is established (see Fig. 14.1).

As these hypertrophic, dysfunctional adipocytes produce a local milieu of insulin resistance, impaired lipid handling and inflammation, the consequence becomes systemic metabolic dysregulation, manifest as systemic insulin resistance, type 2 diabetes, dyslipidaemia and cardiovascular disease. Secondary organ damage occurs in the liver, pancreas, skeletal muscle and brain [4]. A 'spillover' effect likely contributes to a low-grade systemic inflammatory state, with elevated circulating inflammatory markers in the obesity [6].

In addition to resident leucocyte cytokine adipocyte production and secretion of proinflammatory cytokines (e.g. TNF-α, IL-6, MCP-1), adipocytes secrete a multitude of bioactive molecules, known as 'adipokines'. Over 600 have been described. Many adipokines have net proinflammatory effects by promoting and/or maintaining inflammation. These include leptin, resistin, retinol-binding protein 4 (RBP4), lipocalin 2, angiopoietin-like protein 2 (ANGPTL2), visfatin, CC-chemokine ligand 2 (CCL2) and CXC-chemokine ligand 5 (CXCL5) [7]. A smaller family of 'anti-inflammatory' adipokines includes adiponectin and secreted frizzled-related protein 5 (sFRP5) [7].

The role of adipokines in the chronic inflammation of obesity and its associated metabolic perturbations have led to increased interest and awareness of adipokines as potential signalling molecules in the acute inflammatory response.

14.4 Adipose Tissue in Critical Illness

Sepsis induces a state of tissue catabolism, during which fat is the preferred source of energy. Experimental endotoxaemia in humans is associated with increased lipolysis within WAT [8].

It has long been recognised that lipolysis liberates free fatty acids (FFAs) to act as a circulating energy source, but it is now clear that FFAs have direct signalling effects via a range of receptors in multiple tissues. Furthermore, WAT releases a multitude of adipokines that, during catabolism, directly influence multiple organ systems.

The metabolic syndrome and critical illness share several key physiological perturbations, being insulin resistance, dysregulation of the hypothalamic-pituitary and gonadal axes and inflammation as evidenced by increased circulating proinflammatory cytokines [9]. How this includes adipokine dysregulation is the subject of ongoing research.

There is a huge amount of literature reporting on the multitude of adipokines and acute inflammation. Adipokines described here are those whose potential role in sepsis is most clearly defined at this point.

14.5 The Adipokines

14.5.1 Leptin

Leptin is a peptide hormone synthesized and secreted mostly by adipocytes of WAT. Circulating leptin is positively associated with body fat mass and can be considered a reflection of adipose tissue mass.

Encoded in humans by the obese (ob) gene on chromosome 7, leptin is an adipokine belonging to the type I cytokine family, which includes growth hormone and prolactin [10].

Low leptin levels signal starvation. Leptin acts via central and peripheral mechanisms to regulate food intake, appetite, glucose metabolism and energy expenditure. It acts upon the leptin receptor within the hypothalamus to regulate appetite and body weight. During fasting, insulin and then leptin levels decline, which stimulate appetite and feeding. In the fed state, insulin and leptin levels increase, promoting decreased appetite and food intake and increased energy expenditure [10].

In addition to the central nervous system, leptin receptors are widely expressed in peripheral locations, including the pancreas, liver, adipose tissue and various immune cell types (neutrophils, monocytes, macrophages, lymphocytes, mast cells, dendritic cells and NK cells) [11]. Leptin levels act as a signal to the brain regarding the status of available energy for various biological pathways, including those of the reproductive and immune systems.

Alterations in circulating leptin levels contribute to the immune dysfunction that is a feature of both obesity and malnutrition. Interest in a role for leptin in inflammation was in part due to the observation that it may interact with CRP [12].

Leptin acts to promote, maintain and regulate the immune response. Leptin regulates both innate and adaptive immunities. It induces cytokine secretion by inflammatory cells, stimulates macrophage activation and phagocytosis, acts as a chemoattractant and inhibits immune cell apoptosis. Its anti-apoptotic actions on T lymphocytes maintain the thymic parenchyma and it regulates T-cell function [13].

Leptin induces the expression of acute phase proteins such as lipocalin-2, tissue plasminogen activator (tPA) and fibrinogen β [14].

Acute inflammatory states are associated with elevated leptin levels. Leptin stimulates the release of proinflammatory cytokines such as TNF-α and IL-6, which in turn stimulate the release of leptin from adipocytes, thus establishing a proinflammatory cycle.

Animal studies suggest that leptin controls body temperature and duration and extent of the immune response in sepsis [15]. Interestingly, it may be that the elevated levels of leptin seen in the class 1 obese state (BMI 30–34.9) improve the cellular immune response and contribute to improved outcomes [15]. Exogenous leptin treatment has been reported to attenuate the development of acute lung injury in mice [16].

How this translates into the clinical setting of human sepsis remains unclear, so too, is the usefulness of serum leptin concentration as a marker of inflammation or disease severity in sepsis.

Alterations in circulating leptin concentrations in critical illness have not been conclusively defined. Increased leptin levels have been reported in sepsis and may correlate with proinflammatory markers and illness severity and be useful in distinguishing between systemic inflammatory response syndrome (SIRS) and sepsis [17, 18]. Serum leptin levels have been reported to be as effective as a diagnostic marker for sepsis as traditional biomarkers such as CRP, procalcitonin and body temperature [17]. However, not all studies of septic patients have shown significant alterations in serum leptin concentrations [19].

14.5.2 Visfatin/NAMPT/PBEF

Visfatin (the term used in this review) also known as nicotinamide phosphoribosyltransferase (NAMPT) or pre-B-cell colony-enhancing factor (PBEF) is a protein ubiquitously expressed in almost all human tissues. It is, however, highly expressed by adipocytes of visceral WAT.

The major function of intracellular NAMPT is as a biosynthetic enzyme in the pathway responsible for the generation of nicotinamide adenine dinucleotide (NAD). NAMPT generates nicotinamide mononucleotide (NMN) from nicotinamide. NMN is then converted to NAD [20].

NAD is a critical coenzyme which is utilised in cellular redox reactions and as an enzyme substrate.

By the regulation of the cellular pool of NAD, NAMPT is able to influence NAD-dependent enzymes, many of which are involved in mediation of the inflammatory response, cellular metabolism and circadian rhythms [21].

NAMPT was termed 'visfatin' following the observation that it was secreted by visceral fat [22]. Initially believed to be an insulin-mimicking adipokine, further research suggests that visfatin's role in insulin-signalling pathways is far more complex [20].

It is not yet clear if NAMPT has predominantly proinflammatory or anti-inflammatory actions. The expression of NAMPT in adipocytes is upregulated by exposure to proinflammatory cytokines, and NAMPT exposure stimulates the production of proinflammatory cytokines in adipocytes, suggesting a positive feedback loop. It is secreted from neutrophils and macrophages in response to inflammatory stimuli and may act to prolong neutrophil survival by inhibition of apoptosis [23].

There is much interest in the potential role of PBEF in the development of acute lung injury and ventilator-induced lung injury. Increased PBEF expression in inflammatory lung injury is associated with mechanical stretch, proinflammatory cytokine production and inflammatory cell recruitment in the lung [24]. Its proinflammatory actions are mediated in part by activation of pathways involving Toll-like receptors (TLRs) and NF-κB [25], which are involved in innate immune responses.

Increased levels of PBEF in bronchoalveolar fluid, serum and lung tissues from animal and human, acute lung injury (ALI) models [26] suggest it may be used as a biomarker for acute lung injury. In sepsis, elevated levels of circulating visfatin (PBEF) are associated with scores of illness severity [27, 28] and mortality in ventilated patients [28]. Visfatin levels have been shown to be increased in patients admitted to hospital with community-acquired pneumonia, with levels correlating with mortality and scores of illness severity [29].

14.5.3 Lipocalin 2

Lipocalin 2 (LPN2, neutrophil gelatinase-associated lipocalin, siderocalin, uterocalin, p25, 24p3) is an adipokine produced and secreted by both adipocytes and macrophages. It is a 198 amino acid, secreted glycoprotein. Originally isolated from neutrophil granules, LPN2 is a member of the lipocalin family of carrier/transporter proteins. These are small, soluble proteins which are characterised by a unique structure known as the 'lipocalin fold'. This is a cup-shaped fold in the protein to which a ligand binds. Amino acid variations within the fold impart ligand specificity. Lipocalins associate with and act as carriers for various lipophilic or hydrophobic substances such as steroids, bilins and retinoids [30].

Lipocalin 2 is also expressed by a number of sources of adult human tissue including the kidney, liver, trachea, lungs, small intestine, breast and salivary glands [31].

Lipocalin 2 has bacteriostatic functions, mediated through its ability to bind to bacterial siderophores and transport them into mammalian cells. Siderophores are iron-chelating compounds secreted by iron-utilising bacteria into the extracellular environment with the purpose of iron scavenging. Siderophores have a greater affinity for iron than our endogenous chelators (transferrin, ferritin and lactoferrin). Lipocalin 2 is able to bind to siderophores in both their iron-free and iron-laden states and, via the lipocalin 2 receptor, transport the siderophore into mammalian cells. By depriving the bacteria of iron, they are unable to proliferate [31].

In addition to its bacteriostatic functions, LPN2 may act as a chemoattractant for neutrophils, have antioxidant properties and play a key role in the splenic immune response [31].

Increased circulating and urinary LPN2 is a feature of acute and chronic renal impairment.

The precise mechanism underlying this elevation is unknown, but LPN2 is produced along several segments of the nephron in response to stressors such as ischaemia and toxins. Also, as glomerular filtration fails, less LPN2 may be filtered from the blood to the urine. Alternatively, filtered LPN2 may not be reabsorbed by damaged tubules, contributing to elevated urinary levels [31]. Regardless of the mechanism, an elevation in circulating LPN2 is considered a reliable indicator of acute kidney injury and precedes any derangement of plasma creatinine levels [32].

Given the prevalence of acute kidney injury in sepsis, the quantification of LPN2 levels as an indication of impending or developing renal dysfunction may prove to be a useful tool.

There may also be a role for lipocalin 2 as an acute phase protein and biomarker for acute inflammation. However, the wide range of potential tissue sources of LPN2 makes the interpretation of an elevated level in the presence of more than one pathological process challenging.

Mouse studies show that exposure to TNF-α, IL-1β and IL-6 induces LCN2 production in adipocytes, as does prolonged exposure to noradrenaline under fasting conditions [33]. LCN2 attenuates the proinflammatory effects of TNF-α on adipocytes by reducing TNF-α-induced IL-6 and MCP-1 production by adipocytes and is able to reverse the TNF-α-induced suppression of adiponectin and leptin production by adipocytes [34].

Human studies of critical illness show circulating LCN2 levels are significantly elevated during acute peritonitis [35] and severe acute pancreatitis [36].

LCN2 gene expression as measured in whole blood increases in patients with sepsis-related acute respiratory distress syndrome (ARDS) and correlates with

LCN2 plasma levels [37]. Sepsis is associated with higher urinary LCN2 levels [38] and strongly correlates with elevated plasma LCN2 levels, independent of renal dysfunction [39]. It may also be a useful biomarker to distinguish between bacterial sepsis and SIRS [39].

An elevated LCN2 level may confer prognostic significance as an independent predictor of mortality and multiorgan dysfunction in severe sepsis [40].

14.5.4 Adiponectin

Adiponectin, a hormone with structural homology to complement C1q, is secreted almost exclusively from adipocytes. Adiponectin is an insulin-sensitising, proinflammatory and cardioprotective hormone and reduced circulating levels are a marker of metabolic syndrome [41]. Lower levels of adiponectin are observed in obesity and diabetes [42]. The circulating adiponectin fraction comprises several isoforms – high molecular weight (HMW), medium molecular weight (MMW) and low molecular weight (LMW). The HMW fraction is reported to confer the metabolic benefits of adiponectin [43]. The circulating levels of adiponectin vary significantly over a day in both health [44] and in a critical illness [45], and a daily temporal rhythm may exist [46] .

The biological effects of adiponectin are mediated via its association with receptors on a wide variety of target cells.

The two main transmembrane cell receptors for adiponectin are AdipoR1 and AdipoR2. These two receptors are ubiquitous in their distribution. AdipoR1 is most abundantly expressed in the skeletal muscle and AdipoR2 in the liver [47, 48]. However, these receptors are also present in pancreatic beta cells [49], inflammatory cells [50], cardiac tissues [51] and white adipose tissue [52]. Both receptors are expressed widely throughout the central nervous system by neurons within the cortex, hypothalamus, pituitary gland, brainstem and hippocampus [53]. Studies of sections of the human brain show adiponectin localised within the anterior pituitary gland, with AdipoR1 and R2 receptor localisation in the pars distalis. In addition, strong staining for AdipoR1 was identified in neurons of the lateral hypothalamic area and the nucleus basalis of Meynert, which are important central regulators of feeding and energy expenditure [54]. This central expression of adiponectin receptors is of particular interest when considering the role of adiponectin and inflammation.

T-cadherin is also a possible third receptor, or binding protein, for adiponectin. The association between adiponectin and T-cadherin is reported to confer the cardioprotective effects of the hormone [55].

The immune regulatory functions of adiponectin involve multiple pathways [41].

Adiponectin and TNF-α share an opposing physiological relationship, characterised by a cycle of 'negative feedback' [41]. There is an inverse relationship between the expression and secretion of adiponectin and proinflammatory TNF-α by adipocytes and stromal macrophages within adipose tissue, with a negative association between circulating adiponectin and TNF-α levels.

Adiponectin has anti-inflammatory actions mediated partly via its interaction with NF-κB-signalling pathways. Adiponectin inhibits the activity of NF-kB. Treatment with adiponectin of lipopolysaccharidase (LPS)-treated adipocytes downregulates the activated NF-kB pathway and reduces IL-6 release [56]. Adiponectin treatment of macrophages was found to decrease LPS-stimulated TNF-a production [57]. However, short-term exposure of macrophages to globular adiponectin activated NF-KB, producing in a rapid increase in TNF-a, which resulted in IL-10 release, with the eventual result being the 'desensitisation' of macrophages to LPS exposure [57]. Therefore, the attenuation of the inflammatory response by adiponectin may involve complex interplay between short-term and longer term effects.

Adiponectin has direct actions on inflammatory cells. As mentioned above, adiponectin is able to influence signalling pathways of macrophages, with the net effect being downregulation of their inflammatory response. Adiponectin receptors are present on monocytes, T and B lymphocytes and on NK cells [58] and may effect neutrophil migration [59].

Actions of adiponectin within the central nervous system may contribute to its modulation of inflammatory pathways.

The central regulation and response to systemic inflammation occurs via neuronal and humoral pathways. The neural pathway involves communication between visceral sensory afferent fibres of the vagus nerve, the solitary tract nucleus (STN) of the medulla and the hypothalamus. The humoral pathway involves the circumventricular organs (CVOs). The eight circumventricular organs act as communication points between the blood, CSF and brain. These structures lack a blood-brain barrier, rather, demonstrating distinct histological features, with fenestrated capillaries, looser glial cell apposition and larger perivascular spaces [60]. Sensory circumventricular organs – the subfornical organ (SFO), organum vasculosum of the lamina terminalis (OVLT) and the area postrema (AP) – are vital structures in the regulation of metabolic, endocrine and autonomic functions. They have connections with the hypothalamus, autonomic regulatory systems and the dorsal vagal complex. The interaction of circulating inflammatory mediators with Toll-like receptors on macrophage-like cells within the CVOs results in the activation of endothelial cells and microglial cells within the CVOs, which subsequently produce proinflammatory cytokines, including TNF-α and prostaglandin E_2 (PGE_2). Stress activation of the hypothalamic-pituitary axis (HPA) involves inflammatory mediator activation of CVOs, the rostral ventrolateral medulla (RVLM) and the STN, with subsequent release of corticotropin-releasing hormone (CRH) from paraventricular neurons of the hypothalamus [60].

Adiponectin receptors are expressed in circumventricular organs (CVOs) within the brain. Neurons of both the area postrema (AP) and the subfornical organ (SFO) of rats are responsive to adiponectin [61, 62]. Food deprivation alters the neural response of the SFO to adiponectin [62] and exposure of the AP to adiponectin results in cardiovascular changes [61].

Animal models have shown upregulation of AdipoR2 in the hypothalamus following LPS-induced sepsis [63].

Both AdipoR1 and AdipoR2 are expressed in the cells of the STN of rats and adiponectin affects the electrical activity of neurons within the STN [64]. Introduction of adiponectin into the STN has been observed to reduce systemic blood pressure [64].

The role of adiponectin in the acute inflammatory process of sepsis has not been clearly defined.

The observations that adiponectin antagonised the inflammatory effects of TNF-α negatively correlated with plasma TNF-α levels and showed structural homology to complement factor C1q, leading researchers to further investigate the relationship between adiponectin and lipopolysaccharidase (LPS). Adiponectin was found to directly bind LPS and suppress limulus amoebocyte lysate (LAL) in vitro [65]. In rats with induced polymicrobial sepsis, plasma adiponectin levels have been shown to negatively correlate with plasma endotoxin and TNF-α levels [65].

Studies in human subjects are inconclusive. Lower levels of adiponectin have been found in critically ill patients [66–68]. Additionally, Venkatesh et al. described a strong association between plasma cortisol and adiponectin, an inverse correlation between plasma CRP and adiponectin, as well as a linear response between sickness severity and plasma adiponectin [67]. A study of patients following aneurysmal subarachnoid haemorrhage showed lower levels of adiponectin on days 3 and 7 of their admission when compared to controls. Also, those who developed delayed cerebral ischaemia (DCI) due to vasospasm as evidenced by a clinical deterioration or a new cerebral infarct on imaging had significantly lower adiponectin levels during their admission when compared to those who did not develop DCI [69].

No significant changes in circulating adiponectin levels have been observed in studies of induced endotoxaemia in human subjects [70, 71].

In addition, higher levels of adiponectin in critical illness have been associated with increased risk of mortality [72, 73].

14.5.5 Resistin

Resistin is a protein first identified in the circulation of mice in 2001 and associated with insulin resistance in this species. Similarly to adiponectin, resistin circulates in a number of higher-order multimers which may confer different levels of biological activity. However, mouse resistin differs from the human form in two very significant ways. Firstly, there is significant disparity between the genomic organisation and composition of the different species. Secondly, the primary site of production in the mouse is the adipocyte. In humans, the circulating resistin fraction is primarily derived from peripheral blood mononuclear cells, macrophages and the bone marrow [74]. Differences in structure and function between the species add additional complexity to the understanding of the biological role of resistin.

In humans, resistin likely targets a wide range of tissues, including human myeloid cells, monocytes, epithelial cells and endothelial cells, and may include hypothalamic regulation of inflammation. Resistin's mechanism of action involves

Table 14.1 Adipokines in critical illness

Adipokine	Function
Leptin	Proinflammatory Increased in acute inflammation and sepsis Regulates immunity Controls body temperature in inflammatory states Stimulates proinflammatory cytokine release Induces expression acute phase proteins Direct actions on inflammatory cells
Visfatin (NAMPT, PBEF)	Regulation of inflammation Maintains and supports inflammatory response Anti-apoptotic actions on neutrophils Proinflammatory Potential role in development of acute lung injury
Lipocalin 2 (LPN2, neutrophil gelatinase-associated lipocalin, siderocalin, uterocalin, p25, 24p3)	Bacteriostatic functions Chemoattractant for neutrophils Antioxidant properties Role in splenic immunity Elevated in acute and chronic renal impairment Elevated in sepsis Attenuates the proinflammatory effects of TNF-α on adipocytes
Adiponectin	Anti-inflammatory actions Negative relationship with TNF-α Downregulation of NF-κB pathways Direct actions on inflammatory cells. Actions on central pathways of the inflammatory response
Resistin	Modulation of proinflammatory-signalling pathways Elevated in critical illness

the modulation of proinflammatory-signalling pathways (including NF-kB and MAPK), which then mediate the expression of proinflammatory genes of IL-6, TNF-alpha and MCP-1.

Elevated levels of resistin have been observed in patients with non-septic critical illness [75], sepsis and septic shock [76], with correlation between resistin levels and proinflammatory cytokines [75, 76]. However, it remains unclear whether there exists a relationship between resistin levels and disease severity and/or prognosis (Table 14.1).

14.6 Summary

The therapeutic manipulation of circulating biomarkers, including adipokines, for clinical benefit in sepsis remains the ultimate end goal. The functional role and the prognostic significance of adipokine fluctuations in critical illness remain largely undefined. Also, peculiarities and complexities of the molecular structures and circulating forms create additional challenges. For example, there are no current strategies for the therapeutic administration of adiponectin, with its complex structure and very high circulating concentrations making supplementation impractical.

Leptin is the single adipokine approved for therapeutic administration in a clinical setting. This adipokine is administered for therapeutic purposes in rare patients with leptin deficiency associated with lipodystrophy. In the context of critical illness, the administration of leptin may augment immune cell function and optimise central responses to systemic inflammation and infection. There may be a potential, practical use for leptin in the intensive care setting.

As our understanding of adipokines increases, the modulation of these diverse signalling proteins to improve patient outcomes in critical illness may become possible.

References

1. Aherne W, Hull D (1966) Brown adipose tissue and heat production in the newborn infant. J Pathol Bacteriol 91(1):223–234
2. Cypess AM, Lehman S, Williams G et al (2009) Identification and importance of brown adipose tissue in adult humans. N Engl J Med 360(15):1509–1517
3. Smorlesi A, Frontini A, Giordano A, Cinti S (2012) The adipose organ: white-brown adipocyte plasticity and metabolic inflammation. Obes Rev 13(Suppl 2):83–96
4. Kloting N, Bluher M (2014) Adipocyte dysfunction, inflammation and metabolic syndrome. Rev Endocr Metab Disord 15(4):277–287
5. Exley MA, Hand L, O'Shea D, Lynch L (2014) Interplay between the immune system and adipose tissue in obesity. J Endocrinol 223(2):R41–R48
6. Park HS, Park JY, Yu R (2005) Relationship of obesity and visceral adiposity with serum concentrations of CRP, TNF-α and IL-6. Diabetes Res Clin Pract 69(1):29–35
7. Ouchi N, Parker JL, Lugus JJ, Walsh K (2011) Adipokines in inflammation and metabolic disease. Nat Rev Immunol 11(2):85–97
8. Wellhoener P, Vietheer A, Sayk F, Schaaf B, Lehnert H, Dodt C (2011) Metabolic alterations in adipose tissue during the early phase of experimental endotoxemia in humans. Horm Metab Res 43(11):754–759
9. Robinson K, Kruger P, Prins J, Venkatesh B (2011) The metabolic syndrome in critically ill patients. Best Pract Res Clin Endocrinol Metab 25(5):835–845
10. Otero M, Lago R, Lago F et al (2005) Leptin, from fat to inflammation: old questions and new insights. FEBS Lett 579(2):295–301
11. Gheorghita V, Barbu AE, Gheorghiu ML, Caruntu FA (2015) Endocrine dysfunction in sepsis: a beneficial or deleterious host response? Germs 5(1):17–25
12. Chen KK (2006) Induction of leptin resistance through direct interaction of C-reactive protein with leptin. Nat Med 12(4):425–432
13. Paz-Filho G, Mastronardi C, Franco CB, Wang KB, Wong ML, Licinio J (2012) Leptin: molecular mechanisms, systemic pro-inflammatory effects, and clinical implications. Arq Bras Endocrinol Metabol 56(9):597–607
14. Hekerman P, Zeidler J, Korfmacher S et al (2007) Leptin induces inflammation-related genes in RINm5F insulinoma cells. BMC Mol Biol 8:41
15. Siegl D, Annecke T, Johnson BL 3rd et al (2014) Obesity-induced hyperleptinemia improves survival and immune response in a murine model of sepsis. Anesthesiology 121(1):98–114
16. Landgraf MA, Silva RC, Correa-Costa M et al (2014) Leptin downregulates LPS-induced lung injury: role of corticosterone and insulin. Cell Physiol Biochem 33(3):835–846

17. Chen M, Wang B, Xu Y et al (2014) Diagnostic value of serum leptin and a promising novel diagnostic model for sepsis. Exp Ther Med 7(4):881–886
18. Yousef AA, Amr YM, Suliman GA (2010) The diagnostic value of serum leptin monitoring and its correlation with tumor necrosis factor-alpha in critically ill patients: a prospective observational study. Crit Care 14(2):R33
19. Koch A, Weiskirchen R, Zimmermann HW, Sanson E, Trautwein C, Tacke F. Relevance of serum leptin and leptin-receptor concentrations in critically ill patients. Mediators Inflamm. 2010;2010. doi:10.1155/2010/473540
20. Garten A, Petzold S, Schuster S, Korner A, Kratzsch J, Kiess W (2011) Nampt and its potential role in inflammation and type 2 diabetes. Handb Exp Pharmacol 203:147–164
21. Garten A, Schuster S, Penke M, Gorski T, de Giorgis T, Kiess W (2015) Physiological and pathophysiological roles of NAMPT and NAD metabolism. Nat Rev Endocrinol 11(9): 535–546
22. Fukuhara A, Matsuda M, Nishizawa M et al (2005) Visfatin: a protein secreted by visceral fat that mimics the effects of insulin. Science 307(5708):426–430
23. Jia SH, Li Y, Parodo J et al (2004) Pre-B cell colony-enhancing factor inhibits neutrophil apoptosis in experimental inflammation and clinical sepsis. J Clin Invest 113(9):1318–1327
24. Hong SB, Huang Y, Moreno-Vinasco L et al (2008) Essential role of pre-B-cell colony enhancing factor in ventilator-induced lung injury. Am J Respir Crit Care Med 178(6): 605–617
25. Camp SM, Ceco E, Evenoski CL et al (2015) Unique toll-like receptor 4 activation by NAMPT/PBEF induces NFkappaB signaling and inflammatory lung injury. Sci Rep 5:13135
26. Ye SQ, Simon BA, Maloney JP et al (2005) Pre-B-cell colony-enhancing factor as a potential novel biomarker in acute lung injury. Am J Respir Crit Care Med 171(4):361–370
27. Lee KA, Gong MN (2011) Pre-B-cell colony-enhancing factor and its clinical correlates with acute lung injury and sepsis. Chest 140(2):382–390
28. Lee K, Huh JW, Lim CM, Koh Y, Hong SB (2013) Clinical role of serum pre-B cell colony-enhancing factor in ventilated patients with sepsis and acute respiratory distress syndrome. Scand J Infect Dis 45(10):760–765
29. Hu W, Liu CW, Su J, Lu J, Zhu Y, Liu BW (2013) Elevated plasma visfatin concentrations in patients with community-acquired pneumonia. Peptides 43:8–12
30. Ferreira AC, Da Mesquita S, Sousa JC et al (2015) From the periphery to the brain: Lipocalin-2, a friend or foe? Prog Neurobiol 131:120–136
31. Chakraborty S, Kaur S, Guha S, Batra SK (2012) The multifaceted roles of neutrophil gelatinase associated lipocalin (NGAL) in inflammation and cancer. Biochim Biophys Acta 1826(1):129–169
32. Martensson J, Bell M, Oldner A, Xu S, Venge P, Martling CR (2010) Neutrophil gelatinase-associated lipocalin in adult septic patients with and without acute kidney injury. Intensive Care Med 36(8):1333–1340
33. Zhang Y, Foncea R, Deis JA, Guo H, Bernlohr DA, Chen X (2014) Lipocalin 2 expression and secretion is highly regulated by metabolic stress, cytokines, and nutrients in adipocytes. PLoS One 9(5):e96997
34. Zhang J, Wu Y, Zhang Y, Leroith D, Bernlohr DA, Chen X (2008) The role of lipocalin 2 in the regulation of inflammation in adipocytes and macrophages. Mol Endocrinol 22(6):1416–1426
35. Axelsson L, Bergenfeldt M, Ohlsson K (1995) Studies of the release and turnover of a human neutrophil lipocalin. Scand J Clin Lab Invest 55(7):577–588
36. Chakraborty S, Kaur S, Muddana V et al (2010) Elevated serum neutrophil gelatinase-associated lipocalin is an early predictor of severity and outcome in acute pancreatitis. Am J Gastroenterol 105(9):2050–2059
37. Kangelaris KN, Prakash A, Liu KD et al (2015) Increased expression of neutrophil-related genes in patients with early sepsis-induced ARDS. Am J Physiol Lung Cell Mol Physiol 308(11):L1102–L1113
38. Bell M, Larsson A, Venge P, Bellomo R, Martensson J (2015) Assessment of cell-cycle arrest biomarkers to predict early and delayed acute kidney injury. Dis Markers 2015:158658

39. Martensson J, Bell M, Xu S et al (2013) Association of plasma neutrophil gelatinase-associated lipocalin (NGAL) with sepsis and acute kidney dysfunction. Biomarkers Biochem Indicators Expo Response Susceptibility Chem 18(4):349–356
40. Wang B, Chen G, Zhang J, Xue J, Cao Y, Wu Y (2015) Increased NGAL is associated with mortality and multiple organ dysfunction syndrome in severe sepsis and septic shock. Shock 44:234–238
41. Robinson K, Prins J, Venkatesh B (2011) Clinical review: adiponectin biology and its role in inflammation and critical illness. Crit Care 15(2):221
42. Comuzzie AG, Funahashi T, Sonnenberg G et al (2001) The genetic basis of plasma variation in adiponectin, a global endophenotype for obesity and the metabolic syndrome. J Clin Endocrinol Metab 86(9):4321–4325
43. Seino Y, Hirose H, Saito I, Itoh H (2007) High molecular weight multimer form of adiponectin as a useful marker to evaluate insulin resistance and metabolic syndrome in Japanese men. Metabolism 56(11):1493–1499
44. Scheer FA, Chan JL, Fargnoli J et al (2010) Day/night variations of high-molecular-weight adiponectin and lipocalin-2 in healthy men studied under fed and fasted conditions. Diabetologia 53(11):2401–2405
45. Robinson K, Jones M, Ordonez J et al (2013) Random measurements of adiponectin and IL-6 may not be indicative of the 24-h profile in critically ill patients. Clin Endocrinol (Oxf) 79(6):892–898
46. Gavrila A, Peng C-K, Chan JL, Mietus JE, Goldberger AL, Mantzoros CS (2003) Diurnal and ultradian dynamics of serum adiponectin in healthy men: comparison with leptin, circulating soluble leptin receptor, and cortisol patterns. J Clin Endocrinol Metab 88(6): 2838–2843
47. Yamauchi T, Nio Y, Maki T et al (2007) Targeted disruption of AdipoR1 and AdipoR2 causes abrogation of adiponectin binding and metabolic actions. Nat Med 13(3):332–339
48. Yamauchi T, Kamon J, Ito Y et al (2003) Cloning of adiponectin receptors that mediate antidiabetic metabolic effects. Nature 423(6941):762–769
49. Kharroubi I, Rasschaert J, Eizirik DL, Cnop M (2003) Expression of adiponectin receptors in pancreatic beta cells. Biochem Biophys Res Commun 312(4):1118–1122
50. Chinetti G, Zawadski C, Fruchart JC, Staels B (2004) Expression of adiponectin receptors in human macrophages and regulation by agonists of the nuclear receptors PPARalpha, PPARgamma, and LXR. Biochem Biophys Res Commun 314(1):151–158
51. Ding G, Qin Q, He N et al (2007) Adiponectin and its receptors are expressed in adult ventricular cardiomyocytes and upregulated by activation of peroxisome proliferator-activated receptor gamma. J Mol Cell Cardiol 43(1):73–84
52. Nannipieri M, Bonotti A, Anselmino M et al (2007) Pattern of expression of adiponectin receptors in human adipose tissue depots and its relation to the metabolic state. Int J Obes 31(12):1843–1848
53. Thundyil J, Pavlovski D, Sobey CG, Arumugam TV (2012) Adiponectin receptor signalling in the brain. Br J Pharmacol 165(2):313–327
54. Psilopanagioti A, Papadaki H, Kranioti EF, Alexandrides TK, Varakis JN (2009) Expression of adiponectin and adiponectin receptors in human pituitary gland and brain. Neuroendocrinology 89(1):38–47
55. Parker-Duffen JL, Walsh K (2014) Cardiometabolic effects of adiponectin. Best Pract Res Clin Endocrinol Metab 28(1):81–91
56. Lira FS, Rosa JC, Pimentel GD et al (2012) Both adiponectin and interleukin-10 inhibit LPS-induced activation of the NF-kappaB pathway in 3T3-L1 adipocytes. Cytokine 57(1):98–106
57. Park PH, McMullen MR, Huang H, Thakur V, Nagy LE (2007) Short-term treatment of RAW264.7 macrophages with adiponectin increases tumor necrosis factor-alpha (TNF-alpha) expression via ERK1/2 activation and Egr-1 expression: role of TNF-alpha in adiponectin-stimulated interleukin-10 production. J Biol Chem 282(30):21695–21703
58. Pang TT, Narendran P (2008) The distribution of adiponectin receptors on human peripheral blood mononuclear cells. Ann N Y Acad Sci 1150:143–145

59. Lang K, Ratke J (2009) Leptin and Adiponectin: new players in the field of tumor cell and leukocyte migration. Cell Commun Signal 7:27
60. Siso S, Jeffrey M, Gonzalez L (2010) Sensory circumventricular organs in health and disease. Acta Neuropathol 120(6):689–705
61. Fry M, Smith PM, Hoyda TD et al (2006) Area postrema neurons are modulated by the adipocyte hormone adiponectin. J Neurosci 26(38):9695–9702
62. Alim I, Fry WM, Walsh MH, Ferguson AV (2010) Actions of adiponectin on the excitability of subfornical organ neurons are altered by food deprivation. Brain Res 1330:72–82
63. Iwasa T, Matsuzaki T, Matsui S et al (2014) The effects of LPS-induced endotoxemia on the expression of adiponectin and its receptors in female rats. Endocr J 61(9):891–900
64. Hoyda TD, Smith PM, Ferguson AV (2009) Adiponectin acts in the nucleus of the solitary tract to decrease blood pressure by modulating the excitability of neuropeptide Y neurons. Brain Res 1256:76–84
65. Tsuchihashi H, Yamamoto H, Maeda K et al (2006) Circulating concentrations of adiponectin, an endogenous lipopolysaccharide neutralizing protein, decrease in rats with polymicrobial sepsis. J Surg Res 134(2):348–353
66. Jernas M, Olsson B, Sjoholm K et al (2009) Changes in adipose tissue gene expression and plasma levels of adipokines and acute-phase proteins in patients with critical illness. Metabolism 58(1):102–108
67. Venkatesh B, Hickman I, Nisbet J, Cohen J, Prins J (2009) Changes in serum adiponectin concentrations in critical illness: a preliminary investigation. Crit Care 13(4):R105
68. Langouche L, Vander Perre S, Frystyk J, Flyvbjerg A, Hansen TK, Van den Berghe G (2009) Adiponectin, retinol-binding protein 4, and leptin in protracted critical illness of pulmonary origin. Crit Care 13(4):R112
69. Takeuchi S, Wada K, Otani N, Osada H, Nagatani K, Mori K (2014) Temporal profile of plasma adiponectin level and delayed cerebral ischemia in patients with subarachnoid hemorrhage. J Clin Neurosci 21(6):1007–1010
70. Keller P, Moller K, Krabbe KS, Pedersen BK (2003) Circulating adiponectin levels during human endotoxaemia. Clin Exp Immunol 134(1):107–110
71. Anderson PD, Mehta NN, Wolfe ML et al (2007) Innate immunity modulates adipokines in humans. J Clin Endocrinol Metab 92(6):2272–2279
72. Kaplan JM, Denenberg A, Monaco M, Nowell M, Wong H, Zingarelli B (2010) Changes in peroxisome proliferator-activated receptor-gamma activity in children with septic shock. Intensive Care Med 36(1):123–130
73. Walkey AJ, Rice TW, Konter J et al (2010) Plasma adiponectin and mortality in critically ill subjects with acute respiratory failure. Crit Care Med 38(12):2329–2334
74. Codoner-Franch P, Alonso-Iglesias E (2015) Resistin: insulin resistance to malignancy. Clin Chim Acta 438:46–54
75. Koch A, Gressner OA, Sanson E, Tacke F, Trautwein C (2009) Serum resistin levels in critically ill patients are associated with inflammation, organ dysfunction and metabolism and may predict survival of non-septic patients. Crit Care 13(3):R95
76. Sunden-Cullberg J, Nystrom T, Lee ML et al (2007) Pronounced elevation of resistin correlates with severity of disease in severe sepsis and septic shock. Crit Care Med 35(6):1536–1542

Part III
Particular Clinical Situations

Chapter 15
Severe Undernutrition

Pierre Singer and Jonathan Cohen

Abstract Undernutrition in critically ill patients appears to be common, being encountered both at the time of admission and developing during the ICU stay. While many definition criteria for this state are available, loss of muscle mass and strength seem to be the most relevant signs. During the ICU stay, the main reason for undernutrition is underfeeding, a frequent occurrence in ICU practice, together with bed rest. Negative energy and nitrogen balance may result in an increase in morbidity and a prolonged rehabilitation period. While nutritional support is essential for these patients, it is important not to induce the refeeding syndrome. Enteral feeding is the preferred route for providing nutritional support but is not always achievable, usually the result of prolonged feeding interruptions. The calorie target should be reached progressively using the gastrointestinal route or the parenteral route if necessary. Indirect calorimetry remains the best guide for appropriately prescribing nutritional support. Protein administration should follow current guidelines. Careful monitoring of electrolytes (mainly phosphorus, magnesium, and potassium) is mandatory. Nutritional support is of extreme importance not only to provide enough nutrients in a deficiency condition but also to prevent prolonged rehabilitation periods for survivors.

P. Singer, MD (✉)
Intensive Care Department, Rabin Medical Center,
Jabotinsky Street 39, Petah Tikva 49100, Israel

Department of Intensive Care, Institute for Nutrition Research, Rabin Medical Center, Sackler School of Medicine, Tel Aviv University, Petah Tikva, Israel
e-mail: psinger@clalit.org.il

J. Cohen, MD
Department of Intensive Care, Institute for Nutrition Research, Rabin Medical Center, Sackeler School of Medicine, Tel Aviv University, Petah Tikva, Israel

J.-C. Preiser (ed.), *The Stress Response of Critical Illness: Metabolic and Hormonal Aspects*, DOI 10.1007/978-3-319-27687-8_15

15.1 Introduction

Malnutrition among hospitalized patients has been recognized as a major health problem, reaching 30–54 % of all patients [1]. The recent ESPEN definition of malnutrition focused on weight loss and a decrease in lean body mass assessed by measurement of the free fat mass index [2]. However, of more concern than the body mass index, which might be normal in malnutrition, is the loss of lean body mass. The definition describes various categories of undernutrition, including starvation-related underweight, cachexia/disease-related malnutrition, frailty, and sarcopenia [2]. In addition, obesity sarcopenia may also be described as malnutrition, and the larger the loss of weight and the decrease in muscle mass, the more severe the undernutrition. In the intensive care unit (ICU), most patients are recognized during screening as suffering from or at risk of malnutrition, according to the screening tool Nutrition Risk Score 2002 (NRS 2002) [3]. In addition, the concept of frailty in the intensive care has been suggested [4]. Whereas frailty has been strongly correlated with age and disability status as well as the burden of comorbid disease [5], among critically ill patients, decrease in muscle mass, strength and endurance, as well as mobility makes these patients very analogous to the typically frail, geriatric patient. The purpose of this chapter is to define undernutrition and its nutritional profile, evaluate its prevalence in the ICU setting, and suggest a nutritional plan, which also takes into account the problem of refeeding, in this very high-risk population.

15.2 Definitions

Most of the tools described below have been validated in the intensive care setting (Table 15.1). The *Subjective Global Assessment* (SGA) is a well-known tool that includes patient history and physical examination [6]. In an attempt to validate SGA, others have shown a correlation with percentage of weight loss, BMI, ICU stay, and APACHE II score [7]. Sheean et al. compared SGA to the mini-nutritional assessment (*MNA*), NRS 2002, as well as MNA short form (MNA-SF) [8]. SGA and MNA-SF had the highest specificity, while NRS 2002 had the highest sensitivity. According to *the new ESPEN definition*, patients suffering from

Table 15.1 Diagnosis of undernutrition based on nutritional parameters

	SGA	MNA-SF	ESPEN diagnosis	Sarcopenia	Frailty
Weight loss <10 %	+	+	+		
Muscle loss	+		+	+	
Edema	+				
Calf circumference	+	+			
BMI <18.5		+	+		
Muscle function		+		+	+
Clinical frailty score					+

malnutrition include those with a BMI <18.5 kg/m^2 or suffering from an unintentional weight loss >10 % irrespective of time or >5 % over the last 3 months combined with either a BMI <20 if <70 years of age or <22 if >70 years of age or an FFMI <15 and 17 kg/m^2 in women and men, respectively [2]. Validation of this score in the ICU is pending. An additional score, the *Clinical Frailty Score* [9], ranging from 1 (very fit) to 7 (very frail), has been validated in the ICU and is useful mainly in elderly patients [10]. *Sarcopenia* has been defined as a decrease in muscle loss and/or function and is frequent in undernourished patients admitted to the ICU [11]. Muscle mass may also be assessed by various tools such as *handgrip dynamometer* [12] if the patient is conscious, being an especially good prognostic factor in conscious ARDS patients [13]. *Bioelectrical impedance* can be used to assess body composition and mainly lean body mass in a stabile patient not suffering from fluid compartment shifts [14]. However, its use is limited. Finally, recently *CT scan* has been used in the ICU to assess lean body mass and may be a promising tool for patients undergoing abdominal CT [15].

Length of stay and immobility increase catabolism in critically ill patients [16]. In addition, patients are frequently underfed. Thus the nutrition day survey in the ICU revealed that >40 % of patients had not received nutrition on the first hospital day and >20 % remained without nutrition on day 2 [17]. Enteral feeding was prescribed to only 10 % of the patients on the first day but this number increased to more than 40 % after 5 days. Parenteral nutrition was prescribed to around 10 % of the patients and supplemental parenteral nutrition was ordered after 3–5 days in only 15 % of the population studied. Total energy intake appeared to be randomly assigned and ranged from no intake up to 4000 kcals/day. Interestingly, the longer the patients stayed in the ICU, the more calories they received. The mean caloric intake was 1409 kcal/day and many patients failed to reach their caloric target, mainly as assessed by predictive required energy equations.

15.3 Prevalence

Exclusively chronic starvation-related malnutrition is extremely rare. Most patients with undernutrition have an acute disease associated with a small or a large subset of comorbidities. According to Bector et al., the prevalence of malnutrition on the intensive care assessed by SGA was 35 % [6]. Mortality was increased in the moderate (45.5 %) and severely malnourished (55.6 %) groups when compared to the well-nourished (10.8 %) group ($p=0.04$). Another study found a prevalence rate of 40 % in 161 trauma patients according to SGA, and length of stay was found to be related to SGA [18]. Albumin and prealbumin levels are not useful for the diagnosis of undernutrition. Nutrition day data [17] from 9137 patients revealed that the mean BMI was 26.6 ± 6.4 kg/m^2. Heyland et al., in a study of the prevalence of iatrogenic underfeeding in nutritionally at-risk critically ill patients, found that enteral feeding was commenced 39 h in mean after admission and 74 % failed to meet the target of at least 80 % of the energy requirements [19].

15.4 Nutritional Profile

Patients suffering from severely malnutrition are characterized by significant decrease in weight before admission, loss of lean body mass as well as fat mass, and impaired immune function. These alterations in body composition and function are often associated with numerous comorbidities such as renal failure, history of cancer, past surgical history, as well as pulmonary, liver, and cardiac diseases which may further complicate the metabolic profile. Elderly patients are the most vulnerable but the definition of frailty is not limited to admission demographics. This nutritional profile may also be acquired during the ICU stay as a consequence of immobilization, inadequate nutritional supplementation, and the use of neuromuscular blockade and steroids [20].

Stress combined with undernutrition is associated with a negative energy balance and loss of lean body mass. This condition leads to worsening of clinical outcomes, increased complications such as infections and new organ failures, as well as prolonged mechanical ventilation and ICU stay. Positive nitrogen balance, adequacy of caloric administration, upper extremity strength assessed by handgrip dynamometer, and self-reported assessment may be good prognostic factors for this category of patient. On the other hand, albumin and prealbumin are not very useful in the nutritional assessment, since they are the reflect of capillary leakage.

Indirect calorimetry is extremely useful in the evaluation of energy requirements of these complex patients who may also be at risk for overfeeding. De Waele et al. [21] screened 266 ICU patients and found that 86.5 % were at risk of malnutrition. Indirect calorimetry which was assessed in 118 revealed that the measured energy expenditure was 1649 ± 544 kcal/day, which poorly correlated with predictive equations. In 210 malnourished hospitalized patients aged ≥75 years suffering from weight loss of >4 kg in the preceding month, measured resting energy expenditure (REE) was found to be as low as 1473 ± 311 kcal/day, with a fat-free mass of 47.6 ± 8 kg. The study also found that predictive equations were found to have only 40 % accuracy compared to REE [22]. Since predictive equations have such a poor accuracy, there is a risk of both over- and underfeeding which may increase complication rates [23]. Patients with both high-calorie intake and deficient in protein were found less likely to be discharged in 213 surgical ICU patients, confirming that inadequate macronutrient delivery is associated with worse clinical outcomes after critical illness [24].

15.5 Nutritional Needs and Therapy: Risk of Refeeding

After repeated stress and inadequate oral intake, the undernourished patient requires nutritional support which should be provided as early as possible via the digestive tract. The absence of enteral stimulation may negatively affect the gut microbiota, the enteric nervous system, as well as the gut epithelium and gut-associated lymphoid tissue [25]. These systems often interact with each other although the

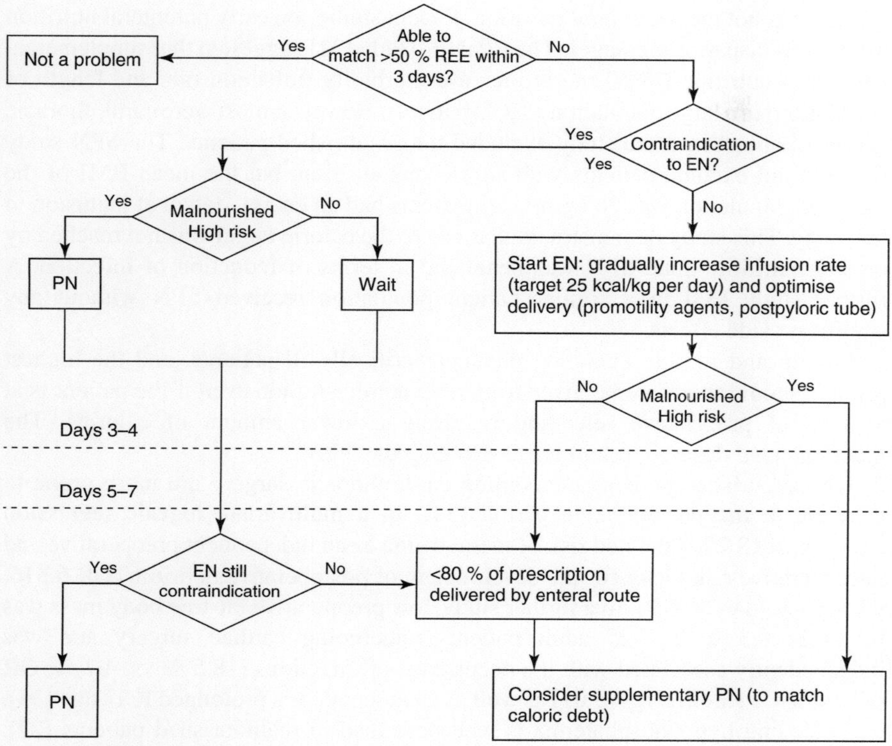

Fig. 15.1 Diagram proposed to optimize nutritional support in malnourished patients. From Weimann and Singer [30]. Proposed framework for starting parenteral nutrition in severely ill patients. *REE* resting energy expenditure, *EN* enteral nutrition, *PN* parenteral nutrition

mechanisms involved are still not fully understood. Early enteral feeding has been demonstrated to decrease infectious complications and may also improve survival [26]. However, early feeding may result in the refeeding syndrome, which is important to avoid [27]. When nutritional therapy is started, intracellular demands for phosphate and potassium are increased due to enhanced glycolysis and Na/K-ATPase pump stimulation. In practice, phosphate and potassium delivery should increase from 15–30 to 30–60 mmol PO_4/day and from 80–120 to 120–200 mmol KCL/day. In many cases, intolerance to enteral feeding is encountered which may be manifested by large gastric residual volumes, intestinal ileus, diarrhea, and abdominal pain [28]. Because of the large energy deficit existing in many patients, some guidelines recommend starting parenteral nutrition early in order to reach nutritional targets as soon as possible [29], while others advise commencing on days 7–10 [26]. An approach (see Fig. 15.1) to determine when to start parenteral nutrition has recently been proposed [30]. In malnourished patients, targeting calorie needs according to indirect calorimetry is preferred if available. If necessary, supplemental or total parenteral nutrition should be prescribed at an early stage if the target is not met by enteral nutrition. Recent studies on early parenteral nutrition have given disparate messages. The EPaNIC study [31] suggested that supplemental parenteral nutrition (SPN) might increase morbidity (infection rate and length of ventilation) in a large population of ICU patients. However, most were cardiothoracic surgical patients and the study excluded undernourished patients. The SPN study [32] did not exclude patients with severe malnutrition, but the mean BMI of the included population was 26 kg/m^2. All patients had an energy deficit at inclusion to the study. This study demonstrated that where the calorie target was not reached by enteral nutrition alone SPN was beneficial in terms of reduction of infection. A further study [33] in a similar patient population received SPN without any significant side effects.

Protein and muscle depletion endanger critically ill patients, and the highest priority should therefore be given to protein administration even if the patient is at a stage of progressive refeeding requiring a lower amount of calories. The recommended dose of protein is 1.2–1.5 g/kg/day [29].

Undernourished patients undergoing cardiothoracic surgery are more prone to delirium in the postoperative period [34]. In a multivariate logistic regression analysis, NRS 2002 defined risk of malnutrition as an independent preoperative and intraoperative risk factor for the development of postoperative delirium (OR 6.316, 95 % CI 1.384–28.819). In a further study, low preoperative fat-free body mass was found in 8.3 % of 325 adult patients undergoing cardiac surgery and was independently associated with the occurrence of infections (18.5 % vs. 4.7 %, OR 6.9, 95 % CI 1.8–27.7, $p=0.01$) as well as a tendency for a prolonged ICU stay [35].

Refeeding hypophosphatemia is well described in malnourished patients [27]. Thus patients with a high NRS score before commencing nutrition support are more at risk of refeeding hypophosphatemia [27]. In particular, patients receiving a continuous parenteral nutrition regimen providing >70 % of the required calorie requirements containing <12 mmol phosphate are at an increased risk of hypophosphatemia [36]. In addition, we found [37] that severe hypophosphatemia was present in 34.3 % of 566 consecutive patients after major cardiac surgery and was associated with prolonged ventilation, increased requirements for cardioactive drugs, and a prolonged hospital stay.

Protein wasting and loss of body weight are associated with immobility and acute illness [16]. Early mobilization should therefore be encouraged. Maintenance of correct posture and passive mobilization of the legs are important. Muscle strength and endurance performance can be improved using cycle ergometry [38]. In addition, a mobilization algorithm comprising waking of the patient, positioning on the bed, sitting on the edge of the bed, transfer to the chair, the use of orthostatic and walking techniques, and finally the implementation of assisted exercises and exercises with resistance and use of the ergometer bicycle on the bed has been described [39]. An elegant demonstration of the importance of muscle mass was shown in a study including a population of 338 mainly cachexic liver transplantation candidates who underwent pre-transplant computed tomography to identify muscle and fat mass [40]. Muscle mass but not fat mass predicted ICU and hospital length of stay, as well as length of ventilation. Muscle mass also predicted survival and disposition to home versus another facility, demonstrating the fundamental importance of this component.

Patients suffering from acute kidney injury represent another patient population where protein-energy wasting is common and is a major negative prognostic factor. Insulin resistance and the release of pro-inflammatory mediators lead to lean body mass wasting and fat mass depletion. In this condition too, targeted calorie intake together with a protein intake of 1.7–2.0 g/kg BW/day in the case of severe catabolism or continuous renal replacement therapy is recommended [41]. Aging has a positive influence on nitrogen accretion in renal failure showing that with each increase in nitrogen intake, there was an increase in nitrogen balance [42].

The paradigm of correcting nutritional deficit using enteral or mainly parenteral nutrition has been recently challenged by Puthacheary et al. who reported that increased protein delivery during the first week in the ICU was associated with more pronounced muscle wasting [43]. Early parenteral nutrition increased the incidence of weakness and decreased recovery potential [44]. However, the 600 patients included in the study were from a study which excluded malnourished patients [31].

15.6 Conclusions

Undernutrition in critically ill patients appears to be common, being encountered both at the time of admission and mainly developing during the ICU stay. Weight loss related to muscle deficiency and decrease in strength are associated with increased morbidity. Numerous tools are available to assess muscle loss and may also be used to assess the response to nutritional therapy. Indirect calorimetry should ideally be used to plan appropriate energy administration. Adequate protein intake is an important goal and should reach 1.2–1.5 g/kg/day. Promising research is being performed to explore the use of physiotherapy together with a high-protein regimen to counteract the anabolic resistance often encountered in the undernourished bedridden patient.

References

1. Norman K, Pichard C, Lochs H, Pirlich M (2007) Prognostic impact of disease related malnutrition. Clin Nutr 27:5–15
2. Cederholm T, Bosaeus I, Barazzoni R et al (2015) Diagnostic criteria for malnutrition- an ESPEN consensus statement. Clin Nutr 34:335–340
3. Kondrup J, Rasmussen HH, Hamberg O, Stanga Z (2003) Nutritional risk screening (NRS 2002); a new method based on analysis of controlled clinical trials. Clin Nutr 22:321–336
4. McDermid RC, Stelfox HT, Bagshaw SM (2011) Frailty in the critically ill: a novel concept. Crit Care 15:301
5. Fried LP, Tangen CM, Walston J et al (2001) Frailty in older adults: evidence for a phenotype. J Gerontol A Biol Sci Med Sci 56:M146–M156

6. Bector S, Vagianos K, Suh M, Duerksen DR (2015) Does the subjective global assessment predict outcome in critically ill medical patients? J Intensive Care. Epud ahead of print.
7. Sungurtekin H, Sungurtekin U, Oner O, Okke D (2008) Nutrition assessment in critically ill patients. Nutr Clin Pract 23:635–641
8. Sheean PM, Peterson SJ, Chen Y, Liu D, Lateef O, Brauschweig CA (2013) Utilizing multiple methods to classify malnutrition among elderly patients admitted to the medical and surgical intensive care units (ICU). Clin Nutr 32:752–757
9. Roclwood K, Song X, MacKnight C, Bergman H, Hogan DB, McDowell I, Mitniski A (2005) A global clinical measure for fitness and frailty in elderly people. CMAJ 173:489–495
10. The Support Principal Investigators (1995) A controlled trial to improve care for seriously ill hospitalized patients. The study to understand prognoses and preferences for outcomes and risks of treatments (SUPPORT). JAMA 274:1591–1598
11. Studenski SA, Peters KW, Alley DE et al (2014) The FNIH sarcopenia project: rationale, study description, conference recommendations and final estimates. J Gerontol A Biol Sci Med Sci 69:547–558
12. Lad UP, Satyanarayana P, Shisode-Lad S, Siri CC, Kumari NR (2013) A study of the correlation between the body mass index, the body fat percentage, the handgrip strength and the handgrip endurance in underweight, normal weight and overweight adolescents. J Clin Diagn Res 7:51–54
13. Fan E, Ciesla ND, Truong AD, Bhoopathi V, Zeger SL, Needham DM (2010) Inter-rater reliability of manual muscle strength testing in ICU survivors and simulated patients. Intesive Care Med 36:1038–1043
14. Savalle M, Gillaizeau F, Maruani G et al (2012) Assessment of body cell mass at bedside in critically ill patients. Am J Physiol Endocrinol Metab 303:E389–E396
15. Braunschweig CA, Sheean PM, Peterson SJ et al (2014) Exploitation of diagnostic computed tomography scans to assess the impact of nutrition support on body composition changes in respiratory failure patients. JPEN J Parenter Enteral Nutr 38:880–885
16. Biolo G (2013) Protein metabolism and requirements. In: Singer P (ed) Nutrition in intensive care: beyond physiology, vol 105, World Review of Nutrition and Dietetics. Karger, Basel, pp 12–20
17. Bedavid I, Singer P, Theilla M, Hiesmayr M, et al. Nutrition day in the Intensive Care: a prevalence study. Submitted Clin Nutr
18. Goiburu ME, Goiburu MM, Bianco H et al (2006) The impact of malnutrition on morbidity, mortality and length of stay in trauma patients. Nutr Hosp 21:604–610
19. Heyland DK, Dhaliwal R, Wang M, Day AG (2015) The prevalence of iatrogenic underfeeding on the nutritionally "at risk" critically ill patient: Results of an international, multicenter, prospective study. Clin Nutr 34:659–666
20. Griffiths RD, Hall JB (2010) Intensive care unit-acquired weakness. Crit Care Med 14:186
21. De Waele E, Spapen H, Honore PM, Mattens S, van Gorp V, Filtoer M, Huygens L (2013) Introducing a new generation indirect calorimeter for estimating energy requirements in adult intensive care patients: feasibility, practical considerations and comparison with a mathematical equation. J Crit Care 28:884
22. Neelemaat F. Van Bokhorst MAE, Thijs A, Seidell JC, Weijs PJM (2012) Resting energy expenditure in malnourished older patients at hospital admission and after three months after discharge; predictive equations versus measurements. Clin Nutr 31:958–966
23. Singer P, Hiesmayr M, Biolo G, Felbinger TW, Berger MM, Goeters C, Kondrup J, Wunder C, Pichard C (2014) Pragmatic approach to nutrition in the ICU: expert opinion regarding which calorie protein target. Clin Nutr 33:246–251
24. Yeh DD, Fuentes E, Quraishi SA et al (2016) Adequate nutrition may get you home: effect of caloric/protein deficits on the discharge destination of critically ill surgical patients. JPEN J Parenter Enteral Nutr 40:37–44
25. Genton L, Cani PD, Schrenzel J (2015) Alterations of gut barrier and gut microbiota in food restriction, food deprivation and protein-energy wasting. Clin Nutr 34:341–349
26. Martindale RG, Warren M (2015) Should enteral nutrition be started in the first week of critical illness? Curr Opin Clin Nutr Metab Care 18:202–206

27. Hiesmayr M (2012) Nutrition risk assessment in the ICU. Curr Opin Clin Nutr Metab Care 15:174–180
28. Reintam Blaser A, Poeze M, Malbrain ML, Bjork M, Oudemans-van Straaten HM, Starkopf J (2013) Gastrointestinal symptoms during the first week of intensive care are associated with poor outcome: a prospective multicenter study. Intensive Care Med 39:899–909
29. Singer P, Berger MM, van den Berghe G et al (2006) ESPEN guidelines on parenteral nutrition: intensive care. Clin Nutr 28:387–400
30. Weimann A, Singer P (2013) Avoiding underfeeding in severely ill patients. Lancet 381:1811
31. Casaer MP, Mesotten D, Hermans G, Wouters PJ, Schetz M, Meyfroidt G, Van Cromphaut S, Ingels C, Meersseman P, Muller J, Vlasselaers D, Debaveye Y, Desmet L, Dubois J, Van Assche A, Vanderheyden S, Wilmer A, Van den Berghe G (2011) Early versus late parenteral nutrition in critically ill adults. N Engl J Med 365:506–517
32. Heidegger CP, Berger MM, Graf S, Zingg W, Darmon P, Costanza MC, Thibault R, Pichard C (2012) Optimization of energy provision with supplemental parenteral nutrition (SPN) improves the clinical outcome of critically ill patients: a randomized controlled clinical trial. Lancet 381:385–393
33. Doig GS, Simpson F, Sweetman EA, Finfer SR, Cooper DJ, Heighes PT, Davies AR, O'Leary M, Solano T, Peake S (2013) Early parenteral nutrition in critically ill patients with short-term relative contraindications to early enteral nutrition: a randomized controlled trial. JAMA 309: 2130–2138
34. Ringaitiene D, Gineityte D, Vicka V et al (2015) Impact of malnutrition on post operative delirium development after on pump coronary arterial bypass grafting. J Cardiothorac Surg 10:74
35. Van Venrooij LM, de Vos R, Zijlstra E, Borgmeijer-Hoelen MM, van Leeuwen PA, de Mol BA (2011) The impact of low preoperative fat-free body mass on infections and length of stay after cardiac surgery: a prospective cohort study. J Thorac Cardiovasc Surg 142:1263–1269
36. Marvin VA, Brown D, Portlock J, Livingstone C (2009) Factors contributing to the development of hypophosphatemia when refeeding using parenteral nutrition. Pharm World Sci 30: 329–335
37. Cohen J, Kogan A, Sahar G, Lev S, Vidne B, Singer P (2004) Hypophosphatemia following open heart surgery: incidence and consequences. Eur J Cardiothorac Surg 26:306–310
38. Nava S, Piaggi G, De Mattia E, Carlucci A (2002) Muscle retraining in the ICU patients. Minerva Anesthosiol 68:341–345
39. Koukoutikos K, Tsaloglidou A, Kourkouta L (2014) Muscle atrophy in intensive care unit patients. Acta Inform Med 22:406–410
40. DiMartini A, Cruz RJ, Dew MA, Myaskovsky L, Goodpaster B, Fox K, Him KH, Fontes P (2013) Muscle mass predicts outcomes following liver transplantation. Liver Transpl 19:1172–1180
41. Fiaccadori E, Regolisti G, Maggiore U (2013) Specialized nutritional support interventions in critically ill patients on renal replacement therapy. Curr Opin Clin Nutr Metab Care 16:217–224
42. Dickerson RN, Maish GO, Croce MA, Minard G, Brown RO (2013) Influence of aging on nitrogen accretion during critical illness. JPEN J Parenteral Enter Nutr 39:282–290
43. Puthucheary ZA, Rawal J, McPhail M, Connolly B, Ratnayake G, Chan P et al (2013) Acute skeletal muscle wasting in critical illness. JAMA 310:1591–1600
44. Hermans G, van den Berghe G (2015) Clinical review: intensive care unit acquired weakness. Crit Care 19:274

Chapter 16
The Stress Response after Traumatic Brain Injury: Metabolic and Hormonal Aspects

Hervé Quintard, Carole Ichai, and Jean-Francois Payen

Abstract The pathophysiology of TBI can be considered as a dual insult composed of primary and secondary injuries. Growing experimental and clinical evidence suggests that disturbances of cerebral energy metabolism are a key factor in the pathogenesis of secondary cerebral damages. In addition, hormonal dysfunction after TBI, such as adrenal insufficiency, vasopressin, growth hormone, or thyrothropin deficiency, can be associated with poor prognosis. A better understanding of energy metabolism and hormonal disturbances after TBI is necessary to improve the care management at the early phase of TBI.

Traumatic brain injury (TBI) is a common cause of death and disability especially for young adults with various neurological consequences ranging from simple physical disabilities to long-term cognitive, behavioural, psychological, and social defects [1]. The pathophysiology of TBI is considered as a dual insult composed of primary and secondary processes. Primary injury corresponds to anatomic tissue damage at the time of insult. This produces vulnerable cells that are further

H. Quintard
Service de Réanimation, Hôpital Pasteur 2, 30 Voie Romaine, Nice, Cedex 1 06001, France

CNRS UMR6097- Université Nice Sophia Antipolis, Nice F-06000, France

C. Ichai
Service de Réanimation, Hôpital Pasteur 2, 30 Voie Romaine, Nice, Cedex 1 06001, France

IRCAN (INSERM U1081, CNRS UMR 7284), Université Nice Sophia Antipolis, Nice F-06000, France

J.-F. Payen (✉)
Pôle Anesthésie Réanimation, Hôpital Michallon, CHU de Grenoble, Grenoble F-38043, France

Université Grenoble Alpes, Grenoble Institut des Neurosciences, Grenoble F-38042, France
e-mail: Jean-Francois.Payen@ujf-grenoble.fr

J.-C. Preiser (ed.), *The Stress Response of Critical Illness: Metabolic and Hormonal Aspects*, DOI 10.1007/978-3-319-27687-8_16

compromised by secondary brain injury. Secondary brain damage occurs at the cellular level and results from a complex biochemical cascade, including excitotoxicity, oxidative stress, inflammation, apoptosis, and mitochondrial dysfunction. Secondary brain damage is a major factor involved in the patient outcome following primary brain insult. Several systemic factors have been found to worsen secondary brain damage [2]. Growing experimental and clinical evidence suggests that disturbances of cerebral energy metabolism are a key factor in pathogenesis of this secondary cerebral damage [3, 4]. In this chapter, we discuss the consequences of TBI on metabolic and hormonal homeostasis.

16.1 Metabolic Disturbances After TBI

16.1.1 Exploration of Brain Metabolism in the ICU

Cerebral microdialysis (CMD) has largely contributed to a better understanding of the pathophysiology of acute brain dysfunction at the bedside [3]. CMD consists in the placement of an intra-parenchymal probe with a semipermeable dialysis membrane. A cerebrospinal fluid-like solution, infused through this catheter, allows hourly sampling of patients' brain extracellular fluid [4]. CMD provides monitoring of dynamic changes of main brain energy substrate (glucose, lactate, and pyruvate). High lactate/pyruvate ratio (LPR) values would reflect either a mitochondrial dysfunction or an imbalance between oxygen supply and its tissue utilisation. A LPR >40 and an extracellular glucose <0.7–1 mmol/L are usually considered as thresholds for abnormality in the clinical setting [5].

16.1.2 Metabolism of Normal Brain

Although brain represents 2 % of the body weight, the cerebral metabolic rate of glucose ($CMR_{glucose}$) accounts for 20 % of the amount of glucose utilised by the body. Brain glucose oxidation is about 4–5 μmol/kg/min. The regulation of glucose metabolism is essential for brain homeostasis in the absence of glycogen storage in the brain. The interaction among neurons, astrocytes, and endothelial cells at the interface blood-brain barrier (BBB) is essential for coupling energy supply with change in neural activity. Neurons and astrocytes are surrounded by interstitial fluid, which contains glucose and lactate, at a concentration of 1 mM. The glucose pool is replenished by blood-derived glucose, whereas lactate is interchanged between astrocytes and glial cells, and cleared by the blood at a low rate [6]. The large blood-brain concentration gradient drives the facilitative transport of glucose across the endothelial membranes via several glucose transporters, in particular glucose transporter 1 (GLUT1). This transporter is localised in astrocyte, while GLUT3 receptors, which have higher affinity and transport capacity for glucose, are localised

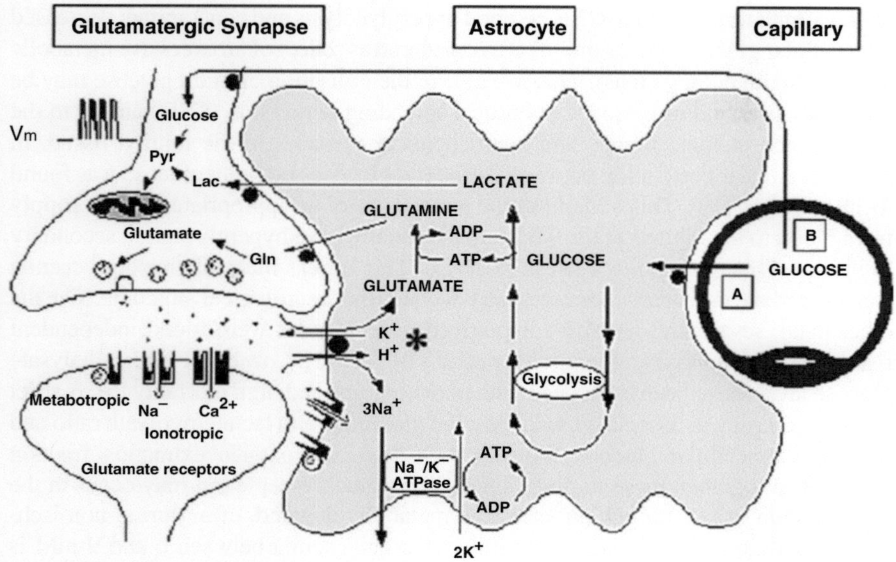

Fig. 16.1 Model for coupling of synaptic activity with glucose utilisation. *A* Glucose uptake by astrocytes in case of neuron activation, *B* direct neuron glucose uptake by resting neuron (Permission conveyed through Copyright Clearance Center, Inc. from [8])

in neurons. The expression of GLUT is regulated by circulating glucose concentration and is upregulated during hypoglycaemia. In resting conditions, blood glucose is raised and metabolised by neurons through the classical glycolytic pathway. During activation, glucose is metabolised by astrocytes, to produce lactate and glutamine. Lactate enters into neurons through the monocarboxylic acid transporter (MCT) to be metabolised by the tricarboxylic acid (TCA) cycle. Glutamine enters into neurons to produce glutamate that is released massively in the synaptic neuronal cleft. Astrocytes reuptake glutamate via a mechanism coupled with sodium reabsorption. ATP produced by glial glycolysis allows the activation of Na/K/ATPase pump to extrude the Na influx coupled to glutamate uptake. This response is illustrative of cell cooperation to metabolic situation. The lactate production is a preferential oxidative fuel when neurons are activated. This interaction between the two types of cells is called "astrocyte to neuron lactate shuttle (ANLS)" [7] (Fig. 16.1). In resting awake brain, brain glucose is mostly oxidised into CO_2 and water, leading to an oxygen/glucose ratio around 5.5–5.8.

16.1.3 Metabolism of Injured Brain

Several studies have found an increased aerobic glycolysis in the acute phase of brain injury, leading to brain lactate accumulation. This hyperglycolysis is reflected by an elevated tissue lactate to glucose ratio using CMD [9]. Because there was no evidence of concomitant reduction in CBF, cerebral hyperglycolysis and concomitant decreased extracellular glucose (<0.2 mmol/l) are considered as reflect of an excessive metabolic demand (brain energy crisis). This increase in the utilisation of brain glucose may be due to seizures and/or episodes of cortical spreading depression (CSD) and/or to the maintenance of ionic pumps and neurochemical cascades in the injured tissue. In addition, a linear correlation between peripheral glucose and brain glucose was found in TBI patients [10]. This underlines the importance of an appropriate glucose supply from blood to the injured brain. TBI patients usually have hyperglycaemia secondary to insulin resistance and to a stress response. This "stress-induced" hyperglycaemia can exacerbate ischaemic damages and worsen the neurological outcome. On the other hand, severe and repetitive hypoglycaemic episodes were found independent risk factors for mortality and morbidity after TBI [11, 12]. Low but also high dialysate glucose levels have been associated with poor outcome and high mortality [5]. A strict glucose control was associated with elevated glutamate and lactate/pyruvate ratio and reduced extracellular glucose, together with increased oxygen extraction fraction [13]. Taken together, these findings suggest that glucose depletion may occur in the injured brain tissue through an excessive metabolic demand, even during non-ischaemic conditions. Therefore, a permissive hyperglycaemia between 6 and 9 mM is recommended to avoid the aggravation of cerebral damages [13, 14].

The brain can use substrates as supplemental fuel other than glucose, e.g., ketone bodies and lactate [15]. Evidence of lactate as an alternative fuel was firstly demonstrated in vitro by limiting neuronal cell death from glucose deprivation induced by ischaemia-reperfusion model [16, 17]. Further studies showed that lactate was preferentially used of lactate by the human brain after TBI [18]. The contribution of lactate to cerebral energy metabolism was increased from 10 to 15 % up to 60 % [19]. Additionally, intracellular lactate inhibits glucose consumption in resting astrocytes in order to redistribute glucose to active areas [20]. Sparing glucose is important to maintain neurotransmission and oxidative stress response in the injured brain. In this context, exogenous lactate supplementation has been studied after trauma. A lactate transfer from blood to brain with a subsequent conversion to pyruvate with spared glucose was described in TBI patients [21]. In a cortical impact model, lactate solution was associated with elevated cerebral blood flow and reduced cortical contusion volume [22]. Besides these metabolic effects, hypertonic sodium lactate administration in severe TBI patients was more effective to lower intracranial hypertension than mannitol [23]. A preventive treatment with hypertonic sodium lactate solution was effective in reducing the number of ICP episodes [24]. Therefore, lactate solution appears as a promising option to treat energetic crisis after TBI by sparing glucose and/or by improving cerebral haemodynamics.

16.2 Hormonal Disturbances After TBI

The hypothalamic-pituitary-adrenal axis (HPA) is altered by numerous causes, particularly after TBI. The primary lesion as well as secondary systemic insults such as arterial hypotension, severe hypoxia, and high intracranial pressure can induce pituitary dysfunction. The pituitary gland is particularly vulnerable to the blood flow conditions because the anterior lobe is tightly dependent on small vessels from the Willis circle. Somatotropic and gonadotropic cells that are located in the lateral part of the anterior pituitary gland are even more exposed to reduce cerebral blood flow. Other mechanisms involved in hypopituitarism include side effects of sedative drugs used in brain-injured patients and autoimmune mechanisms triggered by TBI [25]. The first report of hypopituitarism post trauma was published in 1918. The prevalence of hypopituitarism in the chronic phase after TBI is 30 % of patients [26]. While the literature about chronic posttraumatic hypopituitarism is abundant, there is still limited data regarding the severity, incidence, and risk factors associated with hypopituitarism in the acute phase after TBI. In those studies, the prevalence of posttraumatic hypopituitarism ranged from 9 to 53 % of patients, including secondary adrenal insufficiency (AI), hypothyroidism, and/or hypogonadism [27, 28]. In many cases, hormonal disturbances have a spontaneous resolution within 6 months after TBI. Indeed, hypopituitarism during a long-term follow-up after TBI was diagnosed in 5.4 % of patients [29]. However, acute AI, central hypothyroidism, SIADH, and diabetes insipidus may cause poor neurological outcomes including death, hypo-/hypernatraemia, hypotension, and increased vasoactive drug requirements [30].

16.2.1 Adrenal Insufficiency

Among clinical conditions of AI, brain trauma is responsible for secondary (central) AI, i.e., suppression of the synthesis of corticotrophin-releasing hormone (CRH) or adrenocorticotrophic hormone (ACTH) [31]. According to the definition used, the prevalence of AI has a broad range from 10 % to more than 75 % of severe TBI patients [32, 33]. There is thus a need to define appropriately AI after TBI.

Absolute AI is considered where serum cortisol is less than 15 μg/dL, and relative AI is defined where serum cortisol cannot exceed 9 μg/dL from baseline using the ACTH test [34] In one study exploring AI in the initial phase of TBI, authors considered AI where baseline serum cortisol was less than 15 μg/dL from 2 blood samples or less than 5 μg/dL from 1 blood sample [28]. Because a normal value of serum cortisol cannot rule out AI for all critically ill patients [35], it was proposed to perform a dynamic test, i.e., the ACTH test (250 μg), to explore the capacity of adrenal glands to produce cortisol. However, due to the nature of AI after TBI, and the absence of confounding factors, a random serum cortisol is usually enough to detect AI. Random serum cortisol less than 10 μg/dL is currently recommended to diagnose AI in critically ill patients [36]. Of note was the delayed diagnosis of AI often mistaken for symptoms of head injury. In the presence of unexplained hyponatraemia and /or large requirements for vasopressors after severe TBI, a dosage of serum cortisol should be considered. It has been suggested that severity of TBI, young age, arterial hypotension, barbiturates, and/or the use of vasopressors could predispose to AI post trauma [28, 37, 38]. Another factor of AI could be the use of etomidate to facilitate tracheal intubation in these patients [28]. However, this drug-induced disturbance lasts no more than 48 h after the drug administration [39].

The normalisation of serum cortisol level might be a marker of good outcome [40]. In that context, a replacement therapy with low-dose hydrocortisone (200 mg/day) should be initiated in the presence of acute AI. However this proposal has not to be confounded with the abandon of large doses of corticosteroids at the early phase of TBI [41]. In the large Corticosteroid Randomisation after Significant Head Injury (CRASH) trial, a 48-h infusion of methylprednisolone within 8 h of TBI resulted in higher mortality rate compared with placebo group [42].

16.2.2 Vasopressin Dysfunction

The antidiuretic hormone (ADH, or arginine vasopressin) is secreted by the posterior pituitary gland to promote free water reabsorption in the kidney to concentrate urine. ADH acts on vasopressin receptors with three subtypes V1a, V1b, and V2. The water reabsorption depends on the stimulation of V2 receptors that enhances the expression of specific water channel proteins (aquaporins) on the luminal surface of the collecting duct [43]. The secretion of ADH is triggered by the increase in extracellular fluid tonicity that activates osmoreceptors in the hypothalamus. ADH can be secreted, to a lesser extent, during hypovolaemia via the activation of baroreceptors located in the right atrium and carotid sinus.

A failure of homeostatic release of ADH leads to the development of central diabetes insipidus (DI). DI manifests with loss of large volumes of dilute urine in the presence of normal or high plasma osmolality. The criteria to define DI combine urine volume >300 mL/h, urine osmolality <300 mosm/kg, and hypernatraemia >145 mmol/L. The urine specific gravity is less than 1005 (or 1008 if associated glycosuria). DI is usually transient, secondary to hypoperfusion of the posterior pituitary and/or inflammatory oedema. However DI can persist 1 year after TBI in 12 % of patients [35]. The prevalence of DI after severe TBI is around 3 % and is strongly associated with basal skull fracture. Risk factors for DI include low Glasgow coma scale, brain oedema, and severe injury [35]. The development of DI after TBI is associated with higher mortality [44]. The treatment of DI is based on fluid replacement guided by a constant clinical monitoring and a correction rate of hypernatraemia of less than 10 mmol/day. In the case of high ICP, the correction rate should be lowered to exceed no more than 5 mmol/day in order to prevent secondary brain oedema. In conscious patients with DI, intravenous (0.4 μg) or intranasal (100 μg) desmopressin (DDAVP) can be administered and repeated every 12 h. Unconscious patients are treated with fluid replacement with 2.5 % dextrose or water and concomitant DDAVP administration.

Another disturbance in the ADH secretion corresponds to the inappropriate secretion of ADH (SIADH). The diagnosis criteria of SIADH combine plasma osmolality <275 mOsm/kg, hyponatraemia <135 mmol/L and urinary osmolality >100 mOsm/kg, urine sodium >40 mmol/l, euvolemia, and absence of glucocorticoid or thyroid hormone deficiency. In the presence of hyponatraemia, the differential diagnosis with other conditions may be difficult: secondary AI is classically associated with glucose control disturbances, while the "cerebral salt wasting syndrome" (CSWS) is associated with hypovolaemia and increased serum urea. The presence of SIADH is associated with an increase in length of stay in the ICU. The natural history of SIADH spontaneously resolves after the initial insult. The key issue to manage hyponatraemia in this setting is an accurate diagnosis of the underlying cause. If SIADH is diagnosed, treatment is essentially based in a fluid restriction strategy. Although the use of selective of vasopressin-2 receptor antagonist (vaptan) could be attractive [45], this treatment has not been recommended in recent guidelines [46].

16.2.3 Growth Hormone Deficiency

Growth hormone (GH) deficiency is frequently observed after TBI with an incidence of 2–66 % [47]. Basal serum GH concentrations were increased in TBI patients. Excessive GH response to a stimulation test with GH-releasing hormone (GHRH) was found in patients with poor outcome. Patients with severe and permanent GH deficiency should be treated with hormonal substitution because GH acts on limbic structures with consequences on memory and behaviour. Some studies found benefits of supplementation by GH on motor or cognitive functions at the post-acute phase of trauma [48].

16.2.4 Thyrotropin Deficiency

The incidence of hypothyroidism after TBI varies between 0 and 19 %. A low serum-free T4 concentration (<8 pmol/L) associated with normal or low serum TSH level (<0.1 µUI/mL) is a criterion to diagnose thyrotropin deficiency. No dynamic test is required. Replacement therapy with thyroxine is mandatory, but this treatment requires to rule out CRH deficiency because cortisol clearance is increased by thyroxine. However, there is no evidence that replacement therapy at the acute phase of TBI may improve the outcome. The decrease of thyroid hormonal values was less pronounced during early enteral nutrition compared to delayed enteral nutrition [49].

16.2.5 Gonadotrophin Deficiency

The incidence of gonadal deficiency ranges from 0 to 29 % of TBI patients. A hypothalamic origin has been proposed. The deficit is associated with menstrual irregularities and/or reduced libido. Results between serum testosterone level and prognosis are conflicting. The level of prolactin is also associated with prognosis with a positive correlation [35]. A complete restoration of hormone levels was observed in 85 % of patients at 1-year post-TBI, but persistent deficiency should benefit for replacement therapy for prevention of osteoporosis and cardiovascular disease.

Traumatic brain injury induces various metabolic and hormonal stress responses that could be associated with poor outcome. A better understanding of these dysfunctions could help us in the management of brain-injured patients during the early phase of trauma.

References

1. Zaloshnja E, Miller T, Langlois JA, Selassie AW (2008) Prevalence of long-term disability from traumatic brain injury in the civilian population of the United States, 2005. J Head Trauma Rehabil 23(6):394–400
2. Jeremitsky E, Omert L, Dunham CM, Protetch J, Rodriguez A (2003) Harbingers of poor outcome the day after severe brain injury: hypothermia, hypoxia, and hypoperfusion. J Trauma 54(2):312–319
3. Hutchinson PJ, Jalloh I, Helmy A et al (2015) Consensus statement from the 2014 International Microdialysis Forum. Intensive Care Med 41(9):1517–1528
4. Hillered L, Vespa PM, Hovda DA (2005) Translational neurochemical research in acute human brain injury: the current status and potential future for cerebral microdialysis. J Neurotrauma 22(1):3–41
5. Timofeev I, Carpenter KL, Nortje J et al (2011) Cerebral extracellular chemistry and outcome following traumatic brain injury: a microdialysis study of 223 patients. Brain 134(Pt 2):484–494
6. Barros LF, Deitmer JW (2010) Glucose and lactate supply to the synapse. Brain Res Rev 63(1–2):149–159
7. Pellerin L, Magistretti PJ (2012) Sweet sixteen for ANLS. J Cereb Blood Flow Metab 32(7):1152–1166
8. Magistretti PJ (2009) Role of glutamate in neuron-glia metabolic coupling. Am J Clin Nutr 90(3):875S–880S
9. Sala N, Suys T, Zerlauth JB et al (2013) Cerebral extracellular lactate increase is predominantly nonischemic in patients with severe traumatic brain injury. J Cereb Blood Flow Metab 33(11):1815–1822
10. Magnoni S, Tedesco C, Carbonara M et al (2012) Relationship between systemic glucose and cerebral glucose is preserved in patients with severe traumatic brain injury, but glucose delivery to the brain may become limited when oxidative metabolism is impaired: implications for glycemic control. Crit Care Med 40(6):1785–1791
11. Finfer S, Chittock D, Li Y et al (2015) Intensive versus conventional glucose control in critically ill patients with traumatic brain injury: long-term follow-up of a subgroup of patients from the NICE-SUGAR study. Intensive Care Med 41(6):1037–1047
12. Kalfon P, Le Manach Y, Ichai C et al (2015) Severe and multiple hypoglycemic episodes are associated with increased risk of death in ICU patients. Crit Care 19:153
13. Vespa P, McArthur DL, Stein N et al (2012) Tight glycemic control increases metabolic distress in traumatic brain injury: a randomized controlled within-subjects trial. Crit Care Med 40(6):1923–1929
14. Meierhans R, Bechir M, Ludwig S et al (2010) Brain metabolism is significantly impaired at blood glucose below 6 mM and brain glucose below 1 mM in patients with severe traumatic brain injury. Crit Care 14(1):R 13

15. Valente-Silva P, Lemos C, Kofalvi A, Cunha RA, Jones JG (2015) Ketone bodies effectively compete with glucose for neuronal acetyl-CoA generation in rat hippocampal slices. NMR Biomed 28(9):1111–1116
16. Schurr A, Payne RS, Miller JJ, Rigor BM (1997) Brain lactate, not glucose, fuels the recovery of synaptic function from hypoxia upon reoxygenation: an in vitro study. Brain Res 744(1):105–111
17. Cater HL, Chandratheva A, Benham CD, Morrison B, Sundstrom LE (2003) Lactate and glucose as energy substrates during, and after, oxygen deprivation in rat hippocampal acute and cultured slices. J Neurochem 87(6):1381–1390
18. Gallagher CN, Carpenter KL, Grice P et al (2009) The human brain utilizes lactate via the tricarboxylic acid cycle: a 13C-labelled microdialysis and high-resolution nuclear magnetic resonance study. Brain 132(Pt 10):2839–2849
19. Boumezbeur F, Petersen KF, Cline GW et al (2010) The contribution of blood lactate to brain energy metabolism in humans measured by dynamic 13C nuclear magnetic resonance spectroscopy. J Neurosci 30(42):13983–13991
20. Sotelo-Hitschfeld T, Fernandez-Moncada I, Barros LF (2012) Acute feedback control of astrocytic glycolysis by lactate. Glia 60(4):674–680
21. Bouzat P, Sala N, Suys T et al (2014) Cerebral metabolic effects of exogenous lactate supplementation on the injured human brain. Intensive Care Med 40(3):412–421
22. Berthet C, Castillo X, Magistretti PJ, Hirt L (2012) New evidence of neuroprotection by lactate after transient focal cerebral ischaemia: extended benefit after intracerebroventricular injection and efficacy of intravenous administration. Cerebrovasc Dis 34(5–6):329–335
23. Ichai C, Armando G, Orban JC et al (2009) Sodium lactate versus mannitol in the treatment of intracranial hypertensive episodes in severe traumatic brain-injured patients. Intensive Care Med 35(3):471–479
24. Ichai C, Payen JF, Orban JC et al (2013) Half-molar sodium lactate infusion to prevent intracranial hypertensive episodes in severe traumatic brain injured patients: a randomized controlled trial. Intensive Care Med 39(8):1413–1422
25. Kelly DF, Gonzalo IT, Cohan P et al (2000) Hypopituitarism following traumatic brain injury and aneurysmal subarachnoid hemorrhage: a preliminary report. J Neurosurg 93(5):743–752
26. Schneider HJ, Schneider M, Saller B et al (2006) Prevalence of anterior pituitary insufficiency 3 and 12 months after traumatic brain injury. Eur J Endocrinol 154(2):259–265
27. Agha A, Sherlock M, Phillips J, Tormey W, Thompson CJ (2005) The natural history of post-traumatic neurohypophysial dysfunction. Eur J Endocrinol 152(3):371–377
28. Cohan P, Wang C, McArthur DL et al (2005) Acute secondary adrenal insufficiency after traumatic brain injury: a prospective study. Crit Care Med 33(10):2358–2366
29. Kokshoorn NE, Smit JW, Nieuwlaat WA et al (2011) Low prevalence of hypopituitarism after traumatic brain injury: a multicenter study. Eur J Endocrinol 165(2):225–231
30. Powner DJ, Boccalandro C, Alp MS, Vollmer DG (2006) Endocrine failure after traumatic brain injury in adults. Neurocrit Care 5(1):61–70
31. Prigent H, Maxime V, Annane D (2004) Science review: mechanisms of impaired adrenal function in sepsis and molecular actions of glucocorticoids. Crit Care 8(4):243–252
32. Koiv L, Merisalu E, Zilmer K, Tomberg T, Kaasik AE (1997) Changes of sympatho-adrenal and hypothalamo-pituitary-adrenocortical system in patients with head injury. Acta Neurol Scand 96(1):52–58
33. Bernard F, Outtrim J, Menon DK, Matta BF (2006) Incidence of adrenal insufficiency after severe traumatic brain injury varies according to definition used: clinical implications. Br J Anaesth 96(1):72–76
34. Cooper MS, Thickett DR, Stewart PM (2013) Reduced cortisol metabolism during critical illness. N Engl J Med 369(5):480
35. Agha A, Phillips J, O'Kelly P, Tormey W, Thompson CJ (2005) The natural history of post-traumatic hypopituitarism: implications for assessment and treatment. Am J Med 118(12):1416
36. Marik PE (2009) Critical illness-related corticosteroid insufficiency. Chest 135(1):181–193

37. Bondanelli M, De Marinis L, Ambrosio MR et al (2004) Occurrence of pituitary dysfunction following traumatic brain injury. J Neurotrauma 21(6):685–696
38. Llompart-Pou JA, Perez-Barcena J, Raurich JM et al (2007) Effect of barbiturate coma on adrenal response in patients with traumatic brain injury. J Endocrinol Invest 30(5):393–398
39. Vinclair M, Broux C, Faure P et al (2008) Duration of adrenal inhibition following a single dose of etomidate in critically ill patients. Intensive Care Med 34(4):714–719
40. Barton RN, Stoner HB, Watson SM (1987) Relationships among plasma cortisol, adrenocorticotrophin, and severity of injury in recently injured patients. J Trauma 27(4):384–392
41. Alderson P, Roberts I (2000) Corticosteroids for acute traumatic brain injury. Cochrane Database Syst Rev (2):CD000196
42. Roberts I, Yates D, Sandercock P et al (2004) Effect of intravenous corticosteroids on death within 14 days in 10008 adults with clinically significant head injury (MRC CRASH trial): randomised placebo-controlled trial. Lancet 364(9442):1321–1328
43. Treschan TA, Peters J (2006) The vasopressin system: physiology and clinical strategies. Anesthesiology 105(3):599–612
44. Boughey JC, Yost MJ, Bynoe RP (2004) Diabetes insipidus in the head-injured patient. Am Surg 70(6):500–503
45. Schrier RW, Gross P, Gheorghiade M et al (2006) Tolvaptan, a selective oral vasopressin V2-receptor antagonist, for hyponatremia. N Engl J Med 355(20):2099–2112
46. Spasovski G, Vanholder R, Allolio B et al (2014) Clinical practice guideline on diagnosis and treatment of hyponatraemia. Intensive Care Med 40(3):320–331
47. Bushnik T, Englander J, Katznelson L (2007) Fatigue after TBI: association with neuroendocrine abnormalities. Brain Inj 21(6):559–566
48. Devesa J, Reimunde P, Devesa P, Barbera M, Arce V (2013) Growth hormone (GH) and brain trauma. Horm Behav 63(2):331–344
49. Chourdakis M, Kraus MM, Tzellos T et al (2012) Effect of early compared with delayed enteral nutrition on endocrine function in patients with traumatic brain injury: an open-labeled randomized trial. JPEN J Parenter Enteral Nutr 36(1):108–116

Chapter 17
Sepsis and Multiple Organ Failure

Jean-Charles Preiser and Vincent Fraipont

Abstract Signs of sepsis are systematically present in each critically ill patient after a few days of stay in an intensive care unit. The associated metabolic response includes a rise in expended energy a few after its onset and changes in the use of energy substrates. General recommendations include the preference of the oral or enteral route and a limitation of the caloric intake during the early phase. Nutritional interventions have been assessed to modulate the inflammatory response underlying the metabolic changes, including the addition of supplemental omega-3 fatty acids, glutamine and antioxidants. The beneficial effects of these interventions started during the course of critical illness have not been convincingly confirmed. Hence, no specific diet or nutritional formula is currently recommended.

Among the situations requiring prolonged care in an intensive care unit, sepsis and subsequent organ failures are the commonest. Their clinical burden is huge, as most clinicians are daily facing patients with "sepsis," described as the body's overwhelming and life-threatening response to infection, which can lead to tissue damage, organ failure, and death. The magnitude of the response and the organs and systems involved have been further characterised and embedded into "severe sepsis," "septic shock" or "multiple organ failures." From a metabolic viewpoint, sepsis is viewed as "a failure of homeostasis," i.e., "an inability for the organism or cell to maintain internal equilibrium by adjusting its physiological processes under fluctuating environmental conditions in response to infection or injury."

J.-C. Preiser, MD, PhD (✉)
Department of Intensive Care, Erasme University Hospital, Free University of Brussels, 808 route de Lennik, Brussels 1070, Belgium
e-mail: Jean-Charles.Preiser@erasme.ulb.ac.be

V. Fraipont, MD
Intensive Care, Centre hospitalier regional La Citadelle, Liege, Belgium

J.-C. Preiser (ed.), *The Stress Response of Critical Illness: Metabolic and Hormonal Aspects*, DOI 10.1007/978-3-319-27687-8_17

Table 17.1 Main metabolic changes during sepsis

Metabolism	Energy	Carbohydrates	Lipids	Proteins
Changes	Increased expenditure (late phase)	Increased glucose production from glycogenolysis and gluconeogenesis (glycogénolyse puis néoglucogenèse), increased lactate production, hyperglycaemia, and insulin resistance	Increased lipolysis and lipid oxidation	Increased muscle and splanchnic protein breakdown, synthesis of inflammatory proteins
Likely mechanisms	Fever, epinephrine, cytokines	Cortisol, glucagon, epinephrine, cytokines	Cortisol, epinephrine, growth hormone	Cortisol, cytokines

In this chapter, we will review the typical metabolic patterns occurring during sepsis, the nutritional interventions targeting inflammatory pathways involved in the pathogenesis of sepsis, and the current recommendations for nutrition during sepsis.

17.1 Metabolic Changes During Sepsis

17.1.1 Energy Expenditure

Very typically, the energy expended after the onset of sepsis increases progressively over time, as depicted in Chap. 2 (Fig. 2.2). Several teams [1, 2] reported stepwise increases of metabolic rate from the lowest value during septic shock, progressively increasing during severe sepsis and recovery. The magnitude of the inflammatory response and the common need for sedative agents during the acute early phase contribute to the lower metabolic rate. More recently, mitochondrial dysfunction and cell hibernation have also been suggested as a contributing factor (see Chap. 4).

Facing the demand for energy substrates, insulin resistance has developed and appears as an adaptive mechanism preserved over evolution to provide sufficient amounts of glucose to the immune and inflammatory cells needed to neutralise the invading microorganisms [3, 4].

17.1.2 Use of Substrates

During sepsis, the energy metabolism is characterised by the mobilisation of endogenous substrates as a result of increased glucose production from glycogenolysis and gluconeogenesis, lipolysis and proteins, under the influence of hormonal and inflammatory mediators, including tumour necrosis factor (TNF, interleukin 1 (IL1) and interleukin 6 (IL6)) (Table 17.1) [5, 6]. These changes result in the release of fatty acids from adipose tissues and of amino acids from skeletal muscles in order to provide substrates for gluconeogenesis and synthesis of the acute-phase proteins. Stress hyperglycaemia is a reflection of the increased turnover of the energy substrates [7–9].

17.1.2.1 Lipid Metabolism

During sepsis, the metabolism of lipids is characterised by an increased production of fatty acids from peripheral tissues and by an increased oxidation. However, the circulating levels of free fatty acids are usually unchanged, suggesting an increased uptake in peripheral tissues and/or a decreased activity of the lipoprotein lipase [5, 10, 11].

17.1.2.2 Protein Metabolism

Overall, the rate of protein breakdown is increased during sepsis, proportionally to the magnitude and severity of sepsis; the rate of protein synthesis is also increased to a lesser extent. The protein turnover is in fact massively enhanced [6, 12]. However the optimal provision of proteins during sepsis is unknown; the current recommendations will be discussed at the end of this chapter. Likewise, qualitative changes by additions of specific amino acids will be reviewed in the next section.

17.2 Nutritional Interventions Targeting Inflammatory Pathways Involved in the Pathogenesis of Sepsis

The major steps in the field of sepsis and inflammation allowed the identification of pro- and anti-inflammatory states occurring after the onset of sepsis. Very importantly, and in contrast with the former concept (top panel of Fig. 17.1), the current understanding implies the simultaneous start of the pro- and of the anti-inflammatory status (bottom panel of Fig. 17.1, which also includes the distinction between innate and adaptive immune responses). This concept is very important, when the

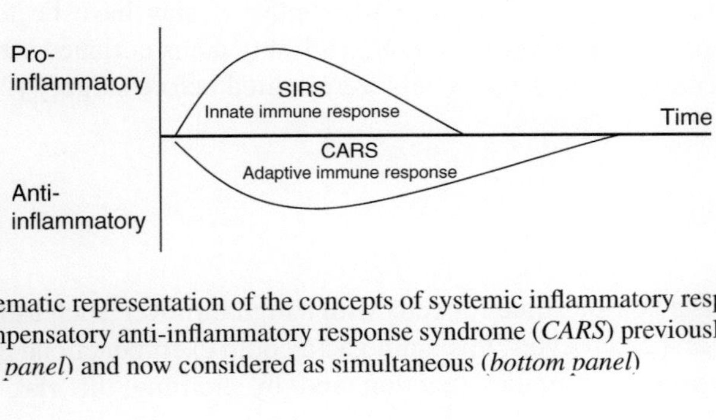

Fig. 17.1 Schematic representation of the concepts of systemic inflammatory response syndrome (*SIRS*) and compensatory anti-inflammatory response syndrome (*CARS*) previously understood as sequential (*top panel*) and now considered as simultaneous (*bottom panel*)

"hyperinflamed" patient is also more susceptible to new infections. Hence any intervention designed to dampen the pro-inflammatory component of sepsis can increase the risk of superinfection. Conversely, immune-enhancing interventions will carry the inherent risk of enhancing the septic response.

In the field of nutrition, several companies marketed "immune-enhancing" or "immunomodulating" formulas, whose composition was based on preclinical findings demonstrating the effects of some nutrients on inflammatory pathways. These "immunonutritive" formulas contained several particular nutrients, implying difficulties in the interpretation of clinical data. Therefore "immunonutrition" is now replaced by "pharmaconutrition," a new wording used to describe solutions containing single nutrients. This chapter will summarise the data related to the commonest nutrients used to modulate the immune response: omega-3 fatty acids, glutamine, and antioxidants (selenium and vitamins), including the results of the large-scale recent trials summarised in Table 17.2.

17.2.1 Omega-3 Fatty Acids

The production of pro-inflammatory lipid mediators as well as the immunosuppressive effects of lipid emulsions is mostly related to ω-6 polyunsaturated fatty acids. Therefore, the proportion of ω-3 fatty acids has been increased. Indeed, experimental data confirm in different settings that the exposure to ω-3 fatty acids results in a decreased production of thromboxane (TX) A2, prostaglandin (PG) E2, and leukotriene (LT) B4 derived from arachidonic acid, while TXA3, PGE3, and LTB5 derived from eicosapentaenoic (EPA) and docosahexaenoic (DHA) acid are increased. These changes reduce the magnitude of the inflammatory response, including the cytokine response [5, 13–16]. Hence, the optimal use of ω-3 fatty acids would be before or at the time of onset of sepsis to prevent a hyperinflammation. This condition is rarely met in clinical practice, when septic patients are usually referred after the development of the clinical picture. Hence, the clinical benefit of parenteral and enteral solutions enriched with ω-3 fatty acids has not been convincingly confirmed in the critically ill septic patient [17–23]. These findings can also be partly related to the design of some studies and to the heterogeneity of the patients' populations and of methodologies used.

In contrast, during the perioperative period of oncologic surgery, several complications including infections and hospital lengths of stay have been consistently avoided or improved in patients receiving ω-3 fatty acids enriched with nutritional solutions, especially when supplements were started before surgery [24].

17.2.2 Glutamine

As glutamine is a key substrate for cells with a high turnover, such as lymphocytes, macrophages, and enterocytes, this amino acid could exert beneficial effects during sepsis, by improving immune function and by limiting the risk of bacterial

Table 17.2 Summary of the recent studies on pharmaconutrition [41–47]

	Glutamine	Sélénium	AOX	Ω3 Entéral	Ω3 IV
Scandinavian Study (40)					
n = 413	ICU mortality (PP)				
SIGNET (30)					
n=502		ICU infections (>5d Se)			
REDOXS (31)	28-d mortality Hospital and 6-month mortality				
n=1223					
MetaPlus (32)					
n=301	6-month mortality (medical patients)				
Grau (41)	Pneumonia – UTI.				
n = 117	Insulin doses				
Valenta (42)					
n=150					
INTERSEPT (22)				Severe sepsis	
n=115				ICU and hosp LOS	
Grau (43)					
n=132				ICU LOS	
Stapleton (44)					
n=90					
OMEGA (45)				Ventilator-free days (VFD)	
n=272				ICU LOS – OF - diarrhoea	
Kagan (OMT) (46)					
n=120				Bacteremia, PRBC	
ICU Lipids (20)					Delta SOFA
n=159					CRP
Hall (47)					Nosocomial infections
n=60					

Summary of the main results of the different studies on pharmaconutritional interventions in critically ill patients

Boxes are coloured in white for significant positive effect on an outcome variable, in grey when the result is neutral (no difference) or in black when a negative effect was retorted for the outcome variable. For each study, the main outcome variable is displayed on the first line and secondary variable on the second line.

ICU intensive care unit, *PP* per protocol, *UTI* urinary tract infection, *LOS* length of stay, *OF* number of organ failures, *PRBC* number of packed red blood cells, *SOFA* sepsis-related organ failure assessment, *CRP* C-reactive protein translocation. Moreover, the plasma levels of glutamine are usually low in the critically ill, as a result of the exhaustion of the endogenous stores. Several animal experiments confirmed these beneficial effects [25]. However, an increase of the inflammatory response could be deleterious during sepsis [26]. Several clinical trials assessed the effects of intravenous glutamine (0.2–0.4 g/kg/day) in patients receiving exclusive parenteral nutrition and confirmed decreases in the rate of infection and even in mortality [27–29]. However, recent and larger studies challenged these encouraging results (Fig. 17.1) [30–32]. In particular, the REDOXS [31] and MetaPlus [32] trials reported an increased mortality in patients randomised to glutamine. Hence, despite the early promises, the use of glutamine is now discouraged in patients with organ failures.

17.2.3 Antioxidant Strategies

As for ω-3 fatty acids and for glutamine, the rationale for using antioxidant nutrients during sepsis is strong. The oxidative stress (an imbalance between reactive oxygen species and antioxidant defence mechanisms) is believed to play a critical role in the development of organ failures [33]. Several strategies have been evaluated (selenium, a key factor of the glutathione peroxidase enzyme), and antioxidant vitamins (vitamins A, C, and E) have been used and successfully improved the antioxidant capacity assessed ex vivo [34], but did not improve the outcome of septic patients (Table 17.2). The important heterogeneity of the antioxidant cocktails and of clinical situations represents additional difficulties when interpreting the available data [35]. The use of biomarkers of oxidative stress could help to identify patients in whom an antioxidant approach is likely to be beneficial [34].

17.3 Recommendations for Clinical Practice

All the aspects of the management of patients with sepsis have been discussed among a board of experts, who issued a set of recommendations [36]. In terms of nutrition, the following recommendations have been issued (available on http://www.survivingsepsis.org/Guidelines/Documents/Other%20supportive%20therapy.pdf):

1. Administer oral or enteral (if necessary) feedings, as tolerated, rather than either complete fasting or provision of only intravenous glucose within the first 48 h after a diagnosis of severe sepsis/septic shock (grade 2C).
2. Avoid mandatory full caloric feeding in the first week but rather suggest low-dose feeding (e.g., up to 500 cal per day), advancing only as tolerated (grade 2B).
3. Use intravenous glucose and enteral nutrition rather than total parenteral nutrition (TPN) alone or parenteral nutrition in conjunction with enteral feeding in the first 7 days after a diagnosis of severe sepsis/septic shock (grade 2B).

4. Use nutrition with no specific immunomodulating supplementation rather than nutrition providing specific immunomodulating supplementation in patients with severe sepsis (grade 2C).

However, the level of evidence supporting these recommendations is low [37]. Other guidelines (www.criticalcarenutrition and 38) suggest the provision of nonprotein energy substrates as carbohydrates (60–70 %) and lipids (30–40 %) with a maximum set at 7 g/kg.d and 1.5 g/kg.d for carbohydrates and lipids, respectively (maximal oxidisable levels).

The recommended protein intakes range between 1.2 and 1.5 g/kg.d, supported by a very low evidence level [37–39]. The various pharmaconutrients are usually not recommended during sepsis, with the notable exception of glutamine, which should be considered during exclusive parenteral nutrition [36, 38].

References

1. Kreymann G, Grosser S, Buggisch P, Gottschall C, Matthaei S, Greten H (1993) Oxygen consumption and resting metabolic rate in sepsis, sepsis syndrome, and septic shock. Crit Care Med 21:1012–1019
2. Plank LD, Connolly AB, Hill GL (1998) Sequential changes in the metabolic response in severely septic patients during the first 23 days after the onset of peritonitis. Ann Surg 228: 146–158
3. Soeters MR, Soeters PB (2012) The evolutionary benefit of insulin resistance. Clin Nutr 31:1002–1007
4. Lena D, Kalfon P, Preiser JC, Ichai C (2011) Glycemic control in the intensive care unit and during the postoperative period. Anesthesiology 114:438–444
5. Tappy L, Chiolero R (2007) Substrate utilization in sepsis and multiple organ failure. Crit Care Med 35:S531–S534
6. Preiser JC, Ichai C, Orban JC, Groeneveld AB (2014) Metabolic response to the stress of critical illness. Br J Anaesth 113:945–954
7. Shaw JH, Klein S, Wolfe RR (1985) Assessment of alanine, urea, and glucose interrelationships in normal subjects and in patients with sepsis with stable isotopic tracers. Surgery 97:557–568
8. Dungan KM, Braithwaite SS, Preiser JC (2009) Stress hyperglycaemia. Lancet 373:1798–1807
9. Mesotten D, Preiser JC, Kosiborod M (2015) Glucose management in critically ill adults and children. Lancet Diabetes Endocrinol 3:723–733
10. Druml W, Fischer M, Ratheiser K (1998) Use of intravenous lipids in critically ill patients with sepsis without and with hepatic failure. JPEN J Parenter Enteral Nutr 22:217–223
11. Siegel JH, Vary TC, Rivkind A, Bilik R, Coleman B, Tall BE, Morris JG (1989) Abnormal metabolic control in the septic multiple organ failure syndrome: pharmacotherapy for altered fuel control mechanisms. Prog Clin Biol Res 308:535–543
12. Weijs PJM, Cynober L, Delegge M, Kreyman G, Wernerman J, Wolfe RR (2014) Proteins and amino acids are fundamental to optimal nutrition support in critically ill patients. Crit Care 18:591
13. Goulet O, Antebi H, Wolf C, Talbotec C, Alcindor LG, Corriol O, Lamor M, Colomb-Jung V (2010) A new intravenous fat emulsion containing soybean oil, medium-chain triglycerides, olive oil, and fish oil: a single-center, double-blind randomized study on efficacy and safety in pediatric patients receiving home parenteral nutrition. JPEN J Parenter Enteral Nutr 34:485–495
14. Han YY, Lai SL, Ko WJ, Chou CH, Lai HS (2012) Effects of fish oil on inflammatory modulation in surgical intensive care unit patients. Nutr Clin Pract 27:91–98

15. Mayer K, Schaefer MB, Seeger W (2006) Fish oil in the critically ill: from experimental to clinical data. Curr Opin Clin Nutr Metab Care 9:140–148
16. Michaeli B, Berger MM, Revelly JP, Tappy L, Chiolero R (2007) Effects of fish oil on the neuroendocrine responses to an endotoxin challenge in healthy volunteers. Clin Nutr 26:70–77
17. Barbosa VM, Miles EA, Calhau C, Lafuente E, Calder PC (2010) Effects of a fish oil containing lipid emulsion on plasma phospholipid fatty acids, inflammatory markers, and clinical outcomes in septic patients: a randomized, controlled clinical trial. Crit Care 14:R5
18. Edmunds CE, Brody RA, Parrott JS, Stankorb SM, Heyland DK (2014) The effects of different IV Fat emulsions on clinical outcomes in critically ill patients*. Crit Care Med 42:1168–1177
19. Friesecke S, Lotze C, Köhler J, Heinrich A, Felix SB, Abel P (2008) Fish oil supplementation in the parenteral nutrition of critically ill medical patients: a randomised controlled trial. Intensive Care Med 34:1411–1420
20. Grau-Carmona T, Bonet-Saris A, García-de-Lorenzo A et al (2015) Influence of n-3 polyunsaturated fatty acids enriched lipid emulsions on nosocomial infections and clinical outcomes in critically ill patients: ICU lipids study. Crit Care Med 43:31–39
21. Jurewitsch B (2012) The evolving utility and emergent uses of novel lipid emulsions: new horizons and rediscovered prospects. JPEN J Parenter Enteral Nutr 36:626–629
22. Pontes-Arruda A, Martins LF, de Lima SM, Isola AM, Toledo D, Rezende E, Maia M, Magnan GB, GLA & Antioxidants Role in Sepsis Treatment Study G. II (2011) Enteral nutrition with eicosapentaenoic acid, gamma-linolenic acid and antioxidants in the early treatment of sepsis: results from a multicenter, prospective, randomized, double blinded and controlled Study – INTERSEPT study. Crit Care 15:R144
23. Santacruz CA, Orbegozo D, Vincent JL, Preiser JC (2015) Modulation of dietary lipid composition during acute respiratory distress syndrome: systematic review and meta-analysis. JPEN J Parenter Enteral Nutr 39(7):837–846
24. Marimuthu K, Varadhan KK, Ljungqvist O (2012) Lobo DN.A meta-analysis of the effect of combinations of immune modulating nutrients on outcome in patients undergoing major open gastrointestinal surgery. Ann Surg 255:1060–1068
25. Cynober L, De Bandt JP (2014) Glutamine in the intensive care unit. Curr Opin Clin Nutr Metab Care 17:98–104
26. Oudemans-van Straaten HM, van Zanten AR (2014) Glutamine supplementation in the critically ill: friend or foe? Crit Care 18:143
27. Dechelotte P, Hasselmann M, Cynober L et al (2006) L-alanyl-L-glutamine dipeptide-supplemented total parenteral nutrition reduces infectious complications and glucose intolerance in critically ill patients: the French controlled, randomized, double-blind, multicenter study. Crit Care Med 34:598–604
28. Goeters C, Wenn A, Mertes N, Wempe C, Van Aken H, Stehle P, Bone HG (2002) Parenteral L-alanyl-L-glutamine improves 6-month outcome in critically ill patients. Crit Care Med 30:2032–2037
29. Griffiths RD, Allen KD, Andrews FJ, Jones C (2002) Infection, multiple organ failure, and survival in the intensive care unit: influence of glutamine-supplemented parenteral nutrition on acquired infection. Nutrition 18:546–552
30. Andrews PJ, Avenell A, Noble DW, Campbell MK, Croal BL, Simpson WG, Vale LD, Battison CG, Jenkinson DJ, Cook JA (2011) Randomised trial of glutamine, selenium, or both, to supplement parenteral nutrition for critically ill patients. BMJ 342:d1542
31. Heyland D, Muscedere J, Wischmeyer PE, Cook D, Jones G, Albert M, Elke G, Berger MM, Day AG (2013) A randomized trial of glutamine and antioxidants in critically ill patients. N Engl J Med 368:1489–1497
32. van Zanten AR, Sztark F, Kaisers UX, Zielmann S, Felbinger TW, Sablotzki AR, De Waele JJ, Timsit JF, Honing ML, Keh D, Vincent JL, Zazzo JF, Fijn HB, Petit L, Preiser JC, van Horssen PJ, Hofman Z (2014) High-protein enteral nutrition enriched with immune-modulating nutrients vs standard high-protein enteral nutrition and nosocomial infections in the ICU: a randomized clinical trial. JAMA 312:514–524

33. Motoyama T, Okamoto K, Kukita I, Hamaguchi M, Kinoshita Y, Ogawa H (2003) Possible role of increased oxidant stress in multiple organ failure after systemic inflammatory response syndrome. Crit Care Med 31:1048–1052
34. Preiser JC (2012) Oxidative stress. JPEN J Parenter Enteral Nutr 36:147–154
35. Manzanares W, Langlois PL, Hardy G (2013) Update on antioxidant micronutrients in the critically ill. Curr Opin Clin Nutr Metab Care 16:719–725
36. Dellinger RP, Levy MM, Rhodes A, Annane D, Gerlach H, Opal SM, Sevransky JE, Sprung CL, Douglas IS, Jaeschke R, Osborn TM, Nunnally ME, Townsend SR, Reinhart K, Kleinpell RM, Angus DC, Deutschman CS, Machado FR, Rubenfeld GD, Webb S, Beale RJ, Vincent JL, Moreno R (2013) Surviving sepsis campaign: international guidelines for management of severe sepsis and septic shock, 2012. Intensive Care Med 39:165–228
37. Preiser J-C, van Zanten ARH, Berger MM et al (2015) Metabolic and nutritional support of critically ill patients: consensus and controversies. Crit Care 19:309
38. Lefrant JY, Hurel D, Cano NJ, Ichai C, Preiser JC, Tamion F (2014) Guidelines for nutrition support in critically ill patient. Ann Fr Anesth Reanim 33:202–218
39. Singer P, Berger MM, Van den Berghe G, Biolo G, Calder P, Forbes A, Griffiths R, Kreyman G, Leverve X, Pichard C (2009) ESPEN guidelines on parenteral nutrition: intensive care. Clin Nutr 28:387–400
40. Wernerman J, Kirketeig T, Andersson B et al (2011) Scandinavian glutamine trial: a pragmatic multi-centre randomised clinical trial of intensive care unit patients. Acta Anaesthesiol Scand 55:812–818
41. Grau T, Bonet A, Miñambres E et al (2011) The effect of L-alanyl-L-glutamine dipeptide supplemented total parenteral nutrition on infectious morbidity and insulin sensitivity in critically ill patients. Crit Care Med 39:1263–1268
42. Valenta J, Brodska H, Drabek T, Hendl J, Kazda A (2011) High-dose selenium substitution in sepsis: a prospective randomized clinical trial. Intensive Care Med 37:808–815
43. Grau-Carmona T, Morán-García V, García-de-Lorenzo A et al (2011) Effect of an enteral diet enriched with eicosapentaenoic acid, gamma-linolenic acid and anti-oxidants on the outcome of mechanically ventilated, critically ill, septic patients. Clin Nutr 30:578–584
44. Stapleton RD, Martin TR, Weiss NS et al (2011) A phase II randomized placebo-controlled trial of omega-3 fatty acids for the treatment of acute lung injury. Crit Care Med 39: 1655–1662
45. Rice TW, Wheeler AP, Thompson BT, de Boisblanc BP, Steingrub J, Rock P, NIH NHLBI Acute Respiratory Distress Syndrome Network of Investigators (2011) Enteral omega-3 fatty acid, gamma-linolenic acid, and antioxidant supplementation in acute lung injury. JAMA 306:1574–1581
46. Kagan I, Cohen J, Stein M et al (2015) Preemptive enteral nutrition enriched with eicosapentaenoic acid, gamma-linolenic acid and antioxidants in severe multiple trauma: a prospective, randomized, double-blind study. Intensive Care Med 41:460–469
47. Hall TC, Bilku DK, Al-Leswas D et al (2015) A randomized controlled trial investigating the effects of parenteral fish oil on survival outcomes in critically ill patients with sepsis: a pilot study. JPEN J Parenter Enteral Nutr 39:301–312

Chapter 18
The Stress Response of Critical Illness: Metabolic and Hormonal Aspects, Hormonal Regulation, Particular Clinical Situations "Morbid Obesity"

Moise Coeffier and Fabienne Tamion

Abstract Obesity is a widespread condition associated with a variety of mechanical, metabolic, and physiologic changes that affect outcomes and delivery of care in ICU. In particular, the metabolic response to critical illness of obese patients is characterized by changes in the metabolism of carbohydrates and fat, and in the utilization of proteins. The endocrine functions of adipose tissue might be involved role in the adaptive changes to critical illness.

18.1 Introduction

Obesity is a worldwide public health issue with extensive medical, social, and economic consequences. Obesity, which is defined by the presence of excess adiposity, negatively impacts health and increases an individual's risk for developing a variety of medical conditions, including cardiovascular disease, certain cancers, and diabetes mellitus. The incidence of adult obesity in the United States has doubled in the past 30 years [1]. Obesity in adults is defined by the World Health Organization (WHO) and the National Institutes of Health (NIH) using the BMI. The

M. Coeffier
Institut National de la Santé et de la Recherche Médicale U1073, Rouen, France

Institute for Research and Innovation in Biomedicine, Rouen, France

Nutrition Department, Rouen University Hospital, Rouen, France

F. Tamion (✉)
Institut National de la Santé et de la Recherche Médicale U1096, Rouen, France

Institute for Research and Innovation in Biomedicine, Rouen, France

Medical Intensive Care Unit, Rouen University Hospital, Rouen, France
e-mail: Fabienne.Tamion@chu-rouen.fr

J.-C. Preiser (ed.), *The Stress Response of Critical Illness: Metabolic and Hormonal Aspects*, DOI 10.1007/978-3-319-27687-8_18

recommended classifications based on BMI are as follows: underweight (BMI <18.49 kg/m^2), normal weight (BMI 18.5–24.9 kg/m^2), overweight (BMI 25.0–29.9 kg/m^2), obesity class I (BMI 30.0–34.9 kg/m^2), obesity class II (BMI 35.0–39.9 kg/m^2), and obesity class III (BMI >40.0 kg/m^2) [2]. This epidemic has reached the ICUs, such that 33 % of ICU patients are obese and 7 % are morbidly obese. Obesity presents the intensive care unit (ICU) team with a unique set of challenges. Sarcopenic obesity (SO) refers to the copresence of sarcopenia and obesity, and the prevalence of SO ranges from 0 to 41 % in older populations. Not only does the greater frequency of comorbid diseases in this population lead to increased complexity of care, but the physical aspect of severe obesity makes routine elements of nursing care and diagnostic/therapeutic interventions extremely demanding. Obesity is a proinflammatory state, and probably this state becomes overwhelmed or exaggerated during critical illness.

18.2 Neuroendocrine Pathophysiology in Obesity

The pathophysiology of obesity is complex, in large part, because of the heterogeneous nature of the pathology. If clinicians focus only on the concept of energy balance, they will not appreciate the interface between the central nervous system and metabolically active organs that is involved in this important law of thermodynamics. In addition, obesity-induced inflammation and its metabolic consequences (e.g., liver disease, type 2 diabetes mellitus, dyslipidemia) further complicate the understanding of obesity, its treatment, and its consequences specially in critical illness. The central nervous system (CNS) receives information from several regulatory loops that help control energy balance [3]. The brain gets additional information about metabolic need from the more metabolically active tissues, such as adipose, liver, stomach, intestine, muscle, and bone. Furthermore, the CNS gets information about current energy availability in the environment through sensory organs and through the stomach, small intestine, pancreas, and liver. Central controls of body weight and appetite that influence food intake and energy expenditure involve satiation/satiety signals and “adiposity” hormones. Satiation/satiety signals induced by agents such as leptin, POMC, cholecystokinin (CCK), and glucagon-like peptide-1 (GLP-1) result in feelings of fullness, which contribute to cessation of food intake (satiation) and/or suppression of appetite after meal intake (satiety). “Adiposity” hormones (e.g., insulin, leptin) are secreted, not in response to a meal but as a result of the amount of adipose tissue present in the host organism. Both satiety/ satiation signals and adiposity hormones represent a complex messaging system between the CNS and the periphery that influence energy homeostasis and intake. In addition to the aforementioned mechanisms, many of these molecules (e.g., leptin) are also important to the maladaptive obesity-induced inflammation and its resultant complications. As macronutrients are consumed, a number of these satiety/satiation signals result in a message delivered to the CNS. The classic satiation signal, CCK, is secreted from I cells in the blood in response to fat and protein as they pass into the duodenum. Systemic CCK then influences a number of gastrointestinal mechanisms such as motility, gastric acid secretion, pancreatic enzyme secretion, and contraction of the gallbladder [4]. Satiation signaling is produced by CCK through a paracrine mechanism via vagal sensory nerves [5]. In opposition to CCK, ghrelin is a potent orexigen that stimulates food intake [6]. In response to fasting, specific endocrine cells in the stomach and duodenum release ghrelin. Ghrelin appears to have several actions, one of which is a direct action on receptors in the hypothalamus to stimulate appetite and increase food intake [7]. Another major effect of ghrelin is stimulating the release of growth hormone [8]. The peripheral actions of GLP-1 are numerous and include an increased release of insulin, inhibition of glucagon secretion, reduction of gastrointestinal (GI) motility and secretions, and stimulation of an anorexic effect [9]. Central actions of GLP-1 include reducing food intake via caloric homeostatic circuits in the hypothalamus and eliciting symptoms of stress/malaise in the amygdale [10]. The satiation actions of GLP-1 stemming from the variety of aforementioned mechanisms have been seen in both animal models and human studies [11]. These actions are further demonstrated with long-acting GLP-1 pharmacotherapy for diabetes mellitus, which results in not only improvement in glucose control but also meaningful weight loss [12]. Several other satiation/satiety signaling molecules, such as glicentin, GLP-2, glucagon, oxyntomodulin, peptide YY, apolipoprotein A-IV, and enterostatin, have been described and have recently been reviewed [3]. These hormones then act centrally (e.g., hypothalamus) to influence energy homeostasis, resulting in decreased food intake and weight loss. The neuroendocrine pathophysiology is incompletely understood, which serves to further complicate patient management for the >60 recognized conditions associated with obesity.

18.3 Obesity and the ICU Conundrum

Despite the aforementioned challenges of obesity in the ICU, as well as having an increased all-cause and cause-specific mortality, obesity has been associated with improved ICU outcomes in numerous studies (including 3 meta-analyses) [13–15]. One meta-analysis included 14 studies with 62,045 total and 15,437 obese patients [14]. Obesity was not associated with an increased risk of ICU mortality (relative risk [RR], 1.00; 95 % confidence interval [CI], 0.86–1.16; $P=0.97$). However, ICU length of stay was 1.08 days longer for obese (95 % CI, 0.27–1.88; $P=0.009$) compared to nonobese individuals. Duration of ventilation was significantly longer in obese individuals by 1.48 days (95 % CI, 0.07–2.89; $P=0.04$) compared to nonobese individuals. In a subgroup analysis, improved survival was observed for class I and class II obesity patients compared with nonobese patients (RR, 0.86; 95 % CI, 0.81–0.91; $P<0.001$), suggesting a protective effect from the obesity [14]. A second meta-analysis evaluated 12 studies and found that overweight, obesity class I, and obesity class II patients had lower rates of mortality compared to patients with normal weight [15]. The pooled average for ICU length of stay (LOS) was significantly increased for underweight, overweight, and obesity class III patients when compared to normal-weight individuals. When multiple organ dysfunction (MOD) was evaluated in six trauma/surgery studies, four reports found increased MOD in obese individuals compared to patients of normal weight. A third meta-analysis evaluated 22 studies, and the pooled analysis found no significant difference in ICU mortality between obese and normal individuals [13]. Hospital mortality was lower in obese individuals (RR, 0.76; 95 % CI, 0.59–0.92) compared to normal-weight individuals. Unlike the previous analyses, there was no difference in ICU LOS or duration of mechanical ventilation between obese and nonobese individuals. There has been no clear explanation for this "ICU conundrum." The reasons given in the meta-analyses to explain the association are not well supported by the available evidence. One such explanation provided suggested that obese individuals have a survival benefit because increased nutritional reserves help the patient respond to inflammation and metabolic stress. This notion of nutritional reserves is based on the assumption that excess adipose tissue is readily available for utilization in critical illness. Another explanation given for the decreased hospital mortality in obesity suggested that an increased release of anti-inflammatory adipokines, IL-10, and leptin would favorably modulate the inflammatory process. This explanation appears to be erroneous, as leptin has strong proinflammatory effects that activate macrophages and induce hepatic tumor necrosis factor (TNF)-α, interleukin (IL)-6, IL-12, and monocyte chemoattractant protein-1 (MCP-1) production [16]. So, no good explanation for these findings is correct.

18.3.1 The Obesity Paradox in the ICU

Three meta-analyses combining in total 25 different studies on BMI and outcome of the critically ill patient were recently published [13–15]. Although largely heterogeneous and working with different obesity definitions, the studies included in the meta-analyses altogether are highly suggestive of a lower mortality risk in overweight (BMI 25–29.9 kg/m^2) and obese (BMI 30–39.9 kg/m^2) patients, whereas underweight (BMI <18.5 kg/m^2) patients appear to suffer from increased risk of mortality. Morbidly obese patients however do suffer from longer duration of mechanical ventilation and longer ICU length of stay [17]. In more detail, the association between BMI and mortality in critically ill patients appears to follow a J-shaped curve. It is possible that overweight and obese individuals have a lower mortality rate during critical illness, only because they have a larger amount of nutritional reserves [18]. This might protect the obese patient from the severe hypercatabolism present in critical illness, which generally evokes a profound decrease of lean body mass. On the other hand, the excessive adipose tissue in overweight and obese patients may play a metabolic role through enhanced triglycerides and glucose storage, which could be protective during critical illness [19]. Cytokines produced in the adipose tissue might be of importance as obese individuals often suffer from chronic adipose tissue inflammation with higher circulating TNF-α levels. So, the initial blood leukocyte inflammatory response to blunt trauma did not differ significantly between patients from different BMI categories [20]. It is possible that the impact of severe injury or illness on acute inflammation overwhelms the metabolic disturbances and subclinical inflammation associated with obesity.

Obese individuals generally have higher circulating levels of lipoproteins and lipids than lean individuals. This could theoretically be beneficial during critical illness because during acute illness, hypocholesterolemia has been associated with severity of illness, morbidity, and mortality [21]. Future studies on the relation between obesity and mortality in critically ill patients are needed to clarify the mechanisms "the obesity paradox."

18.3.2 Metabolic Response to Critical Illness and Obesity

Regardless of the inciting cause of injury or illness, there is a common hypermetabolic, inflammatory response to stress, directed at promoting acute survival, which affects macronutrient (protein, lipid, and carbohydrate) utilization throughout the body. Obesity is a proinflammatory state and probably this process becomes overwhelmed or exaggerated during critical illness.

18.3.2.1 Carbohydrate Metabolism and Hyperglycemia

Stress-induced hyperglycemia is a frequent complication of critical illness and the end product of increased counterregulatory hormone production (glucagon, glucocorticoids, and catecholamines) and inflammatory cytokine release leading to accelerated hepatic gluconeogenesis, lipolysis, and peripheral insulin resistance [22]. Further, circulating levels of proinflammatory cytokines, including IL-6 and tumor necrosis factor, rise dramatically following tissue injury from sepsis or trauma [23]. Lipolytic rate is increased and the ability of insulin to suppress fatty acid release from adipose tissue is impaired, promoting elevated plasma free fatty acid (FFA) concentration, which is strongly associated with rapid development of insulin resistance [24]. Hepatic gluconeogenesis is increased and clearance of glucose from plasma by skeletal muscle is impaired by these factors. Unlike healthy patients, administration of intravenous glucose fails to suppress hepatic glucose output in critical illness and indeed may exacerbate hyperglycemia. And so, hyperglycemia during critical illness is associated with poorer outcomes [25]. Obesity is also strongly associated with insulin resistance, high plasma FFA concentration, and increases in sympathetic nervous system activity, providing a "second hit" to insulin action in critical illness. Obese patients have defects in oxidation of circulating fatty acids during critical illness, further exacerbating elevated plasma FFA concentration and insulin sensitivity [26]. Given the increased prevalence of diabetes and insulin resistance among the obese patients, it is especially important to include glycemic control into the plan for nutrition support. Infusion of insulin will rapidly reduce plasma FFA and lower plasma triglyceride concentration.

18.3.2.2 Fatty Acid Oxidation

Elevations in FFA usually signify insulin resistance, which causes increased lipolysis, impaired skeletal muscle FFA oxidation, and reduced suppression of plasma FFA by insulin [27]. Despite having a relative abundance of serum FFAs and triglyceride-rich adipose stores, it appears the obese individuals are ineffective at mobilizing or using these energy sources during critical illness [28]. Contrary to the general belief that the most abundant supply of adipose tissues will be the primary fuel, the injured obese patients experience a relative block both in lipid mobilization and utilization. Jeevanandam et al. [26] showed major differences in utilization of endogenous fuel sources between starved obese and nonobese trauma patients; lean patients relied largely on fatty acid oxidation for energy [about 61 % of resting energy expenditure (REE)], whereas obese patients derived most energy from catabolism of lean mass (only 39 % of energy from FFA).

18.3.2.3 Protein Utilization

Muscle protein catabolism is a hallmark feature of critical illness, regardless of BMI, with studies showing losses of up to 10–20 % of skeletal muscle after 1 week in the ICU [29]. Obese persons have increased amounts of fat-free mass (FFM) over their height-matched lean counterparts, but are more likely to use this muscle mass as fuel during critical illness when fasted, only accelerating the rate of protein losses. Under stress conditions, obese patients could not take advantage of their most abundant fat fuel sources but have to depend on the efficient use of endogenous glucose synthesized from the breakdown products of body protein. The mechanism responsible for this blunted lipolytic response in subjects with increased adiposity is not known. Body composition contributes to the regulation of lipolysis during fasting, and the decreased rate of lipolysis, in subjects who have excess fat, may reflect the decreased need per unit fat mass for lipolysis to meet the energy requirements of the lean body mass [30]. FFM (protein) catabolism typically persists despite the provision of nutritional support, though administration of either greater total calories or protein calories has been shown to mitigate its rate and improve nitrogen balance. Hypocaloric, high-protein nutrition seems a preferable approach in obese patients, as it can promote endogenous fat oxidation and shift obese patients away from utilization of FFM as the predominant fuel source while simultaneously inducing favorable changes in body composition [31]. Avoidance of overfeeding is also critical because excess caloric load is associated with increased protein turnover and fat storage [32].

18.3.3 Hypocaloric Feeding

In healthy obese humans, with or without type 2 diabetes, even brief periods of calorie restriction may markedly improve insulin sensitivity. Fasting may actually worsen insulin resistance in skeletal muscle and therefore cannot be recommended as an intervention to improve insulin sensitivity. Several studies clearly show that hypocaloric feeding for a limited amount of time is not inferior to eucaloric feeding. There is no standard method for hypocaloric feeding, but generally involves providing 30–70 % estimated daily caloric needs in conjunction with a higher proportion of protein calories (often 50–60 % of total calories) in order to minimize glucose loads while sparing lean body mass from catabolism. Calorie-restricted nutrition (even briefly) can markedly improve insulin sensitivity and glycemic control, in addition to preventing metabolic consequences of overfeeding, such as hypercapnia, fluid retention, and hypertriglyceridemia. Weight loss and reduction in fat mass is another beneficial effect of this intervention, but never be the primary objective for nutritional support during critical illness. Multiple studies have demonstrated positive outcomes in the ICU related to reduced caloric intake. Dickerson et al. [31] showed that hypocaloric enteral feeding in obese surgical patients was associated with improved nitrogen balance, shorter length of stay in the ICU, and decreased use of antibiotics. Although their study was not specific to obese patients, Krishnan et al. [33] found improved ICU outcomes, including mortality, return of spontaneous ventilation, and nosocomial sepsis rates among patients receiving approximately 9–18 kcal/kg/d (33–65 % of the ACCP target). The strongest evidence against hypocaloric feeding was provided by Villet et al. [34], who found a higher rate of infections and poor outcomes associated with increasing negative energy balance in a prospective study of 48 ICU patients. However, only 20 patients (41 %) had BMI more than 27 kg/m^2, and therefore findings may not fully represent the obese subgroup. The 2009 Consensus statement issued jointly by the Society of Critical Care Medicine (SCCM) and the American Society for Parenteral and Enteral Nutrition (ASPEN) recommends hypocaloric feeding of critically ill obese patients with enteral feeds, with the goal to provide, no more than 60–70 % of target energy requirements or 11–14 kcal/kg actual body weight per day [35]. Based on nitrogen balance data from studies on hypocaloric feeding, the ASPEN/SCCM guidelines also recommend administration of protein in the range of at least 2.0 g/ kg IBW per day for class I and II obese patients and at least 2.5 g/kg IBW per day for class III obesity. Otherwise, hypocaloric nutrition adjusted ideal body weight should be considered for the obese ICU patient to minimize the loss of lean body mass.

18.4 Conclusion

Obesity is a widespread condition associated with a variety of mechanical, metabolic, and physiologic changes that affect outcomes and delivery of care in ICU. The endocrine functions of adipose tissue might play a role in the adaptation to critical illness. In the acute phase of illness, the anti-inflammatory adiponectin is reduced, whereas proinflammatory cytokine expression in adipose tissue is upregulated. Several of the changes in adipose tissue observed during critical illness could in theory be adaptive and protective. So, nutritional support is a key element of management during critical illness to improve outcomes, but the optimal caloric and protein requirements for obese hospitalized patients are difficult. The current literature indicates that hypocaloric, high-protein nutrition may be the standard of practice for the metabolic support of the critically ill obese patient to prevent the complications associated with overfeeding. Given the increasing prevalence of obesity, further research is needed to develop nutritional support to prevent metabolic consequences and consider the presence of sarcopenic obesity.

References

1. Ogden CL, Yanovski SZ, Carroll MD, Flegal KM (2007) The epidemiology of obesity. Gastroenterology 132(6):2087–2102
2. Kuczmarski RJ, Flegal KM (2000) Criteria for definition of overweight in transition: background and recommendations for the United States. Am J Clin Nutr 72(5):1074–1081
3. Woods SC, D'Alessio DA (2008) Central control of body weight and appetite. J Clin Endocrinol Metab 93(11)(suppl 1):S37–S50
4. Chandra R, Liddle RA (2007) Cholecystokinin. Curr Opin Endocrinol Diabetes Obes 14(1):63–67
5. Lorenz DN, Goldman SA (1982) Vagal mediation of the cholecystokinin satiety effect in rats. Physiol Behav 29(4):599
6. Wiedmer P, Nogueiras R, Broglio F, D'Alessio D, Tschop MH (2007) Ghrelin, obesity and diabetes. Nat Clin Pract Endocrinol Metab 3(10):705–712
7. Asakawa A, Inui A, Kaga T et al (2001) Ghrelin is an appetite-stimulatory signal from stomach with structural resemblance to motilin. Gastroenterology 120(2):337–345
8. Kreitschmann-Andermahr I, Suarez P, Jennings R, Evers N, Brabant G (2010) GH/IGF-I regulation in obesity—mechanisms and practical consequences in children and adults. Horm Res Paediatr 73(3):153–160
9. Dube PE, Brubaker PL (2004) Nutrient, neural and endocrine control of glucagon-like peptide secretion. Horm Metab Res 36(11–12):755–760
10. Kinzig KP, D'Alessio DA, Seeley RJ (2002) The diverse roles of specific GLP-1 receptors in the control of food intake and the response to visceral illness. J Neurosci 22(23): 10470–10476
11. Hayes MR, De Jonghe BC, Kanoski SE (2010) Role of the glucagon-like-peptide-1 receptor in the control of energy balance. Physiol Behav 100(5):503–510
12. Mafong DD, Henry RR (2008) Exenatide as a treatment for diabetes and obesity: implications for cardiovascular risk reduction. Curr Atheroscler Rep 10(1):55–60
13. Hogue CW Jr, Stearns JD, Colantuoni E et al (2009) The impact of obesity on outcomes after critical illness: a meta-analysis. Intensive Care Med 35(7):1152–1170
14. Akinnusi ME, Pineda LA, El Solh AA (2008) Effect of obesity on intensive care morbidity and mortality: a meta-analysis. Crit Care Med 36(1):151–158
15. Oliveros H, Villamor E (2008) Obesity and mortality in critically ill adults: a systematic review and meta-analysis. Obesity (Silver Spring) 16(3):515–521
16. Cave MC, Hurt RT, Frazier TH et al (2008) Obesity, inflammation, and the potential application of pharmaconutrition. Nutr Clin Pract 23(1):16–34
17. Martino JL, Stapleton RD, Wang M et al (2011) Extreme obesity and outcomes in critically ill patients. Chest 140:1198–1206
18. Caloin M (2004) Modeling of lipid and protein depletion during total starvation. Am J Physiol Endocrinol Metab 287:E790–E798
19. Langouche L, Perre SV, Thiessen S et al (2010) Alterations in adipose tissue during critical illness: an adaptive and protective response? Am J Respir Crit Care Med 182:507–516

20. Winfield RD, Delano MJ, Dixon DJ et al (2010) Differences in outcome between obese and nonobese patients following severe blunt trauma are not consistent with an early inflammatory genomic response. Crit Care Med 38:51–58
21. Dunham CM, Fealk MH, Sever WE 3rd (2003) Following severe injury, hypocholesterolemia improves with convalescence but persists with organ failure or onset of infection. Crit Care 7:R145–R153
22. Dungan KM, Braithwaite SS, Preiser JC (2009) Stress hyperglycemia. Lancet 373: 1798–1807
23. Wolfe RR, Martini WZ (2000) Changes in intermediary metabolism in severe surgical illness. World J Surg 24:639–647
24. Boden G, Shulman GI (2002) Free fatty acids in obesity and type 2 diabetes: defining their role in the development of insulin resistance and beta-cell dysfunction. Eur J Clin Invest 32 (Suppl 3):14–23
25. Van den Berghe G, Wilmer A, Hermans G et al (2006) Intensive medical therapy in the medical ICU. N Engl J Med 354:449–461
26. Jeevanandam M, Young DH, Schiller WR (1991) Obesity and the metabolic response to severe multiple trauma in man. J Clin Invest 87:262–269
27. Abdul-Ghani MA, Muller FL, DeFronzo RA et al (2008) Deleterious action of FA metabolites on ATP synthesis: possible link between lipotoxicity, mitochondrial dysfunction, and insulin resistance. Am J Physiol Endocrinol Metab 295:E678–E685
28. Schiffelers SL, Saris WH, van Baak MA (2001) The effect of an increased free fatty acid concentration on thermogenesis and substrate oxidation in obese and lean men. Int J Obes Relat Metab Disord 25:33–38
29. Reid CL, Campbell IT, Little RA (2004) Muscle wasting and energy balance in critical illness. Clin Nutr 23:273–280
30. Choban PS, Flancbaum L (2000) Nourishing the obese patient. Clin Nutr 19(5):305–311
31. Dickerson RN, Boschert KJ, Kudsk KA (2002) Hypocaloric enteral tube feeding in critically ill obese patients. Nutrition 18:241–246
32. Biolo G, Agostini F, Simunic B et al (2008) Positive energy balance is associated with accelerated muscle atrophy and increased erythrocyte glutathione turnover during 5 wk of bed rest. Am J Clin Nutr 88:950–958
33. Krishnan JA, PArce PB, Martinez A (2004) Caloric intake in medical ICU patients: consistency of care with guidelines and relationship to clinical outcomes. Nutr Clin Pract 19:645–646
34. Villet S, Chiolero RL, Bollmann MD et al (2005) Negative impact of hypocaloric feeding and energy balance on clinical outcome in ICU patients. Clin Nutr 24:502–509
35. McClave SA, Martindale RG, Vanek VW et al (2009) Guidelines for the provision and assessment of nutrition support therapy in the adult critically ill patient: Society of Critical Care Medicine (SCCM) and American Society for Parenteral and Enteral Nutrition (A.S.P.E.N.). JPEN J Parenter Enteral Nutr 33:277–316

Chapter 19
Hypermetabolic Response to Burn Injury

Abdikarim Abdullahi, David Patsouris, Sheila R. Costford, and Marc G. Jeschke

Abstract The stress response to injuries like burns and sepsis entails a number of endocrine, metabolic, and immunological changes. These alterations in the secretion of key hormones and cytokines in the initial stages of the injury are believed to be a necessary and beneficial response. However, an exaggerated and prolonged stress response results in the dysfunction and breakdown of key metabolic tissues of the body. The adverse effects of the stress response also goes beyond the tissue level and has been implicated as a negative predictor of poor outcome, infections, and longer hospital stays in patients. For these reasons, a comprehensive and physiological detail of the hypermetabolic response to injury is warranted to better understand how this pro-survival response transforms into catastrophic response. In addition, the scrutiny of this stress response will enhance our understanding of the different types of therapies available to attenuate this catabolic response. Thus, this chapter aims to review the pathophysiological mechanisms, the clinical consequences, and therapeutic implications of the hypermetabolic response to burn injury.

19.1 Introduction

A hallmark of the metabolic response to burn injury is the development of "hypermetabolism," which is associated with a plethora of pathological alterations in endocrine, metabolic, and inflammatory and immunological responses. During

A. Abdullahi
Institute of Medical Science, University of Toronto, Sunnybrook Health Sciences Centre, Rm M7140, 2075 Bayview Avenue, Toronto, ON M4N 3M5, Canada

D. Patsouris • S.R. Costford
Department of Surgery, University of Toronto, Sunnybrook Health Sciences Centre, Rm M7140, 2075 Bayview Avenue, Toronto, ON M4N 3M5, Canada

M.G. Jeschke (✉)
Division of Plastic Surgery, Department of Surgery, Department of Immunology, Ross Tilley Burn Centre – Sunnybrook Health Sciences Centre, Burn Research, Sunnybrook Research Institute, University of Toronto, Rm D7-04B, 2075 Bayview Avenue, Toronto, ON M4N 3M5, Canada
e-mail: marc.jeschke@sunnybrook.ca

J.-C. Preiser (ed.), *The Stress Response of Critical Illness: Metabolic and Hormonal Aspects*, DOI 10.1007/978-3-319-27687-8_19

the last decades, this hypermetabolic state with its concomitant hyperglycemia, lipolysis, hyperinflammation, and muscle wasting has been implicated as the major contributor of poor outcome and hospital stay. Thus, the quest for an effective therapy that can help to attenuate these deeply rooted metabolic changes has been and still is an unresolved priority in the care of critically ill patients. This chapter will give an overview of what is known from the metabolic and hormonal alterations described in critically ill burn patients. We will also focus on established and on new therapeutic parameters which can be used to attenuate persistent hypermetabolism, as well as the restoration of anabolic function.

19.2 Epidemiology

Burn injuries represent one of the most debilitating forms of trauma and rank fourth among most common types of trauma worldwide following traffic accidents, falls, and interpersonal violence [62]. More than two million people suffer from burn-related injuries each year in the United States alone [6]. According to the World Health Organization, there are 330,000 thermal-related deaths per year worldwide, and this death toll is disproportionately concentrated in Southeast Asia and Africa [62]. It is estimated that at least 300,000, and possibly as many as 17 million, cases of burn trauma occur in Africa each year [46]. Burn injury has a high mortality rate because unlike other forms of trauma, burns result in permanent pathological alterations in nearly every organ system of the human body.

Most thermal injuries in the Western world are caused by heat exposure due to scalding, flame contact with hot objects, and electrical or chemical exposure [20, 21]. Among these, burn injuries resulting from flame contact are most common in children and elderly populations, who are more prone to scalding accidents [6]. Electrical and chemical burn injuries, which are far more serious, occur to a lesser extent. Although thermal injury does not discriminate, groups with the highest risk for burn injury tend to be children, the elderly, the disabled, and individuals who abuse drugs or alcohol.

19.3 Hypermetabolic Response to Burn Injury

Burn injury results in a complex neuroendocrine and metabolic response termed the hypermetabolic response, which is initiated by neuronal and humoral signals from the site of injury. This hypermetabolic response and its associated metabolic changes are critical for survival. The hypermetabolic response perhaps developed through evolution as a survival mechanism to facilitate the mobilization of energy resources for wound repair; however, if this adaptive stress response becomes prolonged and heightened, it can result in significant depletion of fuel sources with detrimental consequences like multiorgan failure or even death [51]. Burn size is one of the major factors that determines the magnitude of the hypermetabolic response [53].

Burn injury that is localized to less than 15 % of total body surface area (TBSA) generally elicits a more subdued response, whereas as a severe burn injury (defined as ≥15 % TBSA) causes a more robust response [43, 51, 53]. In any case, manifestation of the hypermetabolic response upon activation is very complex and results in significant alterations to critical metabolic pathways, such as glycogenesis, gluconeogenesis, lipolysis, and proteolysis. Clinically, it has been shown that there appears to be two distinct phases of metabolic regulation post-burn injury [48, 89]. The first phase is termed the "ebb phase" and generally occurs within the first 48 h of thermal injury. It is characterized by increased oxygen consumption, reduced cardiac output, and a rise in plasma glucose [48]. During this acute ebb phase, energy expenditure tends to remain unchanged or even decreased and is accompanied by a decrease in core body temperature [48]. Progression from the ebb phase to the "flow phase" post-burn injury is associated with a dramatic increase in energy expenditure, the magnitude of which is related to the type, severity, and extent of the burn injury. This highly energy expensive phase can last for days or even months in cases where another insult occurs, such as sepsis, thereby complicating the clinical picture [48, 96]. If the flow phase is not resolved swiftly, it can transform into a persistent catabolic state that has dire consequences for patient outcomes [51]. Furthermore, severe burns have been shown to elicit massive release of inflammatory mediators, such as tumor necrosis factor–α (TNF-α) and interleukin (IL-1, IL-6, and IL-1β). Many of these pro-inflammatory mediators have been proposed to account for prolonging the hypermetabolic response. Most of the changes in the metabolic response to injury are concentrated mainly in the metabolically active tissues, liver, adipose, and skeletal muscle (Fig. 19.1).

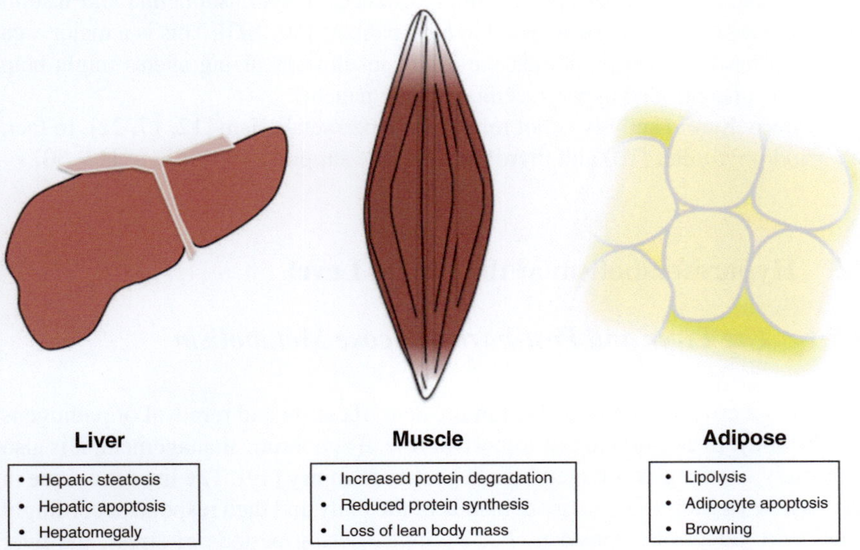

Fig. 19.1 Severe burn injury leads to profound alterations in the liver, muscle, and adipose tissue

19.4 Hormonal Regulation of Hyperglycemia Post-burn

Consisting of mainly dopamine, norepinephrine, and epinephrine, catecholamines are produced by the adrenal glands in response to stress. Catecholamines increase 10- to 20-fold normal in patients post-burn [12, 14, 31, 91] and correlate with energy expenditure [40]. Known for driving the "fight-or-flight" response, catecholamines have significant metabolic effects. They stimulate glycogenolysis in the liver [78], skeletal muscle [23], adipose tissue [83], and heart [44]. The glycogenolytic effect of epinephrine results in a parallel increase in blood glucose and lactate. Catecholamines also stimulate lipolysis post-burn, leading to high circulating free fatty acids (FFA) [99] and ectopic storage of lipid in the liver [8, 9].

Produced by the adrenal glands, the stress hormone cortisol is increased in patient's post-burn injury [14, 50] in proportion to burn size [25, 83]. In fact, the normal circadian fluctuations in plasma cortisol can be blunted [83] or completely abolished [58] following burn trauma. Cortisol stimulates both gluconeogenesis and glycogenolysis in the liver, contributing to hyperglycemia post-burn.

Produced by the alpha cells of the pancreas, glucagon is a catabolic hormone that is normally secreted when circulating glucose is low. It stimulates glycogenolysis in the liver, promoting release of glucose into the circulation. Glucagon levels rise immediately post-burn [3, 11, 90] in proportion to the burn size [84]. The actions of glucagon further complicate the regulation of glycemia in burn patients.

The anabolic hormone insulin is produced by the beta cells in the islets of Langerhans of the pancreas in response to high circulating levels of glucose. Insulin stimulates the uptake of glucose into peripheral tissues and suppresses hepatic glucose output (glycogenolysis and gluconeogenesis) in order to regulate glycemia. If the periphery and the liver become insensitive to the actions of insulin, blood glucose remains high despite hyperinsulinemia, a state termed "insulin resistance." Hyperinsulinemia and insulin resistance have been well-documented in burn patients [50, 103]. This is a major area of study; it has been suggested that the use of insulin-sensitizing agents might help alleviate the uncontrolled hyperglycemia in these patients.

Post-burn thyroid activity is not related to hypermetabolism [12, 17, 22]. In fact, both triiodothyronine (T3) and thyroxine (T4) are suppressed post-burn [13, 50].

19.5 Hypermetabolism at the Organ Level

19.5.1 The Liver and Post-burn Glucose Metabolism

The liver is a critical organ involved in the detoxification and removal of pathogens from the body. In addition to this important role in xenobiotic management, it is also the primary site for glucose metabolism post-burn injury [49]. The liver is unique in that it is able to gauge the energy demands of the body and then respond accordingly to maintain glucose homeostasis. For example, during periods of stress, the liver responds by activating glycogenolysis and gluconeogenesis, two metabolic pathways that generate glucose and ultimately elevate plasma glucose levels [49, 98]. This critical function of the liver to adequately sense and regulate glucose homeostasis becomes impaired post-burn injury. Although burn patients become hyperglycemic, the liver continues to release large amounts of glucose at increased rates, even though there is impaired uptake of glucose in the peripheral tissues [49, 98]. Prolonged, uncontrolled hyperglycemia is detrimental and associated with adverse clinical outcomes post-burn injury [32]. In fact, a number of studies in burn patients have shown that hyperglycemia is associated with increased infections and sepsis, increased incidence of pneumonia, and most importantly, with an increased post-burn risk of mortality [32, 41, 54]. During critical illness or injury, elevated levels of catecholamines promote adipose tissue lipolysis and the release of FFA into the portal circulation. FFA are taken up by the liver for energy production; however, if elevated circulating levels of FFA persist, the hepatic influx of FFA exceeds the liver's ability to generate ATP through fatty acid oxidation, and the result is an accumulation of stored lipid in the liver [49]. Hepatic steatosis has devastating implications for hepatic function. Indeed, postmortem studies of burn patients who died with multiorgan failure have revealed hepatic changes such as hepatomegaly, steatosis, necrosis, and apoptosis [49, 68].

19.5.2 Skeletal Muscle and Post-burn Protein Metabolism

Skeletal muscle is the largest tissue in the body, accounting for 45 % of total body weight [97]. It is also responsible for more than 70 % of postprandial whole body glucose uptake [97]. Skeletal muscle is one of the tissues most affected by burn trauma. During periods of stress or injury, skeletal muscle protein is catabolized to release amino acids that are ultimately used for endogenous glucose production by the liver [66]. Muscle catabolism is further exacerbated by increased circulating proinflammatory cytokines in the critically ill and eventually leads to significant losses in muscle mass [33]. It is believed that this loss of muscle mass results from both a decrease in protein synthesis and an increase in protein degradation [33]. Burn patients experience a 10–15 % loss in muscle mass, which has been linked to poor outcomes [48]. A number of studies have shown that significant losses in muscle mass not only impair immediate healing from the injury, but also have long-term effects on functional capacity even after the immediate injury has been resolved [29, 33, 66].

19.5.3 Adipose Tissue and Browning

For many years, white adipose tissue (WAT) was considered as an inert organ whose only function was the storage of excess energy in the form of triglyceride. It is now known that WAT is a complex endocrine organ that secretes hormones termed "adipokines" and participates in metabolic cross talk with skeletal muscle, liver, and the hypothalamus. Brown adipose tissue (BAT) is a thermogenic organ characterized by multilocular lipid droplets, expression of uncoupling protein-1 (UCP1), and a high density of mitochondria, which account for its brown color [18, 61] (Fig. 19.2). UCP1, a classical mitochondrial uncoupler, is upregulated in response to cold or high levels of circulating free fatty acids [18, 61]. UCP1 allows protons to return to the mitochondrial matrix, bypassing ATP synthase and effectively uncoupling oxidation of the electron transport chain from the phosphorylation of ADP. The energy that is wasted through this "proton leak" is dissipated as heat. For many years, it was believed that the BAT existed only in human infants and disappeared with age; however, BAT has recently been discovered in small pockets in human adults [24, 82, 86]. This discovery is of great interest in the field of obesity, as it represents a mechanism of energy wasting that was previously thought to be impossible in human adults [27, 39].

Cold-induced activation of BAT is mediated by catecholamines that are released from the nerves that innervate BAT. Catecholamines also stimulate lipolysis, releasing FFA from triglyceride, which further activates UCP1 [18, 27]. The thermogenic function of the BAT is necessary for maintenance of core body temperature in human infants, but not in adults. Rather, the function of BAT in adults has rather been associated with increased energy expenditure, as BAT correlates inversely with BMI [57, 85]. Two independent teams have developed a protocol to stimulate BAT in human adults to result in significant weight loss [81, 102]. Research to identify effective and safe drugs to activate these pathways is underway [88].

An intermediate form of adipose tissue has been recently identified and termed "beige" or "brite" adipose tissue [30, 39]. Beige adipose tissue is multilocular like BAT and is rich in UCP1-expressing mitochondria, although to a lower degree than BAT (Fig. 19.2). WAT can be differentiated into beige adipose tissue in rodents, a process referred to as "beiging" or "browning" [10, 15]. While browning of WAT

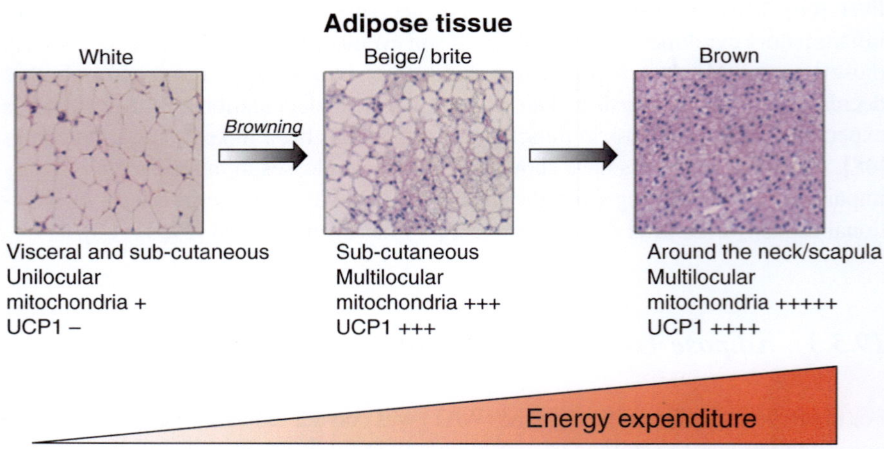

Fig. 19.2 Characteristics of the different classes of adipose tissue found in humans

and increased energy expenditure can be beneficiary in obese or diabetic patients, browning of WAT has been associated with muscle wasting in cachectic patients, a situation in which increased energy expenditure is detrimental [64]. BAT in adult humans is localized around the neck area, whereas the largest depot in mice is interscapular (Fig. 19.3). It is the delocalized subcutaneous WAT that is capable of undergoing browning in humans or the defined inguinal WAT depot in mice.

Recently, Yo et al. discovered that burn injury activates UCP1 in BAT and increases metabolic activity in rats [101]. Furthermore, blockade of BAT activity was sufficient to prevent the burn-induced elevation of metabolic activity. This was a significant finding, as it suggested for the first time that the BAT plays a major role in the increased energy expenditure following thermal injury. In support of these findings, two consecutive publications from the same group demonstrated that burn injury induces the browning of subcutaneous adipose tissue in mice and children [65, 75]. This remodeling of white adipocytes results in multilocularity, increased mitochondrial content, increased expression of UCP1, and increased uncoupling of oxidative phosphorylation, all characteristics of BAT. The browning process requires several days post-burn to become evident at the morphological level. UCP1 expression is first detected 9 days post-burn and increases until 31 days post-burn. This observation is of great importance as it provides an alternative treatment route for hypermetabolism. To date, however, the factors mediating this remodeling have not been identified. The elevated catecholamines that typically follow burn and

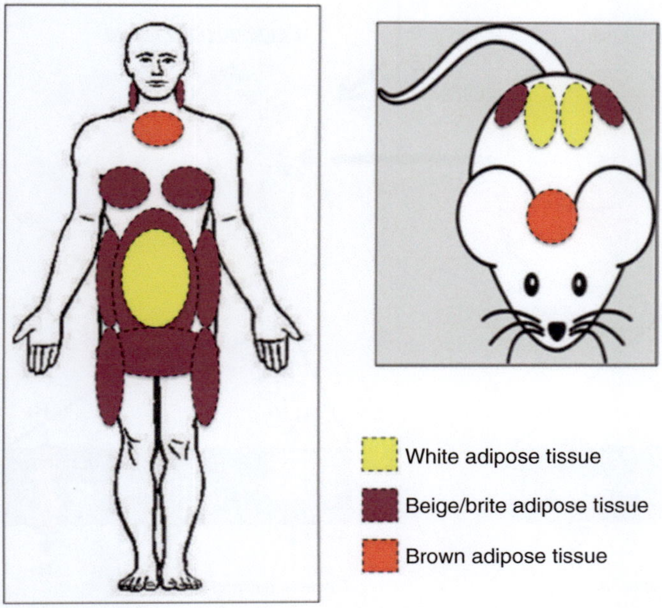

Fig. 19.3 A summary of the location of the different fat depots in rodents and humans

trauma have been implicated in mediating subcutaneous browning; however, this hypothesis has not yet been verified (Fig. 19.4).

19.6 Multiorgan Failure

Although, failure of the metabolic tissues discussed earlier in burn and septic patients has received considerable attention in the context of clinical management and scientific research. It is now clear that several other organs like the brain, the kidneys, and the gut are adversely affected by the stress response to injury.

19.6.1 The Brain

The brain is a critical organ that defines the internal and external response to stress of the body. It accomplishes this by activating the hypothalamic-pituitary-adrenal (HPA) axis, a key adaptive neuroendocrine system that is central to all responses to

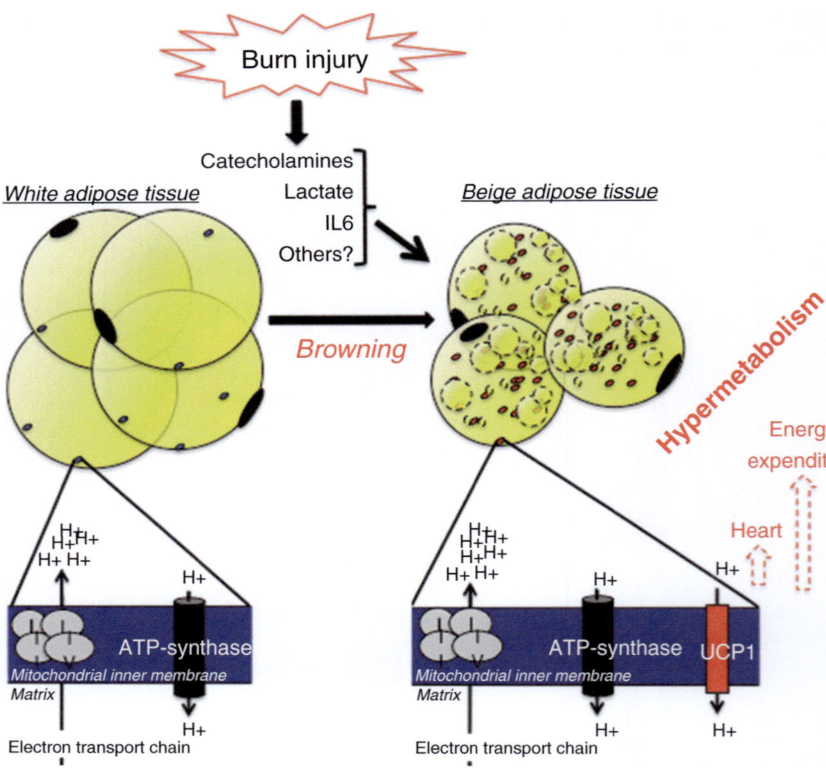

Fig. 19.4 Burn injury results in browning of subcutaneous adipose tissue

stress post injury [63]. In fact, many of the hormonal mediators discussed earlier like cortisol and catecholamines are directly regulated by HPA. Depending on the level of activation (chronic vs. acute) of the HPA axis, it can facilitate a response that is either adaptive or damaging in regard to the injury [63]. Indeed, chronic activation of the HPA axis post injury has been implicated in the structural and functional breakdown of the central nervous system [47, 73]. For instance, postmortem pathology of the brain of severe burn patients has revealed significant hippocampus and prefrontal cortex atrophy, cerebral infarcts and hemorrhages, and metabolic encephalopathies [93]. These alterations in brain function and structure can have long-lasting adverse effects for these patients in terms of memory loss, anxiety, and anger issues, as well as learning deficits.

19.6.2 The Kidney

While the pathophysiology of burn injury leading to renal failure is not fully understood, it likely involves diminished renal blood flow and glomerular filtration rate. In addition, reductions in stress hormones such as angiotensin, aldosterone, and vasopressin post-burn injury have been implicated in the vasoconstriction of renal arteries and further reductions in renal blood supply [2]. Collectively, these hormonal and systemic responses to stress result in oliguria, which if not resolved swiftly manifests into acute tubular necrosis and renal failure [45]. Failure to resolve and restore adequate blood flow to the kidneys and the resultant renal failure has dire consequences for patient outcome and recovery. In fact, studies have shown that severely burned adults have an 88 % mortality rate upon the development of renal failure [45, 60, 95]. Fortunately renal failure can be managed successfully with dialysis until function returns, but the latter is usually linked to the recovery of other organs, especially the liver.

19.6.3 The Gut

The stress response to injury has also been associated with the onset and exacerbation of a number of gastrointestinal disorders like gastroesophageal reflux disease, inflammatory bowel disease, and peptic ulcers. The hormonal context that ensues following the stress response to injuries like burns and sepsis has been associated with altering the amicable relationship between hosts and their bacterial microenvironment. Accordingly, studies in burn patients have shown mucosal atrophy, malabsorption, and increased intestinal permeability [69, 72, 100]. These changes in gut permeability have dire consequences for patient outcome as it facilitates bacterial translocation and ultimately sepsis [26]. It is therefore important to further study the fundamental changes in the gut, induced by stress, in order to find therapeutic interventions to restore correct GI integrity and function.

19.7 Therapeutic Strategies to Curtail the Hypermetabolic Response

It is important to note that the adverse alterations in metabolism and the mechanisms underlying the development of persistent hypermetabolism that occurs post-burn injury are still not completely understood; however, progress has been made in the development of therapeutic strategies to curtail the adverse events associated with this response. Two types of therapeutic interventions, nutritional support and pharmacotherapy, are used to attempt to modulate hypermetabolism (Tables 19.1 and 19.2). It is believed that the increased energy and nutritional requirements post-burn injury can be met by nutritional provision. It is also believed that hormone repletion and drug therapy can restrict catabolism of vital tissues and promote an anabolic state. In both cases, the net goal is to halt catabolism, normalize glycemia, and improve patient outcome.

19.8 Nutritional Support

Due to the metabolic response to injury, most burn and critically ill patients present with complex nutritional needs and require intensive nutritional support. The aim of nutritional provision in burn patients in particular has been to normalize resting energy expenditure, improve lean body mass, and promote successful wound repair [1]. Despite the widespread agreement of the use of nutritional support in critically

Table 19.1 Nutritional recommendations for burn patients

Nutrient	Recommendation
Carbohydrate	5–7 mg/kg/min
Protein	1.5–2 g/kg/day
Lipids	<20 % of nonprotein calories

Nutritional recommendations based on guidelines from the Ross Tilley Burn Center, American Burn Association, American Society for Parenteral and Enteral Nutrition, and European Society for Clinical Nutrition and Metabolism

Table 19.2 Common anabolic agents used in burns

Nutrient	Target tissue	Effect
Insulin	Liver	Decreases proteolysis
	Muscle tissue	Improves lean body mass
	Fat tissue	Decreases fat oxidation
Insulin-like growth factor 1	Muscle tissue	Improves lean body mass
		Decreases proteolysis
Propranolol	Fat tissue	Decreases fat oxidation
		Promotes glucose homeostasis

Commonly used and prescribed anabolic agents utilized in the care of burn patients to modulate the hypermetabolic response ill patients, there still remains a lack of consensus as to what this nutritional support should encompass [79]. The only recommendations that have been put forth are by the American and the European parenteral enteral nutrition societies [56, 71]. In line with these recommendations, we at the Ross Tilley Burn Center recommend the use of high carbohydrate/high glucose, high protein/amino acid intake in the clinical management of hypermetabolism (Table 19.1) [38]. We are also of the opinion that the most physiological method of administering nutritional support is enteral nutrition (EN) as opposed to parenteral nutrition. This is due to the countless studies and trials that have shown that EN has beneficial effects on the patient's immunocompetence as well as on intestinal integrity and gut-associated immune activity [4, 59, 87].

The rationale for high carbohydrate provision in burn patients is not only to improve wound healing, but also to halt further deficits in lean body mass by sparing protein stores. It is important to note that substrate utilization patterns differ markedly from patient to patient depending on the type, the severity, and the duration of injury. Additionally, there seems to be a maximum rate of glucose that can be absorbed and oxidized in most critically ill patients. In burn patients, the minimum baseline adult carbohydrate requirement is 2 g/kg/day, and the maximum rate at which glucose can be absorbed in severely burned patients is 7 g/kg/day [16, 38, 48, 67, 74]. It is important to keep in mind that over-provision of nutrients is just as devastating as under-provision in these critically ill patients; thus, for burn patients, we suggest the delivery of carbohydrate support in the amount of 55–60 % of total energy intake without surpassing 5 mg/kg/min in adults and children, which corresponds to 7 g/kg/day in adult patients [70, 87].

Since significant losses in lean body mass are hallmarks of burn and critical illness, protein and amino acid supplementation have been suggested to remedy such losses. In fact, it has been reported that burn patients can lose up to 150 g/day or one-half pound of lean muscle tissue post injury [33, 66, 89]. The recommended protein intake for healthy individuals is estimated to be 0.8–1 g/kg/day [38, 70]. Given that burn patients oxidize proteins at rates greater than 50 % than their healthier counterparts [48, 76], it is recommended that protein intake be 1.5–2 g/kg/day in burned adults and 2.5–4.0 g/kg/day in burned children [38, 56, 71]. Again, it is important to stress that with all recommendations, the protein needs will vary from individual to individual and will depend on the nature and severity of the injury. Aside from total protein supplementation, many clinical trials have examined the impact of supplementation of specific amino acids, such as glutamine, as part of EN therapy in critically ill patients [92]. These glutamine supplementation trials have shown benefits with regard to wound healing, muscle loss, and infection, thereby reducing length of ICU stay [28, 94].

19.9 Pharmacotherapy

The increased metabolic demands and catabolism that ensue after trauma or burn injury are not always met by a simple increase in energy intake. Successful management of hypermetabolism requires the repletion of hormones that can only be met through pharmacological approaches. Due to their known anti-catabolic effects, three pharmacological agents (insulin, metformin, and propranolol) have received considerable attention in the management of injury-induced hypermetabolism (Table 19.2) [1]. In essence, it is believed that the action of these agents in concert can cease catabolism by putting the brakes on lipolysis, glycogenolysis, and gluconeogenesis.

19.10 Insulin

Insulin is perhaps the most studied and recognized anabolic hormone for its effects on ameliorating protein breakdown and normalizing plasma glucose levels in critically ill patients. In fact, it is the loss of the actions of insulin, in particular the development of insulin resistance, that is the main culprit of the series of pathological alterations and the consequent hypermetabolic state that occurs in response to injury. As such, intensive insulin therapy in burn patients has been shown to lower infection rates and improves survival [41]. A number of other clinical trials have also confirmed these findings, in which intensive insulin therapy in burn patients was associated with a reduced incidence of pneumonia, ventilator-associated pneumonia, and urinary tract infection [41, 52, 80]. Although insulin may have some anabolic effects, it is also a double-edged sword in that it becomes detrimental when it causes an episode of hypoglycemia [5]. It is therefore imperative to find another agent that can achieve glucose control without the adverse effects of hypoglycemia.

19.11 Metformin

Metformin is a commonly prescribed antidiabetic drug from the biguanide class of oral hypoglycemic agents and has been shown to have several beneficial effects on human metabolism [36, 77]. Metformin's main action is to normalize glycemia by decreasing hepatic glucose production and improving insulin sensitivity in the periphery, promoting glucose uptake and utilization in skeletal muscle and adipose tissue [77]. Interestingly, metformin has also gained recent recognition for its effects on slowing down aging and increasing life span [55]. Most of what is known about metformin has been revealed through studies in diabetic patients. As such, there is little information regarding the use of metformin in severely burned patients. Given the issues surrounding insulin and the alarming rate of hypoglycemia in critically ill patients [5], metformin is currently being investigated as a safe alternative means to correct hyperglycemia in these patients. In fact, a few studies have already shown promising evidence that metformin improves lean body mass and attenuates muscle catabolism in severely burned patients [34, 36, 37]; however, the appropriate dose, timing, mechanism of action, and clinical settings for the use of metformin in place of insulin are largely unknown.

19.12 Propranolol

Recently, the unspecific beta-blocker propranolol has been shown to be effective in improving hypermetabolism in burned pediatric patients, which supports the notion that catecholamines mediate burn-induced browning and lipolysis of the subcutaneous fat; however, IL6 and lactate are also known inducers of browning whose concentrations are elevated post-burn, and these factors could also stimulate the remodeling of WAT post-burn [19, 64]. The beneficial effects of propranolol on reducing muscle wasting, increasing lean body mass, and preventing hepatic steatosis post-burn injury are well characterized [7, 35, 42]. Unfortunately, WAT browning is a mechanism that has only been described recently, and there is little information available describing the effects of propranolol on WAT browning. In the context of cachexia, Petruzzeli et al. showed that beta-adrenergic signaling blockade interfered with cancer-induced WAT browning [19]; however, although plausible, it is uncertain whether this holds true in burned patients. In summary, more work will be necessary to determine the effects of propranolol and other beta-blockers on WAT browning.

As a result of the complexity of the metabolic response, a number of these therapeutic strategies have failed when used exclusively as a strategy to curtail this adverse metabolic response. Instead, success has occurred when these distinct therapeutic strategies (nutritional support and pharmacotherapy) have been combined in the clinical management of hypermetabolism [1]. Furthermore, new promising therapeutic agents are being tested such as the anabolic steroid analogue oxandrolone that is believed to attenuate muscle wasting, as well as the glucagon-like peptide that aims to target post-burn hyperglycemia.

19.13 Conclusion

The primary aim of this chapter was to acquire knowledge concerning the metabolic, endocrine, inflammatory, and hormonal stress responses in the context of burn injury. It must be kept in mind that this response is not a uniform response across the organs, but regulated by a number of mediators with many interlaced parts that often work together in a nonlinear fashion. It is encouraging, however, that this complex hypermetabolic response to injury is gradually becoming better understood and studied at the microscopic level. With a better understanding of the mediators of persistent hypermetabolism, healthcare providers may stand a chance at curtailing the adverse effects of this response on patient outcome. Despite the difficulties in selecting the appropriate therapy for each patient, nutrition and pharmacotherapy have become the most popular and widely used in the care of burn patients. Ideally, comprehensive-based therapeutic approaches that utilize both avenues of therapy offer the best chance of success in curbing this hypermetabolic response.

References

1. Abdullahi A, Jeschke MG (2014) Nutrition and anabolic pharmacotherapies in the care of burn patients. Nutr Clin Pract 29(5):621–630
2. Aikawa N, Wakabayashi G, Ueda M, Shinozawa Y (1990) Regulation of renal function in thermal injury. J Trauma 30(12 Suppl):S174–S178
3. Alberti KG, Batstone GF, Foster KJ, Johnston DG (1980) Relative role of various hormones in mediating the metabolic response to injury. JPEN J Parenter Enteral Nutr 4(2):141–146
4. Alverdy J, Chi HS, Sheldon GF (1985) The effect of parenteral nutrition on gastrointestinal immunity. The importance of enteral stimulation. Ann Surg 202(6):681–684
5. Arabi YM, Tamim HM, Rishu AH (2009) Hypoglycemia with intensive insulin therapy in critically ill patients: predisposing factors and association with mortality. Crit Care Med 37(9):2536–2544. doi:10.1097/CCM.0b013e3181a381ad
6. Association AB (2012) Burn Incidence and Treatment in the United States. http://www.ameriburn.org/resources_factsheet.php
7. Baron PW, Barrow RE, Pierre EJ, Herndon DN (1997) Prolonged use of propranolol safely decreases cardiac work in burned children. J Burn Care Rehabil 18(3):223–227
8. Barret JP, Jeschke MG, Herndon DN (2001) Fatty infiltration of the liver in severely burned pediatric patients: autopsy findings and clinical implications. J Trauma 51(4):736–739
9. Barrow RE, Mlcak R, Barrow LN, Hawkins HK (2004) Increased liver weights in severely burned children: comparison of ultrasound and autopsy measurements. Burns 30(6):565–568. doi:10.1016/j.burns.2004.01.027
10. Bartelt A, Heeren J (2014) Adipose tissue browning and metabolic health. Nat Rev Endocrinol 10(1):24–36. doi:10.1038/nrendo.2013.204
11. Batstone GF, Hinks L, Whitefoot R, Bloom S, Laing JE (1976) Proceedings: hormonal changes after thermal injury. J Endocrinol 68(3):38P–39P
12. Becker RA, Vaughan GM, Goodwin CW Jr, Ziegler MG, Harrison TS, Mason AD Jr, Pruitt BA (1980) Plasma norepinephrine, epinephrine, and thyroid hormone interactions in severely burned patients. Arch Surg 115(4):439–443
13. Becker RA, Vaughan GM, Ziegler MG, Seraile LG, Goldfarb IW, Mansour EH, McManus WF, Pruitt BA Jr, Mason AD Jr (1982) Hypermetabolic low triiodothyronine syndrome of burn injury. Crit Care Med 10(12):870–875
14. Birke G, Duner H, Liljedahl SO, Pernow B, Plantin LO, Troell L (1958) Histamine, catecholamines and adrenocortical steroids in burns. Acta Chir Scand 114(2):87–98
15. Bonet ML, Oliver P, Palou A (2013) Pharmacological and nutritional agents promoting browning of white adipose tissue. Biochim Biophys Acta 1831(5):969–985. doi:10.1016/j.bbalip.2012.12.002
16. Burke JF, Wolfe RR, Mullany CJ, Mathews DE, Bier DM (1979) Glucose requirements following burn injury. Parameters of optimal glucose infusion and possible hepatic and respiratory abnormalities following excessive glucose intake. Ann Surg 190(3):274–285
17. Caldwell FT Jr (1960) The role of the thyroid gland in the production of the hypermetabolic state occurring in rats with full-thickness burns. Endocrinology 67:363–367. doi:10.1210/endo-67-3-363
18. Cannon B, Nedergaard J (2004) Brown adipose tissue: function and physiological significance. Physiol Rev 84(1):277–359. doi:10.1152/physrev.00015.2003
19. Carriere A, Jeanson Y, Berger-Muller S, Andre M, Chenouard V, Arnaud E, Barreau C, Walther R, Galinier A, Wdziekonski B, Villageois P, Louche K, Collas P, Moro C, Dani C, Villarroya F, Casteilla L (2014) Browning of white adipose cells by intermediate metabolites: an adaptive mechanism to alleviate redox pressure. Diabetes 63(10):3253–3265. doi:10.2337/db13-1885
20. Clouatre E, Gomez M, Banfield JM, Jeschke MG (2013) Work-related burn injuries in Ontario, Canada: a follow-up 10-year retrospective study. Burns 39(6):1091–1095. doi:10.1016/j.burns.2012.12.020

21. Clouatre E, Pinto R, Banfield J, Jeschke MG (2013) Incidence of hot tap water scalds after the introduction of regulations in Ontario. J Burn Care Res 34(2):243–248. doi:10.1097/BCR.0b013e3182789057
22. Cope O, Nardi GL, Quijano M, Rovit RL, Stanbury JB, Wight A (1953) Metabolic rate and thyroid function following acute thermal trauma in man. Ann Surg 137(2):165–174
23. Cori GT, Illingworth B (1956) The effect of epinephrine and other glycogenolytic agents on the phosphorylase A content of muscle. Biochim Biophys Acta 21(1):105–110
24. Cypess AM, Lehman S, Williams G, Tal I, Rodman D, Goldfine AB, Kuo FC, Palmer EL, Tseng YH, Doria A, Kolodny GM, Kahn CR (2009) Identification and importance of brown adipose tissue in adult humans. N Engl J Med 360(15):1509–1517. doi:10.1056/NEJMoa0810780
25. Dolecek R (1985) The endocrine response after burns: its possible correlations with the immunology of burns. J Burn Care Rehabil 6(3):281–294
26. Earley ZM, Akhtar S, Green SJ, Naqib A, Khan O, Cannon AR, Hammer AM, Morris NL, Li X, Eberhardt JM, Gamelli RL, Kennedy RH, Choudhry MA (2015) Burn injury alters the intestinal microbiome and increases gut permeability and bacterial translocation. PLoS One 10(7):e0129996. doi:10.1371/journal.pone.0129996
27. Fedorenko A, Lishko PV, Kirichok Y (2012) Mechanism of fatty-acid-dependent UCP1 uncoupling in brown fat mitochondria. Cell 151(2):400–413. doi:10.1016/j.cell.2012.09.010
28. Garrel D, Patenaude J, Nedelec B, Samson L, Dorais J, Champoux J, D'Elia M, Bernier J (2003) Decreased mortality and infectious morbidity in adult burn patients given enteral glutamine supplements: a prospective, controlled, randomized clinical trial. Crit Care Med 31(10):2444–2449. doi:10.1097/01.CCM.0000084848.63691.1E
29. Gauglitz GG, Herndon DN, Kulp GA, Meyer WJ 3rd, Jeschke MG (2009) Abnormal insulin sensitivity persists up to three years in pediatric patients post-burn. J Clin Endocrinol Metab 94(5):1656–1664. doi:10.1210/jc.2008-1947
30. Giralt M, Villarroya F (2013) White, brown, beige/brite: different adipose cells for different functions? Endocrinology 154(9):2992–3000. doi:10.1210/en.2013-1403
31. Goodall M, Stone C, Haynes BW Jr (1957) Urinary output of adrenaline and noradrenaline in severe thermal burns. Ann Surg 145(4):479–487
32. Gore DC, Chinkes D, Heggers J, Herndon DN, Wolf SE, Desai M (2001) Association of hyperglycemia with increased mortality after severe burn injury. J Trauma 51(3):540–544
33. Gore DC, Chinkes DL, Hart DW, Wolf SE, Herndon DN, Sanford AP (2002) Hyperglycemia exacerbates muscle protein catabolism in burn-injured patients. Crit Care Med 30(11):2438–2442. doi:10.1097/01.CCM.0000034728.52842.EB
34. Gore DC, Herndon DN, Wolfe RR (2005) Comparison of peripheral metabolic effects of insulin and metformin following severe burn injury. J Trauma 59(2):316–322; discussion 322–323
35. Gore DC, Honeycutt D, Jahoor F, Barrow RE, Wolfe RR, Herndon DN (1991) Propranolol diminishes extremity blood flow in burned patients. Ann Surg 213(6):568–573; discussion 573–574
36. Gore DC, Wolf SE, Herndon DN, Wolfe RR (2003) Metformin blunts stress-induced hyperglycemia after thermal injury. J Trauma 54(3):555–561. doi:10.1097/01.TA.0000026990.32856.58
37. Gore DC, Wolf SE, Sanford A, Herndon DN, Wolfe RR (2005) Influence of metformin on glucose intolerance and muscle catabolism following severe burn injury. Ann Surg 241(2):334–342
38. Hall KL, Shahrokhi S, Jeschke MG (2012) Enteral nutrition support in burn care: a review of current recommendations as instituted in the Ross Tilley Burn Centre. Nutrients 4(11):1554–1565. doi:10.3390/nu4111554
39. Harms M, Seale P (2013) Brown and beige fat: development, function and therapeutic potential. Nat Med 19(10):1252–1263. doi:10.1038/nm.3361
40. Harrison TS, Seaton JF, Feller I (1967) Relationship of increased oxygen consumption to catecholamine excretion in thermal burns. Ann Surg 165(2):169–172

41. Hemmila MR, Taddonio MA, Arbabi S, Maggio PM, Wahl WL (2008) Intensive insulin therapy is associated with reduced infectious complications in burn patients. Surgery 144(4):629–635. doi:10.1016/j.surg.2008.07.001; discussion 635–637
42. Herndon DN, Hart DW, Wolf SE, Chinkes DL, Wolfe RR (2001) Reversal of catabolism by beta-blockade after severe burns. N Engl J Med 345(17):1223–1229. doi:10.1056/NEJMoa010342
43. Herndon DN, Tompkins RG (2004) Support of the metabolic response to burn injury. Lancet 363(9424):1895–1902. doi:10.1016/S0140-6736(04)16360-5
44. Hess ME, Haugaard N (1958) The effect of epinephrine and aminophylline on the phosphorylase activity of perfused contracting heart muscle. J Pharmacol Exp Ther 122(2):169–175
45. Holm C, Horbrand F, von Donnersmarck GH, Muhlbauer W (1999) Acute renal failure in severely burned patients. Burns 25(2):171–178
46. Hyder A, Kashyap K, Fishman S, Wali S (2004) Review of Childhood Burn Injuries in Sub-Saharan Africa: A Forgotten Public Health Challenge. African Safety Promotion Vol 2:43–58.
47. Isao T, Masaki F, Riko N, Seiichi H (2005) Delayed brain atrophy after electrical injury. J Burn Care Rehabil 26(5):456–458
48. Jeschke MG, Kamolz LP, Sjoberg F, Wolf SE (2012) Handbook of burns, vol 1. Springer, Wien/New York
49. Jeschke MG (2009) The hepatic response to thermal injury: is the liver important for postburn outcomes? Mol Med 15(9–10):337–351. doi:10.2119/molmed.2009.00005
50. Jeschke MG, Chinkes DL, Finnerty CC, Kulp G, Suman OE, Norbury WB, Branski LK, Gauglitz GG, Mlcak RP, Herndon DN (2008) Pathophysiologic response to severe burn injury. Ann Surg 248(3):387–401. doi:10.1097/SLA.0b013e3181856241
51. Jeschke MG, Gauglitz GG, Finnerty CC, Kraft R, Mlcak RP, Herndon DN (2013) Survivors versus nonsurvivors postburn: differences in inflammatory and hypermetabolic trajectories. Ann Surg. doi:10.1097/SLA.0b013e31828dfbf1
52. Jeschke MG, Kulp GA, Kraft R, Finnerty CC, Mlcak R, Lee JO, Herndon DN (2010) Intensive insulin therapy in severely burned pediatric patients: a prospective randomized trial. Am J Respir Crit Care Med 182(3):351–359. doi:10.1164/rccm.201002-0190OC
53. Jeschke MG, Mlcak RP, Finnerty CC, Norbury WB, Gauglitz GG, Kulp GA, Herndon DN (2007) Burn size determines the inflammatory and hypermetabolic response. Crit Care 11(4):R90. doi:10.1186/cc6102
54. Kraft R, Herndon DN, Mlcak RP, Finnerty CC, Cox RA, Williams FN, Jeschke MG (2013) Bacterial respiratory tract infections are promoted by systemic hyperglycemia after severe burn injury in pediatric patients. Burns. doi:10.1016/j.burns.2013.07.007
55. Martin-Montalvo A, Mercken EM, Mitchell SJ, Palacios HH, Mote PL, Scheibye-Knudsen M, Gomes AP, Ward TM, Minor RK, Blouin MJ, Schwab M, Pollak M, Zhang Y, Yu Y, Becker KG, Bohr VA, Ingram DK, Sinclair DA, Wolf NS, Spindler SR, Bernier M, de Cabo R (2013) Metformin improves healthspan and lifespan in mice. Nat Commun 4:2192. doi:10.1038/ncomms3192
56. Martindale RG, McClave SA, Vanek VW, McCarthy M, Roberts P, Taylor B, Ochoa JB, Napolitano L, Cresci G, American College of Critical Care Medicine; A.S.P.E.N. Board of Directors (2009) Guidelines for the provision and assessment of nutrition support therapy in the adult critically ill patient: Society of Critical Care Medicine and American Society for Parenteral and Enteral Nutrition: executive summary. Crit Care Med 37(5):1757–1761. doi:10.1097/CCM.0b013e3181a40116
57. Matsushita M, Yoneshiro T, Aita S, Kameya T, Sugie H, Saito M (2014) Impact of brown adipose tissue on body fatness and glucose metabolism in healthy humans. Int J Obes (Lond) 38(6):812–817. doi:10.1038/ijo.2013.206
58. Molteni A, Warpeha RL, Brizio-Molteni L, Albertson DF, Kaurs R (1979) Circadian rhythms of serum aldosterone, cortisol and plasma renin activity in burn injuries. Ann Clin Lab Sci 9(6):518–523
59. Moore EE, Jones TN (1986) Benefits of immediate jejunostomy feeding after major abdominal trauma – a prospective, randomized study. J Trauma 26(10):874–881

60. Mustonen KM, Vuola J (2008) Acute renal failure in intensive care burn patients (ARF in burn patients). J Burn Care Res 29(1):227–237. doi:10.1097/BCR.0b013e31815f3196
61. Oelkrug R, Polymeropoulos ET, Jastroch M (2015) Brown adipose tissue: physiological function and evolutionary significance. J Comp Physiol B 185(6):587–606. doi:10.1007/s00360-015-0907-7
62. Organization, W. H. (2012). Burns. http://www.who.int/mediacentre/factsheets/fs365/en/
63. Palmieri TL, Levine S, Schonfeld-Warden N, O'Mara MS, Greenhalgh DG (2006) Hypothalamic-pituitary-adrenal axis response to sustained stress after major burn injury in children. J Burn Care Res 27(5):742–748. doi:10.1097/01.BCR.0000238098.43888.07
64. Petruzzelli M, Schweiger M, Schreiber R, Campos-Olivas R, Tsoli M, Allen J, Swarbrick M, Rose-John S, Rincon M, Robertson G, Zechner R, Wagner EF (2014) A switch from white to brown fat increases energy expenditure in cancer-associated cachexia. Cell Metab 20(3):433–447. doi:10.1016/j.cmet.2014.06.011
65. Porter C, Herndon DN, Bhattarai N, Ogunbileje JO, Szczesny B, Szabo C, Toliver-Kinsky T, Sidossis LS (2015) Severe burn injury induces thermogenically functional mitochondria in murine white adipose tissue. Shock 44(3):258–264. doi:10.1097/SHK.0000000000000410
66. Porter C, Herndon DN, Sidossis LS, Borsheim E (2013) The impact of severe burns on skeletal muscle mitochondrial function. Burns 39(6):1039–1047. doi:10.1016/j.burns.2013.03.018
67. Prelack K, Dylewski M, Sheridan RL (2007) Practical guidelines for nutritional management of burn injury and recovery. Burns 33(1):14–24. doi:10.1016/j.burns.2006.06.014
68. Price LA, Thombs B, Chen CL, Milner SM (2007) Liver disease in burn injury: evidence from a national sample of 31,338 adult patients. J Burns Wounds 7:e1
69. Ramzy PI, Wolf SE, Irtun O, Hart DW, Thompson JC, Herndon DN (2000) Gut epithelial apoptosis after severe burn: effects of gut hypoperfusion. J Am Coll Surg 190(3):281–287
70. Rodriguez NA, Jeschke MG, Williams FN, Kamolz LP, Herndon DN (2011) Nutrition in burns: Galveston contributions. JPEN J Parenter Enteral Nutr 35(6):704–714. doi:10.1177/0148607111417446
71. Rousseau AF, Losser MR, Ichai C, Berger MM (2013) ESPEN endorsed recommendations: nutritional therapy in major burns. Clin Nutr 32(4):497–502. doi:10.1016/j.clnu.2013.02.012
72. Ryan CM, Yarmush ML, Burke JF, Tompkins RG (1992) Increased gut permeability early after burns correlates with the extent of burn injury. Crit Care Med 20(11):1508–1512
73. Scholz T, Rippmann V, Wojtecki L, Perbix W, Rothschild MA, Spilker G (2006) Severe brain damage by current flow after electrical burn injury. J Burn Care Res 27(6):917–922. doi:10.1097/01.BCR.0000245646.80680.26
74. Sheridan RL, Yu YM, Prelack K, Young VR, Burke JF, Tompkins RG (1998) Maximal parenteral glucose oxidation in hypermetabolic young children: a stable isotope study. JPEN J Parenter Enteral Nutr 22(4):212–216
75. Sidossis LS, Porter C, Saraf MK, Borsheim E, Radhakrishnan RS, Chao T, Ali A, Chondronikola M, Mlcak R, Finnerty CC, Hawkins HK, Toliver-Kinsky T, Herndon DN (2015) Browning of subcutaneous white adipose tissue in humans after severe adrenergic stress. Cell Metab 22(2):219–227. doi:10.1016/j.cmet.2015.06.022
76. Stinnett JD, Alexander JW, Watanabe C, MacMillan BG, Fischer JE, Morris MJ, Trocki O, Miskell P, Edwards L, James H (1982) Plasma and skeletal muscle amino acids following severe burn injury in patients and experimental animals. Ann Surg 195(1):75–89
77. Stumvoll M, Nurjhan N, Perriello G, Dailey G, Gerich JE (1995) Metabolic effects of metformin in non-insulin-dependent diabetes mellitus. N Engl J Med 333(9):550–554. doi:10.1056/NEJM199508313330903
78. Sutherland EW, Cori CF (1951) Effect of hyperglycemic-glycogenolytic factor and epinephrine on liver phosphorylase. J Biol Chem 188(2):531–543
79. Todd SR, Kozar RA, Moore FA (2006) Nutrition support in adult trauma patients. Nutr Clin Pract 21(5):421–429
80. Van den Berghe G, Wouters PJ, Bouillon R, Weekers F, Verwaest C, Schetz M, Vlasselaers D, Ferdinande P, Lauwers P (2003) Outcome benefit of intensive insulin therapy in the critically ill: Insulin dose versus glycemic control. Crit Care Med 31(2):359–366. doi:10.1097/01.CCM.0000045568.12881.10

81. van der Lans AA, Hoeks J, Brans B, Vijgen GH, Visser MG, Vosselman MJ, Hansen J, Jörgensen JA, Wu J, Mottaghy FM, Schrauwen P, van Marken Lichtenbelt WD (2013) Cold acclimation recruits human brown fat and increases nonshivering thermogenesis. J Clin Invest 123(8):3395–3403. doi:10.1172/JCI68993
82. van Marken Lichtenbelt WD, Vanhommerig JW, Smulders NM, Drossaerts JM, Kemerink GJ, Bouvy ND, Schrauwen P, Teule GJ (2009) Cold-activated brown adipose tissue in healthy men. N Engl J Med 360(15):1500–1508. doi:10.1056/NEJMoa0808718
83. Vaughan GM, Becker RA, Allen JP, Goodwin CW Jr, Pruitt BA Jr, Mason AD Jr (1982) Cortisol and corticotrophin in burned patients. J Trauma 22(4):263–273
84. Vaughan GM, Becker RA, Unger RH, Ziegler MG, Siler-Khodr TM, Pruitt BA Jr, Mason AD Jr (1985) Nonthyroidal control of metabolism after burn injury: possible role of glucagon. Metabolism 34(7):637–641
85. Vijgen GH, Bouvy ND, Teule GJ, Brans B, Schrauwen P, van Marken Lichtenbelt WD (2011) Brown adipose tissue in morbidly obese subjects. PLoS One 6(2):e17247. doi:10.1371/journal.pone.0017247
86. Virtanen KA, Lidell ME, Orava J, Heglind M, Westergren R, Niemi T, Taittonen M, Laine J, Savisto NJ, Enerbäck S, Nuutila P (2009) Functional brown adipose tissue in healthy adults. N Engl J Med 360(15):1518–1525. doi:10.1056/NEJMoa0808949
87. Wasiak J, Cleland H, Jeffery R (2006) Early versus delayed enteral nutrition support for burn injuries. Cochrane Database Syst Rev (3):CD005489. doi:10.1002/14651858.CD005489.pub2
88. Weyer C, Gautier JF, Danforth E Jr (1999) Development of beta 3-adrenoceptor agonists for the treatment of obesity and diabetes – an update. Diabetes Metab 25(1):11–21
89. Wilmore DW, Aulick LH (1978) Metabolic changes in burned patients. Surg Clin North Am 58(6):1173–1187
90. Wilmore DW, Lindsey CA, Moyland JA, Faloona GR, Pruitt BA, Unger RH (1974) Hyperglucagonaemia after burns. Lancet 1(7847):73–75
91. Wilmore DW, Long JM, Mason AD Jr, Skreen RW, Pruitt BA Jr (1974) Catecholamines: mediator of the hypermetabolic response to thermal injury. Ann Surg 180(4):653–669
92. Windle EM (2006) Glutamine supplementation in critical illness: evidence, recommendations, and implications for clinical practice in burn care. J Burn Care Res 27(6):764–772. doi:10.1097/01.BCR.0000245417.47510.9C
93. Winkelman MD, Galloway PG (1992) Central nervous system complications of thermal burns. A postmortem study of 139 patients. Medicine (Baltimore) 71(5):271–283
94. Wischmeyer PE, Lynch J, Liedel J, Wolfson R, Riehm J, Gottlieb L, Kahana M (2001) Glutamine administration reduces Gram-negative bacteremia in severely burned patients: a prospective, randomized, double-blind trial versus isonitrogenous control. Crit Care Med 29(11):2075–2080
95. Wolf SE, Rose JK, Desai MH, Mileski JP, Barrow RE, Herndon DN (1997) Mortality determinants in massive pediatric burns. An analysis of 103 children with > or = 80% TBSA burns (> or = 70% full-thickness). Ann Surg 225(5):554–565; discussion 565–569
96. Wolfe RR (1981) Review: acute versus chronic response to burn injury. Circ Shock 8(1):105–115
97. Wolfe RR (2006) The underappreciated role of muscle in health and disease. Am J Clin Nutr 84(3):475–482
98. Wolfe RR, Herndon DN, Jahoor F, Miyoshi H, Wolfe M (1987) Effect of severe burn injury on substrate cycling by glucose and fatty acids. N Engl J Med 317(7):403–408. doi:10.1056/NEJM198708133170702
99. Wolfe RR, Herndon DN, Peters EJ, Jahoor F, Desai MH, Holland OB (1987) Regulation of lipolysis in severely burned children. Ann Surg 206(2):214–221
100. Xiao SC, Zhu SH, Xia ZF, Lu W, Wang GQ, Ben DF, Wang GY, Cheng DS (2008) Prevention and treatment of gastrointestinal dysfunction following severe burns: a summary of recent 30-year clinical experience. World J Gastroenterol 14(20):3231–3235

101. Yo K, Yu YM, Zhao G, Bonab AA, Aikawa N, Tompkins RG, Fischman AJ (2013) Brown adipose tissue and its modulation by a mitochondria-targeted peptide in rat burn injury-induced hypermetabolism. Am J Physiol Endocrinol Metab 304(4):E331–E341. doi:10.1152/ajpendo.00098.2012
102. Yoneshiro T, Aita S, Matsushita M, Kayahara T, Kameya T, Kawai Y, Iwanaga T, Saito M (2013) Recruited brown adipose tissue as an antiobesity agent in humans. J Clin Invest 123(8):3404–3408. doi:10.1172/JCI67803
103. Zauner A, Nimmerrichter P, Anderwald C, Bischof M, Schiefermeier M, Ratheiser K, Schneeweiss B, Zauner C (2007) Severity of insulin resistance in critically ill medical patients. Metabolism 56(1):1–5. doi:10.1016/j.metabol.2006.08.014

MIX
Papier aus verantwortungsvollen Quellen
Paper from responsible sources
FSC® C105338

If you have any concerns about our products,
you can contact us on
ProductSafety@springernature.com

In case Publisher is established outside the EU,
the EU authorized representative is:
Springer Nature Customer Service Center GmbH
Europaplatz 3, 69115 Heidelberg, Germany

Printed by Libri Plureos GmbH
in Hamburg, Germany